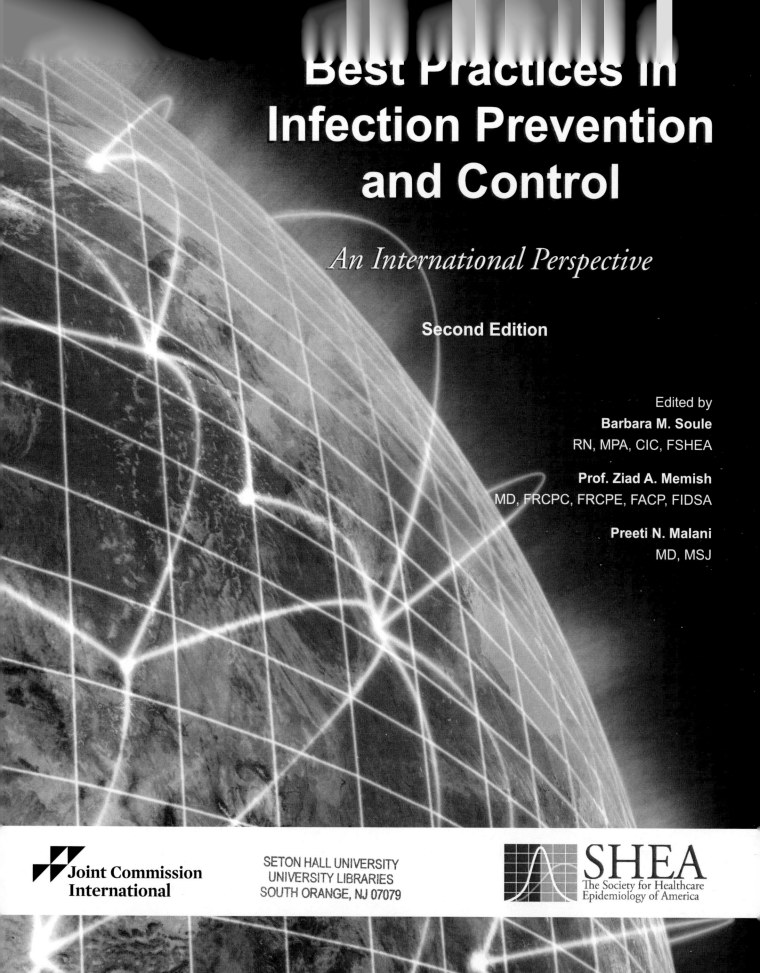

Best Practices in Infection Prevention and Control

An International Perspective

Second Edition

Edited by

Barbara M. Soule
RN, MPA, CIC, FSHEA

Prof. Ziad A. Memish
MD, FRCPC, FRCPE, FACP, FIDSA

Preeti N. Malani
MD, MSJ

Manager, Publications: Paul Reis
Senior Project Manager: Christine Wyllie, MA
Production Manager: Johanna Harris
Executive Director: Catherine Chopp Hinckley, MA, PhD
Reviewers: Ann K. Jacobson, MSN, RN, CNAA; Claudia Jorgenson, RN, MSN; Virginia Maripolsky, MSW, BSN, RNC; Siew Lee Cheng, RN, MSN, CCNS

Content Editors:
Barbara M. Soule, RN, MPA, CIC, FSHEA
Practice Leader, Infection Prevention and Control Services
Joint Commission Resources/Joint Commission International

Prof. Ziad Memish, MD, FRCPC, FRCPE, FACP, FIDSA
Assistant Deputy Minister of Health for Preventative Medicine, Kingdom of Saudi Arabia
Adjunct Professor, Emory University

Preeti N. Malani, MD, MSJ
Associate Professor of Medicine, University of Michigan Medical School
Research Scientist, VA Ann Arbor Healthcare System GRECC

Joint Commission International
The mission of Joint Commission International is to improve the quality of care in the international community through the provision of education and consultation services.

Joint Commission Resources educational programs and publications support, but are separate from, the accreditation activities of Joint Commission International. Attendees at Joint Commission Resources educational programs and purchasers of Joint Commission Resources publications receive no special consideration or treatment in, or confidential information about, the accreditation process.

Joint Commission Resources, Inc. (JCR), a not-for-profit affiliate of The Joint Commission on Accreditation of Healthcare Organizations (Joint Commission), has been designated by The Joint Commission to publish publications and multimedia products. JCR reproduces and distributes these materials under license from The Joint Commission.

Printed in the USA 5 4 3 2 1

Requests for permission to make copies of any part of this work should be mailed to
    Permissions Editor
    Department of Publications
    Joint Commission Resources
    One Renaissance Boulevard
    Oakbrook Terrace, Illinois 60181 USA
    permissions@jcrinc.com

ISBN: 978-1-59940-619-0
Library of Congress Control Number: 2011941312

For more information about Joint Commission International, please visit http://www.jointcommissioninternational.org.

For more information about Joint Commission Resources, please visit http://www.jcrinc.com.

This book is dedicated to the memory of Professora Silma Pinheiro Ribeiro, RN, PhD (1967–2011) of Belo Horizonte, Brazil. A 2010 Society for Healthcare Epidemiology of America (SHEA) International Ambassador, Professora Pinheiro's leadership and vision for infection prevention and control will be deeply missed.

Contents

Foreword

The term *best* is used in many personal and professional settings. Within the Joint Commission enterprise, we use the term frequently. For example, the Joint Commission enterprise strives to make its accreditation programs the best in the world. We aim to be the best at setting standards for health care organizations' performance and the best at assessing performance through on-site surveys and other ongoing evaluation methods.

Being the best is a laudable goal, but even the finest health care providers have no guarantees against adverse events, such as health care–associated infections (HAIs). In fact, the World Health Organization's (WHO's) May 2011 *Report on the Burden of Endemic Health Care-Associated Infection Worldwide* shows that HAIs continue to be the most frequent adverse event in health care delivery worldwide.[1] That same study reports that for every 100 of the world's hospitalized patients, somewhere between 7 and 10 will acquire at least one HAI.[1]

Clearly, in terms of infection prevention and control (IPC), we have not arrived at *best*. Even if we are trying, we are not yet achieving it. That means we must make IPC better—*much better*. This is the urgent, intermediate goal we must achieve.

Achieving and maintaining consistently high levels of safety and quality over time and across all health care services and settings—what we call *high reliability*—must be the ultimate goal. Our challenge is to create a learning and performance environment that turns health care into a high-reliability industry with rates of preventable adverse events that are equal to or better than the highest-reliability industries in the world. IPC is a key factor in whether we succeed or fail in this work.

Incremental steps must be taken to make health care better, and the Joint Commission enterprise is developing a road map to help health care organizations more consistently deliver high levels of performance with no variability or lapses in care. In the area of IPC, our enterprise sets requirements—standards and an International Patient Safety Goal (Reduce the Risk of Health Care–Associated Infections)—to guide caregivers toward a safe, reliable IPC methodology. The Joint Commission Center for Transforming Healthcare, which has forged partnerships with top US hospitals to develop solutions for health care's most critical safety and quality problems—including hand hygiene and surgical site infections—is scheduled to broaden its scope in 2012 to include hospitals outside the United States. And our Joint Commission International Library of Measures has begun tasking organizations with establishing core data measures—particularly, for the audience of this book, screening for and administering pneumococcal vaccination as well as proper use of prophylactic antibiotics for surgical patients—to drive focused, evidence-based clinical and management practices.

This book's task, as the title's reference to *best* makes clear, is to do for IPC what the Joint Commission enterprise strives to do more broadly for health care—to help health care organizations make major strides toward unprecedented levels of safety and quality for all patients and staff.

As improvement tools spread and targeted solutions become much more widely used, the reliability of health care in protecting patients and their families from infection will increase dramatically.

And that's *better*.

—**Mark R. Chassin, MD, FACP, MPP, MPH**
President, The Joint Commission

Reference

1. World Health Organization. Report on the Burden of Endemic Health Care-Associated Infection Worldwide. 2011. Accessed 26 May 2011. http://whqlibdoc.who.int/publications/2011/9789241501507_eng.pdf.

Foreword

The recently updated world population estimates from the United Nations provides a strategic projection of the world population as it continues on a path toward aging and growth.[1] The world population will likely increase from the current 7 billion to 9.2 billion in 2050. This increase will be absorbed mostly by the *less developed regions* (from 5.6 to 7.9 billion) and will include 1.6 billion older adults (> 60 years) and 3.6 billion in the 25- to 59-year-old cohort. Therefore, strategies for employment creation in the developing countries will be key to combating poverty, with its attendant lack of basic hygiene and sanitation and access to health care, and to promoting health and wellness.

Access to adequate health care remains a key concern globally. Among the 234 million surgical procedures performed annually, the wealthiest one third of the global population accounts for 75% of the procedures, while the poorest one third accounts for only 4%.[2] Worldwide estimates suggest that 11% of disability-adjusted life years are attributable to diseases potentially treated with surgery.

A recent World Health Organization (WHO) report on the burden of health care–associated infections (HAIs) is a reminder that access to care does not necessarily imply safe care.[3] Health care–associated conditions are those harms patients acquire while receiving treatment and include HAIs. The WHO report estimated the prevalence for HAIs occurring among patients in developed countries to be 7.6 per 100 patients but highlighted the fact that estimates for developing countries are sparse (two thirds of the 147 developing countries have no published data). I experienced the complications of care first hand with one of my initial outbreak investigations as an Epidemic Intelligence Officer at the US Centers for Disease Control and Prevention (US CDC), which involved a cluster of iatrogenic bacterial meningitis among children in India receiving outpatient itrathecal chemotherapy extrinsically contaminated with bacteria.[4]

The prescription for decreasing the HAI burden, especially in settings with limited resources, is complex and will require innovation. The contribution of poverty (malnutrition, inadequate resources and infrastructure) adds to the barriers of lack of surveillance and use of standardized case definitions.

Tools and skill building for developing surveillance systems using planning, implementation, analysis, and intervention are crucial for execution of infection prevention in developing countries. This second edition of *Best Practices in Infection Prevention and Control: An International Perspective* provides practical strategies for creating a learning and performance environment for HAI prevention that is centered on patient care. The Society for Healthcare Epidemiology of America (SHEA) is pleased to partner with Joint Commission International (JCI) to support this important work. SHEA shares JCI's commitment to patient safety and HAI prevention. Those involved in infection control and prevention understand the power of data-driven, patient-centered interventions and the need for science to inform interventions. SHEA has a strong and growing international membership and a commitment to infection prevention in developing world.[5] For example, SHEA has developed an International Ambassadors Program targeting emerging leaders from resource-limited regions to provide peer-to-peer networking and opportunities to connect with SHEA leadership (http://www.shea-online.org). The primary goal is to improve patient outcomes with solutions based on the realities of the local situations in these developing countries. Several ambassadors have contributed content to this book, highlighting the continued engagement the program seeks to foster.

Finally, money and foreign aid alone will not solve the problems. Alex Perry describes how the success of distributing 300 million mosquito nets with a drop in malaria morbidity and mortality required an execution strategy uniting political leadership, business leadership, media, and engagement of the population.[6] The global challenges to achieve systems for patient-centered health care throughout the world will require strategies that are innovative (for example, cell phones connecting to cloud databases can serve as tools for meaningful surveillance and data collection), evidence-based, and built on commitment and accountability. HAIs, like other health care–associated conditions, must be treated as a priority.

—**Steven M. Gordon, MD**
President, Society for Healthcare Epidemiology of America, 2011
Cleveland Clinic Foundation

References

1. United Nations Department of Economic and Social Affairs, Population Division. World Population Prospects, the 2010 Revision. Accessed 23 Aug 2011. http://www.unpopulation.org.
2. Funk LM, et al. Global operating theatre distribution and pulse oximetry supply: An estimation from reported data. *Lancet.* 2010 Sep 25;376(9746):1055–1061.
3. World Health Organization. Report on the Burden of Endemic Health Care-Associated Infection Worldwide. 2011. Accessed 20 Aug 2011. http://whqlibdoc.who.int/publications/2011/9789241501507_eng.pdf.
4. Kelkar R, et al. Epidemic iatrogenic *Acinetobacter* spp. meningitis following administration of intrathecal methotrexate. *J Hosp Infect.* 1989 Oct;14(3):233–243.
5. Malani PN. Addressing poverty and human development—Synonymous with infection control. *Infect Control Hosp Epidemiol.* 2007 Dec;28(12): 1321–1322.
6. Perry A. *Lifeblood: How to Change the World One Dead Mosquito at a Time.* New York: PublicAffairs, 2011.

Introduction

Unfortunately, in the four years since this book's first edition, the numbers of infection prevention and control (IPC) challenges facing today's health care providers have not diminished. Health care–associated infections (HAIs) continue to plague patients and the organizations that treat them, resource and infrastructure limitations and misappropriations create unnecessary obstacles for effective IPC initiatives, emerging and reemerging diseases are still in evidence, and threats of pandemics and even bioterrorism continue to demand organizational diligence. More than ever, IPC must be a priority in every health care setting in every corner of the globe.

This new edition, developed and published by Joint Commission International (JCI) in partnership with The Society for Healthcare Epidemiology of America (SHEA), gives health care organizations everywhere more and better tools and strategies for battling infections, whether the infection started outside or inside their facilities. The book outlines JCI's requirements for meeting IPC accreditation standards and its IPC–related International Patient Safety Goal. It offers concrete examples of compliance via several case studies in which organizations in a variety of settings have achieved sustained IPC improvements, and it offers a glimpse of future issues all organizations should be planning to address sooner rather than later.

The Content

Chapter 1—Infection Prevention and Control: A Global Perspective on a Health Care Crisis
Anucha Apisarnthanarak, MD; M. Cristina Ajenjo, MD; Linda M. Mundy MD, PhD
This chapter examines the sweeping, global scope of IPC, including the global burden of HAIs, emerging infectious diseases, occupational risk for blood-borne pathogens, and bioterrorism.

Chapter 2—The World Health Organization Approach to Health Care–Associated Infection Prevention and Control
Benedetta Allegranzi, MD; Carmen Lúcia Pessoa-Silva, MD; Didier Pittet, MD

Three World Health Organization (WHO) IPC experts describe their organizational approaches to HAIs, including their guidelines, global campaigns, and practical tools.

Chapter 3—Joint Commission International's Infection Prevention and Control Standards and Requirements: A Detailed Study
This chapter takes an in-depth look at the current IPC standards (and other related requirements) for JCI accreditation and certification programs. It also examines the International Patient Safety Goal that pertains to hand hygiene.

Chapter 4—Surveying Infection Prevention and Control: The Role of Infection Prevention and Control in the Accreditation Survey Process
This chapter walks organizations through the accreditation process as it relates to IPC, including how surveyors check standards and International Patient Safety Goal compliance during the JCI on-site accreditation survey.

Chapter 5—Developing an Effective Infection Prevention and Control Program: Strategies for Success
Barbara M. Soule, RN, MPA, CIC, FSHEA; Preeti N. Malani, MD, MSJ; Prof. Ziad A. Memish, MD, FRCPC, FRCPE, FACP, FIDSA
Chapter 5 discusses some of the challenges to building an effective IPC program, from assessing risk and developing goals and objectives to developing practical IPC plans. Case studies from organizations around the country and some tools offer real-world examples and provide lessons learned; field-tested tips and tools give readers leverage and direction to solve IPC issues.

Chapter 6—Maintaining and Sustaining an Effective Infection Prevention and Control Program
Barbara M. Soule, RN, MPA, CIC, FSHEA; Prof. Ziad A. Memish, MD, FRCPC, FRCPE, FACP, FIDSA; Preeti N. Malani, MD, MSJ
Remaining effective against IPC challenges after some initial

improvements can be as or more difficult than making the initial gains. Chapter 6 discusses the challenges in continuing organizational improvement over time and offers several more case studies, tips, and tools.

Chapter 7—Future Issues in Infection Prevention and Control

Jaffar A. Al-Tawfiq, MD, DipHIC, FACP, FCCP; Prof. Ziad A. Memish, MD, FRCPC, FRCPE, FACP, FIDSA

This chapter explores a few selected issues that will affect the future of the practice over the next years, including setting the target for zero infections, implementing and sustaining evidence-based practices in organizations, reducing multidrug-resistant organisms and antimicrobial resistance, the role of social marketing in health care worker behavior change, developing future IPC staffing resources, environmental design for IPC, data mining and information technology, and emerging diseases and pathogens.

Appendix 1

Appendix 1 includes JCI's IPC requirements for every accreditation and certification program.

Appendix 2

Appendix 2 features Web-based resources from and for IPC–related organizations around the world., compiled and edited by Nizam Damani, MBBS, MSc, MRCPI, FRCPath, CIC, DipHIC.

Audience

This book is intended to benefit IPC and quality-improvement professionals, organization leaders, clinical leaders, nursing leaders, and other staff involved in IPC in every area of health care.

A Note About Health Care Workers and Other Terms

The term *health care workers* (HCWs) is used throughout the text to indicate those persons who provide care, treatment, and services in the organization (for example, medical staff and nursing staff), including those receiving pay (permanent, temporary, and part-time personnel as well as contract employees), volunteers, and health profession students. The term *staff* is also used; unless *staff* is modified by another term (for example, *infection control staff*), consider it the equivalent of *health care worker*. Both *health care worker* and *staff* are used in the text of JCI requirements.

The term *infection prevention and control professional* (or *IPC professional*) is used primarily to denote an HCW responsible for controlling and preventing the spread of infectious diseases in a hospital or other health care setting.[1] *Infection prevention and control practitioner* (or *IPC practitioner*) is also used to describe the same health care role. In some areas of the world, the preferred term for the same role is *infection preventionist*. Similarly, the term *health care epidemiologist* is used to denote a health care professional specializing in the transmission and control of epidemic diseases, and it is interchangeable with *medical director*.

Acknowledgments

Publications of this nature are the result of the important contributions of many individuals. As a result, JCI is grateful to all those who contributed to the success of this publication, most particularly Mark R. Chassin, President, The Joint Commission; and Steven M. Gordon, President, Society for Healthcare Epidemiology of America, for contributing forewords; and to the publication's content editors, Barbara M. Soule, Ziad A. Memish, and Preeti N. Malani, for their dedication. We thank chapter authors M. Cristina Ajenjo, Jaffar A. Al-Tawfiq, Benedetta Allegranzi, Anucha Apisarnthanarak, Linda M. Mundy, Carmen Lúcia Pessoa-Silva, and Didier Pittet for their strong contributions to the literature. Thanks also to content reviewers Ann Jacobson, Siew Lee Cheng, and Claudia Jorgenson of JCI Accreditation and Virginia Maripolsky of Bangkok Medical Center for their time, effort, and expertise. Thanks also to the contributing case study lead authors listed below—and their coauthors, whose names are listed with their contributions—for their practical documentation of their journeys to improved IPC performance.

Case Study Lead Authors

SHEA International Ambassadors

SHEA launched its International Ambassadors Program in 2009, which is dedicated to building collaborative relationships between US and other global health care professionals with expertise in health care epidemiology and infection prevention. Between 2009 and 2011, SHEA welcomed 32 Ambassadors representing 17 countries (Brazil, Chile, China, Columbia, Ghana, India, Ireland, Israel, Japan, Kenya, Malaysia, Mexico, Morocco, Nigeria, Philippines, Thailand, and Vietnam). SHEA Ambassadors who have contributed case studies are recognized below.

Ícaro Boszczowski, MD, MSc
Hospital das Clínicas University of São Paulo, Brazil

Romanee Chaiwarith, MD, MHS
Chiang Mai University, Thailand

Matan J. Cohen, MD, MPH
Hadassah-Hebrew University Medical Center, Israel

Ana Lucia Correa, MD
Andrea Restrepo, MD
Hospital Pablo Tobon Uribe, Medellín, Antioquia, Colombia

Ndegwa Linus, MPHE, HCS, PhD
Centres for Disease Control (CDC), Kenya

Zhiyong Zong, PhD, MBBS
West China Hospital, Sichuan University, China

Other Lead Case Study Authors
Other lead case study authors are listed below.

Hanan H. Balkhy, MD
King Abdulaziz Medical City, Saudi Arabia

Michael A. Borg, MD, MSc (Lond), DipHIC, FRCPath, PhD
Mater Dei Hospital, Malta

Pola Brenner, RN, MSc
Universidad de Valparaíso, Chile

Sandra Callery, RN, MHSc, CIC
Sunnybrook Health Sciences Centre, Canada

Mamoun Elsheikh, MD
Hamad Medical Corporation, Qatar

Petra Gastmeier, MD
Charité Universitätsmedizin Berlin, Germany

Nguyen Viet Hung, MD, PhD
Bach Mai Hospital, Vietnam

Shaheen Mehtar, MBBS, MRCPath (UK), FRCPath (UK), FCPath (SA), MD (Lon)
Tygerberg Academic Hospital, South Africa

Cathryn Murphy, RN, PhD, CIC
Gold Coast Health Service District, Australia

Ossama Rasslan, MD, PhD
Ain Shams University, Egypt

Victor D. Rosenthal, MD, CIC, MSc
International Nosocomial Infection Control Consortium, Argentina

Arisara Suwanarit, RN, BSN, MS
Bangkok Hospital Medical Center, Thailand

Özlem Yıldırım, PhD, MSEM, BSIE
American Hospital, Turkey

Reference
1. US Centers for Disease Control and Prevention. Self-Study Modules on Tuberculosis 6-9: Glossary. http://www.cdc.gov/tb/education/ssmodules/glos%206-9.htm.

Infection Prevention and Control

A Global Perspective on a Health Care Crisis

By
Anucha Apisarnthanarak, MD
M. Cristina Ajenjo, MD
Linda M. Mundy, MD, PhD

Chapter One

nfectious diseases have been around for thousands of years with resultant acute and chronic illnesses that have impacted human and animal health. Health professionals diagnose and treat infection and have attempted to reduce, if not eliminate, infection risk. Infection prevention and control (IPC) strategies are critical to safe, high-quality health care via implementation of effective infrastructure and systems that identify, address, and prevent the spread of infections.

Health care–associated infections (HAIs) are infections that occur during the processes of health care delivery and are restricted to infections that were not present or incubating prior to the onset of care.[1] These HAIs occur in patients who receive care in hospitals and other health care facilities and in health care professionals and staff who are identified with infections as a result of occupational exposures.[1] There is increasing global concern and prioritization of HAIs as a patient-safety issue, particularly because these adverse events are associated with morbidity, if not mortality, and excess costs.[2,3] Improved global communications have enhanced public awareness of health risks, infectious diseases, and HAI burden.[4] Infections that have resulted in international headlines include, but are not limited to, viral infections from pandemic influenza H1N1 and West Nile virus, and bacterial infections from methicillin-resistant *Staphylococcus aureus* (MRSA) and multidrug-resistant (MDR) gram-negative organisms. From a global health perspective, effective IPC strategies for HAIs are readily applicable to preparedness plans and infrastructure for population health challenges, such as widespread epidemics, natural disasters, and bioterrorist threats.

HAIs

One of the primary responsibilities of care providers and health care organizations is to do no harm to the patient or to the health care worker (HCW).[5] Yet health care delivery has inherent risks, the serious nature of HAIs is undeniable, and the safety risks for patients and providers are considerable. Care settings may be reservoirs for infections despite advanced technology, environmental health and cleanliness standards, and well-intentioned staff. There is increased pressure for health care organizations to do more with fewer resources, which creates strategic challenges amid treating increased numbers of patients over shorter inpatient stays, staffing shortages combined with ongoing staff training, lack of or limited supplies, and administrative requests to reduce costs. Historically, concern for HAIs has primarily been a focus only for hospitals. Now health care that traditionally was provided in hospitals has become increasingly provided in subacute and rehabilitation facilities, ambulatory clinics, other care areas,

and the home. This shift in sites of care has heightened the risk of infection at all points along the care continuum, making IPC a priority in all health care settings.[2,6] An abundance of challenges as well as opportunities exist for IPC strategies conducted by knowledgeable, well-trained health care epidemiologists (also called *medical directors* in some areas) and IPC professionals (also known as *IPC practitioners* or *infection preventionists*). The following sections discuss the components of the IPC crisis and identify some future challenges.

Infections pose a significant threat to patient safety, and organizations must work to minimize risk for HAIs and to mitigate adverse effects when prevention has not been achieved. A recent systematic review and meta-analysis reported that the burden of endemic HAIs—the normal or expected incidence of infections in a population—was higher in developing countries (pooled prevalence 15.5 per 100 patients, 95% confidence interval [CI] 12.6–18.9) than proportions reported from Europe and the United States (*see* Sidebar 1-1).[7] Although it is true that some patients who acquire infections in a health care institution are frail, elderly, or immunocompromised, there are also many healthy people who enter hospitals or alternative care sites for elective procedures, fully expecting to return home in good health. When health care encounters include acquisition of infection, the consequences undoubtedly involve excess morbidity, if not mortality, and excess costs. Such infections include, but are not limited to, catheter-associated bloodstream infections (CABSIs), catheter-associated urinary tract infections (CAUTIs), surgical site infections (SSIs), skin and soft tissue infections (SSTIs), and ventilator-associated bacterial pneumonia (VABP). The key criteria to addressing HAIs are early case detection and effective IPC strategies (*see* Sidebar 1-2).

The many reasons that infections occur in a health care setting include

- lack of infrastructure to support the IPC program, such as ineffective or absent leadership support, insufficient staffing levels, insufficient staff training about IPC, and lack of supplies;*
- inadequate hand hygiene and aseptic or sterile technique;
- the emergence of MDR organisms due in part to the inappropriate use of antimicrobial agents;
- increasing number of immunocompromised patients;

---

* *Joint Commission International (JCI) defines* leadership *as an individual(s) who sets expectations, develops plans, and implements procedures to assess and to improve the quality of the organization's governance, management, clinical, and support functions. This includes at least the leaders of the governing body; the chief executive officer and other senior managers; departmental leaders; the elected and the appointed leaders of the medical staff, the clinical departments, and other medical staff members in organizational administrative positions; and the nurse executive and other senior nursing leaders.*

- inappropriate or inadequate procedures and techniques of care;
- ineffective cleaning and disinfection of the patient care environment or medical equipment; and
- public health issues, such as contaminated water supplies, inadequate management of medical waste, and inadequate preparedness plans for natural disasters, bioterrorist threats, and bioterrorist events.

Emerging and Reemerging Diseases, Epidemics, and Bioterrorism

When designing IPC programs to reduce risk of infections in health care settings, organizations must integrate community-based surveillance data and public awareness of infectious-disease threats. Many persons who acquire infections in the community must be seen in clinics, hospitalized, or cared for in the home by family or friends who have little to no training in IPC.[8] Therefore, IPC professionals in health care organizations must incorporate and design strategies that permit uptake and diffusion of IPC into alternative care settings. Below is a discussion of infection clusters, epidemics, and pandemics, as well as selected emerging infectious diseases, blood-borne infections, and bioterrorist threats that are of global interest.

Infection Clusters, Epidemics, and Pandemics

The majority of HAIs are endemic infections—normal or expected incidence of infections in a population—that occur on a continual basis and require ongoing attention to ensure low incidence and prevalence. Evidence-based recommendations to reduce or to prevent endemic HAIs and endorsed by the Society of Healthcare Epidemiology of America (SHEA) target CABSIs, CAUTIs, SSIs, and VABP.[9–12] Periodically, health care organizations experience HAI clusters, if not outbreaks, also known as epidemics. *Epidemics* are a greater-than-expected number of infections in a given population during a defined period. Well-designed procedures and protocols are available to investigate these occurrences in a systematic manner, to determine the cause, and to quickly initiate interventions.[13] System-based improvements and practices from one cluster or outbreak can be incorporated into strategies to prevent future untoward events and outbreaks.

Organizations must have appropriate IPC strategies in place should an outbreak attributed to an infectious etiology be identified or suspected in the community or a health care setting. Standardized practices and policies will minimize the potential interpersonal transmission of infection, optimize effective communication, and standardize reporting.[14] During a crisis, there is typically insufficient time to educate health

Sidebar 1-1. The Global Burden of HAIs

Estimates of HAIs vary widely, and a fragmented picture of the endemic burden of HAIs in developing countries, defined for lower- and middle-income countries, was recently published.[1] As of 2010, only 23 of 147 developing countries (15.6%) had an operational national surveillance system for HAIs, and there were no published data on HAIs' endemic burden from the majority (66%) of developing countries.[1] When HAIs were reported from investigators in developing countries, almost half the published studies were related to SSIs, presumably because cases can be more easily defined and associated with the health care that was delivered. In Europe, annual estimates of HAIs have been associated with 16 million extra days of hospital stay and 37,000 attributable deaths.[2] As assessment of HAIs includes the occupational health and safety of HCWs, the global preparedness and response to the severe acute respiratory syndrome (SARS) pandemic in 2003 remains highly informative, given that between 20% and 60% of HCWs became infected with viruses during routine patient care.[3]

References

1. Allegranzi B, et al. Burden of endemic health-care associated infection in developing countries: Systematic review and meta-analysis. *Lancet.* 2011 Jan 15;377(9761):228–241.
2. European Centre for Disease Prevention and Control (ECDC). *Annual Epidemiological Report on Communicable Diseases in Europe 2008. Report on the State of Communicable Diseases in the EU and EEA/EFTA Countries.* Stockholm: ECDC, 2008.
3. Cherry, JD. The chronology of the 2002–2003 SARS mini pandemic. *Paediatr Respir Rev.* 2004 Dec;5(4):262–269.

Sidebar 1-2. Key Infection Prevention and Control Strategies to Minimize Risk for HAIs

- Strong, supportive leadership
- Evidence-based hand-hygiene practices and policies
- Antimicrobial stewardship
- Sufficient, well-trained staff
- Surveillance for patterns of infections and a system to identify areas that need specific interventions
- Evidence-based infection risk-reduction strategies inclusive of HCW occupational health and safety[1]

Reference

1. Deuffic-Burban S, et al. Blood-borne viruses in health care workers: Prevention and management. *J Clin Virol.* 2011 Sep;52(1):4–10.

care professionals about the warning signs of certain diseases and the appropriate actions to undertake in order to minimize, if not to interrupt, the spread of transmissible infections. These challenges compel health care organizations to develop and to promote preparedness plans in advance of infection clusters, outbreaks (epidemics), and pandemics—epidemics that spread worldwide, or at least across a large region. This goal can be accomplished through a proactive and ongoing risk-assessment process. Practical tips on how to develop such IPC programs are further detailed in Chapters 5 and 6.

Exemplary preparedness plans were executed during the 2003 severe acute respiratory syndrome (SARS) epidemic that occurred in many countries.[15] The multicountry SARS epidemic was associated with transmission dynamics that began in a hotel, spread via global air travel, and subsequently resulted in patient-to–HCW transmission. As noted from the SARS epidemic, when epidemics occur, organizations at point-of-care sites must be prepared to respond rapidly, efficiently, and with transparency. Preparedness plans must include health care administrative support, mechanisms to rapidly create temporary isolation facilities, systems to restrict access to exposed HCWs, and plans to involve specialists to establish case definitions, to screen and to promptly identify cases, to provide for continuous monitoring to ensure adherence to optimal infection control practices, and to provide regular feedback to HCWs and health care administrators.[14]

Most infectious diseases are not associated with pandemics. It is more common for a microorganism to infect a relatively small number of people in routine clinical care than for outbreaks to occur. In some cases, an infectious disease can spread rapidly and affect large populations on multiple continents.[16] If left unchecked, such infections can become epidemics or pandemics. The severity of a pandemic depends on the organism's virulence, how rapidly it is able to spread from population to population, resistance to available drug treatments, immunity within the population, and effectiveness of response efforts. The global impact of prior influenza pandemics has been informative yet devastating (*see* Sidebar 1-3 for more information on influenza pandemics).[17]

Emerging Infectious Diseases

Since 1973 more than 30 new diseases have been characterized that have either viral or bacterial etiologies.[18] Infectious diseases now comprise a mix of acute and chronic infections, and rapid transmission of infections has been further expedited by global travel. The emergence and spread of West Nile virus (WNV) infections in 1994–1999, the worldwide pandemic influenza A (H1N1) in 2009–2010, the ongoing emer-

gence and global spread of MDR bacterial infections, and MDR tuberculosis portray how infectious diseases continue to thrive, how new strains emerge, and how dissemination occurs.[19] These diseases highlight the importance of vigilance, preparedness plans, early case identification, and open communication, which together contribute to effective IPC and preserve patient safety in community and health care–delivery settings.

West Nile Virus (WNV)

WNV has now been reported in most regions of the world. Outbreaks of WNV encephalitis in humans occurred in Algeria in 1994, Romania in 1996–1997, the Czech Republic in 1997, the Democratic Republic of the Congo in 1998, Russia in 1999, Israel in 2000, and the United States in 1999–2003.[20] The US public health experience with the emergence, monitoring, and control strategies for WNV illustrates the importance of strong communication networks and coordinated collection of information not only between health care organizations and government agencies but also among physicians, veterinarians, public health providers, and wildlife experts. Sharing of information and transparent data collection can help enhance case detection, optimize clinical decision making, and contribute to disruption of viral transmission.

The Pandemic Influenza—A H1N1

The 2009 pandemic influenza A H1N1 was first detected in Mexico in late March 2009, followed by prompt case detection in the United States and several other countries. This virus was a unique combination of six influenza virus genes never previously identified in animals or humans.[21] There was triple-reassortant of North American swine virus lineages and two genes encoding neuraminidase and matrix proteins from Eurasian swine virus lineages.[22]

After the initial case detection, the World Health Organization (WHO) declared the 2009 influenza A H1N1 outbreak a public health emergency of international concern, raising the level of influenza pandemic alert from phase 3 to phase 4, and recommended that countries intensify surveillance for unusual outbreaks of influenza-like illness and severe pneumonia. In June 2009 WHO signaled that a global pandemic of 2009 influenza A H1N1 was under way by further raising the worldwide pandemic alert level to phase 6.[23–25] The global pandemic was associated with millions of case infections, more than 19,000 deaths, and several million dollars in health care expenditures.

The mechanisms of person-to-person transmission of the 2009 H1N1 virus appeared similar to those of seasonal

Sidebar 1-3. Influenza Pandemics

Three types of influenza viruses infect humans: Types A, B, and C. Only influenza A has been associated with pandemics; influenza B viruses do not cause pandemics, and type C influenza viruses cause mild infection.

Historical Perspective

The 1918–1919 Spanish influenza pandemic was due to the emergence of H1N1 in humans and resulted in an estimated 50 million deaths worldwide.[1] The 1957–1958 Asian influenza pandemic was due to the emergence of H2N2 in humans and associated with more than 1 million deaths worldwide; this virus no longer circulates in humans. The 1968–1969 Hong Kong influenza pandemic, due to H3N2, was associated with an estimated 34,000 excess deaths in the United States.[2] H3N2 viruses continue to circulate worldwide and have been associated with tremendous morbidity and mortality.

Recent Influenza Epidemiology

The natural reservoirs for new human influenza A virus subtypes are wild aquatic waterfowl, ducks, and geese. Since 2003 the transmission dynamics of avian influenza viruses have involved complex, rapid viral exchange of highly virulent virus in poultry flocks, with infection among humans in Azerbaijan, Cambodia, China, Djibouti, Egypt, Indonesia, Iraq, Thailand, Turkey, and Vietnam.[3]

Minor viral mutations evolve through a process called antigenic drift, which drives seasonal epidemics. But antigenic shift results from the replacement of the hemagglutinin (HA) and sometimes the neuroaminidase (NA), with novel subtypes that have not been present in human viruses for a long time. The introduction of new HA into human viruses usually results in a pandemic. The reemergence of avian influenza A (H5N1) in 2003, together with seasonal influenza vaccine shortages throughout the world, has heightened awareness of the unmet needs related to pandemic preparedness plans. The global response to the 2009 pandemic influenza A H1N1 exemplified well-coordinated IPC strategies and effective response plans at the international, federal, state, local, and community levels.

Relevance to IPC

Influenza pandemics evolve quickly, take an immense human toll, and have tremendous social and economic consequences. Early case detection, effective IPC strategies, and global communication efforts are relevant to minimizing risk of a future viral pandemic. The US Centers for Disease Control and Prevention (US CDC) estimates that another influenza pandemic could cause up to 7.4 million human deaths worldwide and excess health care utilization in outpatient visits and hospital admissions.[3] Risk of human-to-human transmission of influenza A H5N1 was explored in two studies, neither of which confirmed transmission to HCWs exposed to confirmed and probable cases with H5N1 infection.[4,5] WHO published interim IPC recommendations for suspected H5N1 patients in 2004 and updated them in 2006.[6] Full barrier precautions are recommended, when possible, in provision of care for suspected or confirmed avian influenza patients with close patient contact and during aerosol generating procedures. Such precautions are defined as standard, contact, and airborne precautions inclusive of eye protection. Because some elements of full barrier precautions (particularly airborne precautions) may not be available in all health care facilities, minimal requirements for caring for H5N1 patients should include standard, contact, and droplet precautions. In addition, active surveillance for viral infection in HCWs and annual influenza vaccination of HCWs is recommended to potentially reduce the risk of coinfection with H5N1 and human influenza A viruses and to reduce the risk of viral reassortment.

References

1. Taubenberger JK, Morens DM. 1918 influenza: The mother of all pandemics. *Emerg Infect Dis*. 2006 Jan;12(1):15–22.
2. Pan American Health Organization. Hurrying toward disaster? Peters C. 23 Aug 2002. Accessed 7 Oct 2011. http://www.paho.org/common/Display.asp?Lang=E&RecID=4609.
3. World Health Organization. Cumulative Number of Confirmed Human Cases of Avian Influenza A (H5N1) Reported to WHO, 2003-2011. 10 Oct 2011. Accessed 7 Oct 2011. http://www.who.int/influenza/human_animal_interface/EN_GIP_LatestCumulativeNumberH5N1cases.pdf.
4. Apisarnthanarak A, et al. Seroprevalence of anti-H5 antibody among Thai health care workers after exposure to avian influenza (H5N1) in a tertiary care center. *Clin Infect Dis*. 2005 Jan 15;40(2):e16–18.
5. Liem NT, Lim W, World Health Organization International Avian Influenza Investigation Team, Vietnam. Lack of H5N1 avian influenza transmission to hospital employees, Hanoi, 2004. *Emerg Infect Dis*. 2005 Feb;11(2):210–215.
6. World Health Organization. Avian Influenza. (Updated Apr 2011) Accessed 14 Sep 2011. http://www.who.int/mediacentre/factsheets/avian_influenza/en/.

influenza, but the relative contributions of small-particle aerosols, large droplets, and fomites are uncertain.[22] Rates of secondary outbreaks of illness varied according to the setting and the exposed population, yet estimates ranged from 4% to 28%.[23] Household transmission was highest among children and lowest among adults over 50 years of age.[23]

WHO announced the end of the pandemic period in August 2010.[23] The 2009 pandemic influenza A H1N1 occurred against a backdrop of pandemic response planning after years of developing, refining, and regularly exercising preparedness response plans at the international, federal, state, local, and community levels.[26] This emergent disease was a major challenge for health care institutions and HCWs, particularly health care epidemiologists and IPC professionals who invested significant resources to control the pandemic.

Community-Associated MRSA

Staphylococcus aureus is an important cause of infections in health care settings and in communities. MRSA results from the production of an alternate penicillin-binding protein, PBP2a, which has a low affinity for all β-lactam agents and generates resistant strains susceptible only to other antibiotic families, such as glycopeptides. Clinical isolates of MRSA were increasingly reported in the 1980s among patients primarily in hospitals and other health care environments. Since the mid- to late 1990s, however, there has been an explosion in the number of MRSA infections reported in persons lacking exposure to health care systems. These infections have been linked to MRSA clones known as community-associated MRSA (CA-MRSA).[27] Strains of CA-MRSA differ in phenotype from the older, health care–associated MRSA (HA-MRSA) strains and carry a smaller, more mobile, and less physiologically burdensome chromosomal element, termed SCCmec type IV. This genetic element usually carries only the mecA gene, with no other resistance determinants, differentiating it from genetic elements traditionally found in HA-MRSA strains.[27] These CA-MRSA strains differ in antimicrobial susceptibility patterns from HA-MRSA strains, often spread among healthy people in the community, and have been associated with severe skin and respiratory infections.[28]

MDR Gram-Negative Pathogens

Infections caused by MDR gram-negative pathogens are an increasing problem worldwide. Resistance dramatically limits therapeutic options, and, in contrast to new drugs for gram-positive organisms, there has been a paucity of new antimicrobial agents approved for gram-negative bacilli (GNB) in recent years.[29] Furthermore, many GNB are resistant to multiple agents and in some instances are pan-resistant to all commercially available antimicrobial agents.[30] Notably, carbapenemases are categorized by hydrolytic mechanisms that permit drug resistance and include β-lactamases in the molecular Class A, B, and D. Epidemiological investigation suggests complex and differential patterns of emergence of carbapenem-resistant bacteria. As an example, introduction of the plasmid-mediated *Klebsiella pneumoniae* carbapenemase (KPC) gene into several geographic regions has been due to intercountry patient transfer. Israel was the first nation outside the United States to report a large outbreak of KPC–producing *K. pneumoniae* attributed to health care–associated transmission of a strain linked to North America.[31] Greece later identified widespread clonal KPC pathogens that were indistinguishable from contemporary Israeli clones.[32] In Germany, the likely index case in a single-center outbreak was a patient who had been previously hospitalized in Greece.[33] The United Kingdom, France, and other countries have also reported episodes of colonization or infection of patients with KPC pathogens transferred from endemic countries. For additional case studies and outbreaks of carbapenem-resistant *K. pneumoniae* (CRKP) *see* Chapter 5 (Case Study 5-9) and Chapter 6 (Case Study 6-2).

New Delhi metallo-β-lactamase (NDM) is a plasmid-mediated, class B metallo-β-lactamase that has been identified in a broad range of enterobacteriaceae and non-enterobacteriaceae. Isolates are resistant to carbapenems, aminoglycosides, fluoroquinolones, and most antimicrobial drug classes. Of concern, some isolates have also exhibited resistance to tigecycline and colistin. The index case with an NDM–producing pathogen was a man in Sweden who previously received health care in India.[34] Subsequent case reports and case series suggest health care contact in India, Bangladesh, and some Balkan nations has been associated with case detection in the United States, Australia, Canada, Japan, and several European nations.[35,36] These epidemiological observations require further elucidation but highlight the potential risk of intercountry transmission of MDR GNB.

Tuberculosis

Tuberculosis (TB) is the most common infectious disease worldwide. It affects one third of the global population and is the leading cause of death from a potentially curable infectious disease. The 2009 global estimate for TB was 9.4 million incident cases (range 8.9–9.9), for a rate of 137 cases per 100,000 population (range 131–145).[37] TB rates vary widely by geographic region, with 22 low- and middle-income countries accounting for more than 80% of active TB cases worldwide.[38] Prevalence rates of TB are highest in Africa and lowest in the Americas and Europe due to the high prevalence of HIV in some African countries and the effect of HIV on susceptibility to TB.[38] Case infection with MDR-TB is defined as a person with *Mycobacterium tuberculosis* resistant to at least two antitubercular drugs—isoniazid and rifampicin. Recent surveillance data have revealed that prevalence of MDR-TB has risen to the highest rate ever recorded worldwide.[38] The MDR-TB strain generally arises through the selection of resistance mutations that emerge during inadequate treatment. Prior TB treatment, shortage of α-tuberculous drugs, and treatment costs have been the most common reasons for the inadequacy of the initial anti-TB regimen.[39] Other factors that play an important role in the development of MDR-TB include limited administrative control of purchase and distribution of the drugs, inadequate mechanism for quality control and bioavailability tests, poor patient follow-up, and inadequate administrative infrastructure.

Many other infectious diseases not discussed above (for example, cholera, meningococcal disease, and dengue hemorrhagic fever) present ongoing challenges to IPC worldwide. Regional IPC strategies should focus on the infections prevalent in the geographic setting and include preparedness plans that can be implemented should an emerging infectious pathogen or outbreak occur.

Occupational Risk for Blood-Borne Pathogens

Twenty-six different viruses have been reported as occupational transmission risks to HCWs.[17] The majority of occupational health-related cases are due to one of three viruses—hepatitis B virus (HBV), hepatitis C virus (HCV), and human immunodeficiency virus (HIV). In the year 2000, incident HCW infections worldwide due to percutaneous injuries were estimated to be 16,000 for HCV, 66,000 for HBV, and 1,000 for HIV.[40] The highest proportion of blood-borne viral transmission occurs through percutaneous injuries with hollow-bore needles for vascular access, although postexposure risk of infection to HCWs also exists for splashes of blood to skin and mucous membranes.[17] Pathogen-specific postexposure risk related to percutaneous injuries is estimated to be 30% for HBV in susceptive HCWs without post-exposure prophylaxis or adequate HBV vaccination, 0.5% after viremic HCV exposure, and less than 0.3% for HIV.[17]

From a historical perspective, WHO first established the Safe Injection Global Network in 1989 as an international alliance of all organizations concerned with achieving safer use of injections. Current standard precautions and preventive methods to minimize risk for blood-borne pathogens include hand hygiene, use of barrier methods, minimal manual manipulation of sharp instruments and devices, proper disposal of sharp instruments and devices in specific resistant containers, and occupational health and safety programs that promote HCW vaccination and the reporting of percutaneous injuries. Regular and renewed training sessions are relevant to new and long-term HCWs, students, physician trainees, and physicians. A prospective active surveillance program has recently reported lower rates of percutaneous injuries at a large teaching hospital in Saudi Arabia relative to the United States Exposure Prevention Information Network.[41] Improved practices and decreased occupational exposures have been associated with safety training compliance and with safety-engineered devices, such as retractable syringes, needle-free intravenous systems, and winged butterfly needles. In addition, reuse of cheap single-use devices (such as needles, syringes, and surgical gloves) remains common in several resource-limited health care settings, leading to large numbers of preventable infections and opportunities for implementation of effective IPC strategies to minimize risk for HBV, HCV, HIV, and other blood-borne infections.[42,43]

Reports of HCW–to-patient transmission of HBV, HCV, and HIV exist. Although uncommon, patients with blood-exposure to HCWs with HBV, HCV, or HIV should systematically receive the same postexposure assessment and management as HCW protocols.

HIV/AIDS

Acquired immune deficiency syndrome (AIDS) has no cultural, social, or economic boundaries. According to a joint international program of the United Nations and WHO, as of 2009, an estimated 49.2 million people worldwide were living with HIV, 2.6 million of whom were infected in 2009.[44] From a historical perspective, the term *AIDS* was first used in 1982, when public health officials reported the occurrence of opportunistic infections in otherwise healthy people. Public fear, international distrust, and limited understanding of the natural history of disease, disease progression, and the transmission dynamics led to delays in identification of the viral etiology until 1985, when there was global consensus that a pandemic attributed to HIV infection resulted in AIDS.[44] In the United States and elsewhere, AIDS was initially identified in men who had sex with men, and subsequent case detection expanded to include women, injecting drug users, hemophiliacs, newborns, and unscreened blood supplies. Unsafe injection practices, unprotected sex, and the unnecessary use of injections in resource-limited settings continue to contribute to the burden of preventable HIV infection. Initial and ongoing training of HCWs regarding occupational risks for HIV infection and effective IPC strategies to minimize risk of blood-borne infection remains a key component of a sustainable and safe health care environment.

Bioterrorism

Release, or threats of release, of biological agents or materials as weapons of mass destruction has the potential to evoke widespread public fear and panic, human injury, and destruction of physical plant structures. The health care community in each country must work closely with public health officials, law enforcement, and the military to ensure public safety related to deliberate epidemics and bioterrorism.[45] A significant challenge in preparing for a potential bioterrorism event is anticipating the nature of the event and predicting what

IPC issues will come up. The type of organism, the location of the release, the composition of the infected population, and the use of health care organizations by infected people to get treatment will influence how the specific events of a bioterrorist act unfold. Although a multitude of potential bioterrorism agents exists, following is a brief discussion of anthrax and smallpox, two pathogens that have received major media attention over the past decade. Suggestions regarding how to facilitate communication and prompt response to a biological emergency appear in Chapter 5.

Anthrax

Anthrax infection occurs after direct exposure to *Bacillus anthracis* spores, not after direct person-to-person contact. In a bioterrorism event, it is most likely that only the individuals coming in contact with spores would be affected. However, massive air-borne dissemination of *B. anthracis* spores could prove catastrophic if early identification and a rapid response does not occur. If untreated, the clinical progression of anthrax includes septicemia, meningitis, and death. In persons exposed to anthrax, infection can be prevented with antibiotic prophylaxis therapy; early antibiotic treatment can also help increase a person's chance of survival.[45] Early identification of an anthrax bioterrorist attack would lead to rapid antimicrobial distribution and containment, improved case detection, and heightened surveillance.

Smallpox

Smallpox infection occurs after direct, fairly prolonged face-to-face contact with someone infected with variola virus, after direct contact with variola virus in infected bodily fluids, or on contaminated objects, such as bedding and clothing.[46] As a potential biological weapon, transmission of smallpox via person-to-person contact could involve suicide terrorists who used interpersonal transmission dynamics to disseminate the virus.[46] Multiple countries could be affected, and these nations would need to work cooperatively to interrupt the transmission dynamics under way. Although antiviral agents have been identified and are being actively assessed in human trials, none has reached the licensure stage. As of today, there is no specific treatment for smallpox, and the only prevention is vaccination. Notably, a worldwide vaccination program that started in the 1950s has all but eradicated the disease. By 1984 the only known stocks of smallpox virus were in two WHO–approved laboratories—one in Atlanta and the other in Moscow.[47] Destruction of these viral stocks was originally planned for 1987 but postponed to permit further studies on the virus genome. Because the disease has been eliminated, in many parts of the world, routine vaccination no longer occurs. People who received the smallpox vaccine prior to 1980 probably have little to no immunity to smallpox today and in the case of an epidemic would require vaccination.[46] If a bioterrorist event involving smallpox were to occur, early case identification and isolation would be essential, and HCWs would need evidence of vaccination to safely provide care to infected cases. Transmission would need to be minimized via targeted vaccination of close contacts of the index cases.[46] Depending on the nature of the attack, a large-scale vaccination might be necessary, in which case public health organizations and other health care organizations, such as ambulatory clinics, would have to anticipate and plan for the logistics of vaccinating the entire community.

Conclusion

Infection prevention and control strategies are critical to safe, high-quality health care. Organizations that embrace IPC and implement systems to identify, to address, and to prevent the spread of infections help create health care cultures based on safety and organizations rooted in quality. To create such a culture, organizations must continually examine, evaluate, and act on IPC issues and view IPC as an integral component of patient safety and HCW occupational health and safety. Successful strategies to prevent or mitigate infections require ongoing collaboration between the professionals and officials in the public health sector, hospitals, and other health care settings.

References

1. World Health Organization (WHO). *Prevention of Hospital-Acquired Infections: A Practical Guide*, 2nd ed. Geneva: WHO, 2002.
2. Bates DW, et al. Global priorities for patient safety research. *BMJ.* 2009 May 14;338:b1775.
3. Pada SK, et al. Economic and clinical impact of nosocomial meticillin-resistant *Staphylococcus aureus* infections in Singapore: A matched case-control study. *J Hosp Infect.* 2011 May;78(1):36–40.
4. Rubin GJ, Potts HW, Michie S. The impact of communications about swine flu (influenza A H1N1v) on public responses to the outbreak: Results from 36 national telephone surveys in the UK. *Health Technol Assess.* 2010 Jul;14(34):183–266.
5. Smith CM. Origin and uses of primum non nocere—Above all, do no harm! *J Clin Pharmacol.* 2005 Apr;45(4):371–377.
6. Sansoni D, et al. Infection control in the outpatient setting. *Ig Sanita Pubbl.* 2007 Sep–Oct;63(5):587–598.
7. Allegranzi B, et al. Burden of endemic health-care-associated infection in developing countries: Systematic review and meta-analysis. *Lancet.* 2011 Jan 15;377(9761):228–241.
8. Flanagan E, Chopra T, Mody L. Infection prevention in alternative health care settings. *Infect Dis Clin North Am.* 2011 Mar;25(1):271–283.
9. Marschall J, et al. Strategies to prevent central line-associated bloodstream infections in acute care hospitals. *Infect Control Hosp Epidemiol.* 2008 Oct;29 Suppl 1:S22–30.

10. Lo E, et al. Strategies to prevent catheter-associated urinary tract infections in acute care hospitals. *Infect Control Hosp Epidemiol.* 2008 Oct;29 Suppl 1:S41–50.

11. Anderson DJ, et al. Strategies to prevent surgical site infections in acute care hospitals. *Infect Control Hosp Epidemiol.* 2008 Oct;29 Suppl 1:S51–61.

12. Coffin SE, et al. Strategies to prevent ventilator-associated pneumonia in acute care hospitals. *Infect Control Hosp Epidemiol.* 2008 Oct;29 Suppl 1:S31–40.

13. Apisarnthanarak A, et al. Pseudo-outbreak of *Acinetobacter lwoffii* infection in a tertiary care center in Thailand. *Infect Control Hosp Epidemiol.* 2007 May;28(5):637–639.

14. Apisarnthanarak A, Mundy LM. Infection control for emerging infectious diseases in developing countries and resource-limited settings. *Infect Control Hosp Epidemiol.* 2006 Aug;27(8):885–887.

15. Peiris JS, et al. The severe acute respiratory syndrome. *N Engl J Med.* 2003 Dec 18;349(25):243–241.

16. Perez-Padilla R, et al. Pneumonia and respiratory failure from swine-origin influenza A (H1N1) in Mexico. *N Engl J Med.* 2009 Aug 13;361(7):680–689.

17. Deuffic-Burban S, et al. Blood-borne viruses in health care workers: Prevention and management. *J Clin Virol.* 2011 Sep;52(1):4–10.

18. Morens DM, Taubenberger JK, Fauci AS. The persistent legacy of the 1918 influenza virus. *N Engl J Med.* 2009 Jul 16;361(3):225–229.

19. Rogers BA, et al. Country-to-country transfer of patients and the risk of multi-resistant bacterial infection. *Clin Infect Dis.* 2011 Jul 1;53(1):49–56.

20. US Centers for Disease Control and Prevention. West Nile Virus: Background: Virus History and Distribution. Accessed 14 Sep 2011. http://www.cdc.gov/ncidod/dvbid/westnile/background.htm

21. US Centers for Disease Control and Prevention. The 2009 H1N1 Pandemic: Summary Highlights, April 2009–April 2010. (Updated 16 Jun 2010) Accessed 14 Sep 2011. http://www.cdc.gov/h1n1flu/cdcresponse.htm.

22. de León-Rosales SP, et al. Prevalence of infections in intensive care units in Mexico: A multicenter study. *Crit Care Med.* 2000 May;28(5):1316–1321.

23. World Health Organization. Swine Influenza. 25 Apr 2009. Accessed 14 Sep 2011. http://www.who.int/mediacentre/news/statements/2009/h1n1_20090425/en/index.html.

24. World Health Organization. World Now at the Start of 2009 Influenza Pandemic. Chan M. 11 Jun 2009. Accessed 14 Sep 2011. http://www.who.int/mediacentre/news/statements/2009/h1n1_pandemic_phase6_20090611/en/index.html.

25. World Health Organization. Current WHO Phase of Pandemic Alert (Avian Influenza H5N1). Accessed 14 Sep 2011. http://www.who.int/influenza/preparedness/pandemic/h5n1phase/en/index.html.

26. Schuchat A, Bell BP, Redd SC. The science behind preparing and responding to pandemic influenza: The lessons and limits of science. *Clin Infect Dis.* 2011 Jan 1;52 Suppl 1:S8–12.

27. David MZ, Daum RS. Community-associated methicillin-resistant *Staphylococcus aureus*: Epidemiology and clinical consequences of an emerging epidemic. *Clin Microbiol Rev.* 2010 Jul;23(3):616–687.

28. Shilo N, Quach C. Pulmonary infections and community associated methicillin resistant *Staphylococcus aureus*: A dangerous mix? *Paediatr Respir Rev.* 2011 Sep;12(3):182–189.

29. Boucher HW, et al. Bad bugs, no drugs: No ESKAPE! An update from the Infectious Diseases Society of America. *Clin Infect Dis.* 2009 Jan 1;48(1):1–12.

30. Paterson DL, Doi Y. A step closer to extreme drug resistance (XDR) in gram-negative bacilli. *Clin Infect Dis.* 2007 Nov 1;45(9):1179–1181.

31. Navon-Venezia S, et al. First report on a hyperepidemic clone of KPC-3-producing *Klebsiella pneumoniae* in Israel genetically related to a strain causing outbreaks in the United States. *Antimicrob Agents Chemother.* 2009 Feb;53(2):818–820.

32. Giakoupi P, et al. KPC-2-producing *Klebsiella pneumoniae* infections in Greek hospitals are mainly due to a hyperepidemic clone. *Euro Surveill.* 2009 May 28;14(21):69–73.

33. Wendt C, et al. First outbreak of *Klebsiella pneumoniae* carbapenemase (KPC)-producing *K. pneumoniae* in Germany. *Eur J Clin Microbiol Infect Dis.* 2010 May;29(5):563–570.

34. Yong D, et al. Characterization of a new metallo-beta-lactamase gene, bla(NDM-1), and a novel erythromycin esterase gene carried on a unique genetic structure in *Klebsiella pneumoniae* sequence type 14 from India. *Antimicrob Agents Chemother.* 2009 Dec;53(12):5046–5054.

35. US Centers for Disease Control and Prevention. Detection of Enterobacteriaceae isolates carrying metallo-beta-lactamase–United States, 2010. *MMWR Morb Mortal Wkly Rep.* 2010 Jun 25;59(24):750.

36. Struelens MJ, et al. New Delhi metallo-beta-lactamase 1-producing Enterobacteriaceae: Emergence and response in Europe. *Euro Surveill.* 2010 Nov 18;15(46):11–16.

37. World Health Organization. Tuberculosis (TB). Accessed 15 Apr 2011. http://www.who.int/tb/country/data/download/en/index.html.

38. Lawn SD, Zumia AI. Tuberculosis. *Lancet.* 2011 Jul 2;378(9785):57–72.

39. Marahatta SB. Multi-drug resistant tuberculosis burden and risk factors: An update. *Kathmandu Univ Med J (KUMJ).* 2010 Jan–Mar;8(29):116–125.

40. Prüss-Ustün A, Rapiti E, Hutin Y. Estimation of the global burden of disease attributable to contaminated sharps injuries among health-care workers. *Am J Ind Med.* 2005 Dec;48(6):482–490.

41. Balkhy HH, et al. Benchmarking of percutaneous injuries at a teaching tertiary care center in Saudi Arabia relative to United States hospitals participating in the Exposure Prevention Information Network. *Am J Infect Control.* 2011 Sep;39(7):560–565.

42. Popp W, et al. What is the use? An international look at reuse of single-use medical devices. *Int J Hyg Environ Health.* 2010 Jul;213(4):302–307.

43. Okwen MP, et al. Uncovering high rates of unsafe injection equipment reuse in rural Cameroon: Validation of a survey instrument that probes for specific misconceptions. *Harm Reduct J.* 2011 Feb 7;8(1):4.

44. UNAIDS. UNAIDS Report on the Global AIDS Epidemic 2010. Accessed 1 Jun 2011. http://www.unaids.org/globalreport/Global_report.htm.

45. World Health Organization. Preparedness for Deliberate Epidemics: Programme of Work for the Biennium 2004–2005. 2004. Accessed 14 Sep 2011. http://www.who.int/csr/resources/publications/deliberate/WHO_CDS_CSR_LYO_2004_8.pdf.

46. US Centers for Disease Control and Prevention. Anthrax. Accessed 1 Jun 2011. http://www.bt.cdc.gov/agent/anthrax.

47. US Centers for Disease Control and Prevention. Smallpox. Accessed 14 Sep 2011. http://www.bt.cdc.gov/agent/smallpox.

The World Health Organization Approach to Health Care–Associated Infection Prevention and Control

By
Benedetta Allegranzi, MD
Carmen Lúcia Pessoa-Silva, MD
Didier Pittet, MD

Please note: The authors are staff members of the World Health Organization. The authors alone are responsible for the views expressed in this publication, and they do not necessarily represent the decisions or the stated policy of the World Health Organization.

Health care–associated infections (HAIs) represent a major patient-safety issue worldwide. They are the most frequent adverse event during health care delivery and potentially result in prolonged hospital stays, long-term disability, increased antimicrobial resistance, high additional costs for the health care system, financial and human-suffering burdens for patients and their families, and excess deaths.[1] Through the Fifty-fifth World Health Assembly Resolution (WHA 55.18), the World Health Organization (WHO) has recognized the need to promote patient safety as a fundamental principle of all health systems and urged Member States to take action, including the prevention of HAIs.[2,3] Regional Offices and Committees across all six WHO regions (Africa, the Americas, Eastern Mediterranean, Europe, South-East Asia, and Western Pacific) formally committed to respond to this call through official documents and clear mention of HAIs as being among the most serious threats to patient safety in their health care settings.[2]

The emergence of life-threatening infections, such as severe acute respiratory syndrome (SARS) and viral hemorrhagic fevers (for example, Ebola and Marburg viral infections), highlight the urgent need for efficient infection control practices in health care. Among many important lessons learned from the SARS and viral hemorrhagic fever epidemics is the fact that health care settings can act as amplifiers of disease. HAI prevention and control can be enforced also by WHO through International Health Regulations,[4] an international legal instrument that is binding on 194 United Nations (UN) Member States across the globe and that entered into force in June 2007. An essential element for the implementation of the International Health Regulations is the early detection and contention of events that may constitute public health emergencies of international concern. To enable a timely public health response to infectious threats, hospital-based surveillance and infection prevention and control (IPC) practices must be in place for early reporting and containment purposes. International Health Regulations represent an excellent opportunity for the prevention and control of HAIs internationally.

HAIs may represent serious occupational hazards. Health care workers (HCWs) have been heavily affected during epidemics[5,6] and are frequently victims of occupational exposure to blood-borne pathogens. Prüss-Ustün et al.[7] estimate the global burden of disease attributable to occupational exposure among HCWs to be 40% hepatitis B and C infections and 2.5% human immunodeficiency virus (HIV) infections.

Antimicrobial resistance is a global threat, which is accelerating with the emergence of new multiresistance mechanisms and is fast outpacing available solutions. It challenges the control of infectious diseases, jeopardizes progress on health outcomes by increasing morbidity and mortality, and imposes huge costs on societies. It is clear that comprehensive global action by all stakeholders is needed. In response to this growing threat, WHO introduced a policy package on World Health Day on 7 April 2011 to combat antimicrobial resistance and to reframe critical actions to be taken by governments, including the need to enhance IPC measures.[8]

HAI prevention and control is now an important area of work for WHO, particularly over the last decade, with several World Health Assembly and Regional Committee resolutions[2,9–15] emphasizing the need to enhance its capacity worldwide, and WHO has committed to focusing on this aspect by providing leadership, technical expertise, and coordination. Beyond its key role in reaction and support to emergency situations, WHO develops and promotes standards and essential infection control recommendations (for example, hand-hygiene best practices) and supports countries to build and to strengthen long-term capacities—to be better prepared to prevent and to respond to potential outbreaks and to reduce the burden of endemic HAIs.

Given its leading role in international health among UN Member States, WHO is in a unique position to encourage and to strengthen HAI prevention and control through its Regional and Country Offices and WHO Collaborating Centres, to coordinate efforts with ministries of health and other key players, and to create partnerships at local and international levels. Regional and Country Offices have multiple critical roles, including ensuring that the specific needs of Member States in their regions are known and addressed; adapting global standards, directions, plans, and tools appropriate for the region; and coordinating regional initiatives. Country offices have the lead role in coordinating communications and other critical activities with national authorities and WHO efforts to provide local assistance. WHO headquarters collaborates closely with Regional Offices and plays a key role in the coordination of global initiatives and the development of global standards.

As a result of this commitment, the following examples can be cited to illustrate the global scope and reach of some WHO headquarters' initiatives in the field of HAI prevention and control. By developing and testing the Guidelines on Hand Hygiene in Health Care[16] and the Multimodal Hand Hygiene Improvement Strategy and Toolkit[17] over the past five years, WHO has emphasized the importance of hand hygiene as the most effective measure to prevent the transmission of health care–associated pathogens. However, evidence has shown that for many reasons, this basic procedure is often neglected by HCWs, and average compliance is estimated at less than 40% worldwide.[18] Although overcoming this reality (and behavioral issue) initially appeared to be a massive challenge in 2005, WHO has now succeeded in establishing a global campaign, with 124 governments formally committed to reducing HAIs through hand-hygiene best practices and other measures. Among these, 43 have initiated national/subnational hand-hygiene campaigns.[19] Since its launch in 2009, the WHO *SAVE LIVES: Clean Your Hands* global initiative has snowballed, with the participation of almost 14,000 hospitals from 153 countries in 2011.[20] One of the key success factors of this global campaign has been the strong and continuous support of all key players in the field of infection control worldwide as well as of WHO Collaborating Centres and Regional and Country Offices.

Another example of global spread is the Safe Injection Global Network (SIGN) launched by WHO in 1999.[21] SIGN is a network of stakeholders aiming to ensure the safe and rational use of injections worldwide and includes prominent international organizations, government bodies, scientific societies, universities, and industry representatives. A greater awareness of the need for safe injections has been achieved in almost every country since the SIGN launch, and by 2008, two thirds of the 96 low- and middle-income countries for which information is available had implemented safe-injection programs under its guidance. More than 90 countries have built the capacity to identify infection control breaches in injection practices and to implement the needed strategies to address the gaps by using SIGN tools to assess injection practices and to support the development of evidence-based injection-safety strategies.

A very important development is the fact that WHO has recently taken up the task of coordinating efforts for HAI prevention and control around the globe by launching the Global Infection Prevention and Control (GIPC) Network in June 2011.[22] The overall aim is to enhance IPC practices as tools for promoting safer care, containing infectious-disease outbreaks, and fighting antimicrobial resistance. Of note, the Regional and Country Offices are crucial to its functioning. The GIPC Network is expected to assist WHO in providing technical support to Member States through a broad dissemination of IPC policies and guidance documents. In addition, it will contribute to WHO efforts to build IPC capacity, particularly in low- and middle-income countries. The network will take advantage of already-established collaborations with institutions, organizations, agencies, and professional societies with demonstrated influence and experience in international infection control capacity building. Other WHO programs focused on HAI prevention and control will also contribute to its activities.

Since WHO has actively demonstrated its high commitment to HAI prevention and control, the topic of patient safety has finally attracted attention in the developing world. This represents a major change, as the scientific evidence and tradition of IPC have grown in industrialized nations where the vast majority of studies are conducted and key recommendations are issued. With its global perspective, WHO works to raise awareness of the fact that no country or health care setting worldwide can claim to be exempt or to have resolved the problem of HAIs. This not only means that recommendations and standards must be rigorously based on high-quality evidence and valid guidelines developed for use in any country but also implies significant efforts to facilitate implementation and adaptation according to available resources and the local culture and conditions. The work of WHO and others has demonstrated that the burden of HAIs in low- and middle-income countries is much higher and has some implications that differ from those of high-income countries, although other health problems are usually prioritized in settings with limited resources.[1–3] Another aspect indicating the global perspective of WHO's approach is the commitment to translate and to disseminate tools and documents as widely as possible to achieve the best audience reach and adoption.

Within WHO headquarters, two programs are focused only on HAI prevention and control (*Clean Care Is Safer Care* and *Infection Prevention and Control in Health Care*) and tackle different aspects of the problem. Other programs are related to specific topics of infection prevention or environmental health that are relevant for the community and health care settings or include some specific areas of work that have related implications. All collaborate and interact in a complementary manner. Most of these programs are reflected at the regional level with coordinated, but also partially independent, activities. In Table 2-1 these programs are listed in alphabetical order together with the main topics tackled, the main objectives, and the key documents produced to date. Refer to the specific website pages for more details. This list may not be exhaustive, as HAI prevention and control as well as patient-safety aspects might also be included within additional WHO programs. In general, all programs aim to raise awareness among governments, HCWs, and other key players to develop guidelines, standards, policies, and implementation and monitoring tools to support systems and resource strengthening for infection control, to engage with stakeholders and experts, to support training activities, and to facilitate field implementation, monitoring, research, and sharing of results and local experiences.

Acknowledgments

The authors thank Dr. Neelam Dhingra, Blood Transfusion Safety, WHO; Dr. Selma Khamassi, Injection Safety, WHO; and the members of the infection prevention and infection control working group at WHO Headquarters for their contributions to the chapter.

References

1. World Health Organization. Report on the Burden of Endemic Health Care–Associated Infection Worldwide. 2011. Accessed 26 Sep 2011. http://whqlibdoc.who.int/publications/2011/9789241501507_eng.pdf.

2. World Health Organization. Quality of Care: Patient Safety (Resolution WHA55.18). 18 May 2002. Accessed 26 Sep 2011. http://apps.who.int/gb/archive/pdf_files/WHA55/ewha5518.pdf.

3. World Health Organization. Quality of Care: Patient Safety. 23 Mar 2002. Accessed 26 Sep 2011. http://apps.who.int/gb/archive/pdf_files/WHA55/ea5513.pdf.

4. World Health Organization. International Health Regulations. 2008. Accessed 26 Sep 2011. http://www.who.int/ihr/9789241596664/en/index.html.

5. Feldmann H, Geisbert T, Kawaoka Y. Filoviruses: Recent advances and future challenges. *J Infect Dis.* 2007 Nov 15;196 Suppl 2:S129–130.

6. Jeffs B, et al. The Médecins Sans Frontières intervention in the Marburg hemorrhagic fever epidemic, Uige, Angola, 2005. I. Lessons learned in the hospital. *J Infect Dis.* 2007 Nov 15;196 Suppl. 2:S154–161.

7. Prüss-Ustün A, Rapiti E, Hutin Y. Estimation of the global burden of disease attributable to contaminated sharps injuries among health-care workers. *Am J Ind Med.* 2005 Dec;48(6):482–490.

8. World Health Organization. World Health Day 2011: Policy Briefs. Accessed 26 Sep 2011. http://www.who.int/world-health-day/2011/policybriefs/en/index.html.

9. World Health Organization. Emerging and Other Communicable Diseases: Antimicrobial Resistance (Resolution WHA51.17). 11–16 May 1998. Accessed 26 Sep 2011. http://apps.who.int/medicinedocs/index/assoc/s16334e/s16334e.pdf.

10. World Health Organization. Améliorer l'endiguement de la résistance aux antimicrobiens (Résolution WHA58.27). 25 May 2005. Accessed 26 Sep 2011. http://apps.who.int/gb/ebwha/pdf_files/WHA58/WHA58_27-fr.pdf.

11. World Health Organization. Prevention and Control of Influenza Pandemics and Annual Epidemics (Resolution WHA56.19). 28 May 2003. Accessed 26 Sep 2011. http://www.who.int/immunization/sage/1_WHA56_19_Prevention_and_control_of_influenza_pandemics.pdf.

12. World Health Organization. Strengthening Pandemic-Influenza Preparedness and Response (WHA58.5). 23 May 2005. Accessed 26 Sep 2011. http://apps.who.int/gb/ebwha/pdf_files/WHA58/WHA58_5-en.pdf.

13. World Health Organization. Prevention and Control of Multidrug-Resistant Tuberculosis and Extensively Drug-Resistant Tuberculosis (WHA62.15). 22 May 2009. Accessed 26 Sep 2011. http://apps.who.int/gb/ebwha/pdf_files/A62/A62_R15-en.pdf.

14. World Health Organization. Viral Hepatitis (WHA 63.18). 21 May 2010. Accessed 26 Sep 2011. http://www.worldhepatitisalliance.org/Libraries/Documents/2010_WHO_Viral_Hepatitis_Resolution.sflb.ashx.

15. World Health Organization. Infection Prevention and Control in Health Care: Time for Collaborative Action (Em/RC57/6). Oct 2010. Accessed 26 Sep 2011. http://www.emro.who.int/rc57/resolutions.htm.

16. World Health Organization. WHO Guidelines on Hand Hygiene in Health Care. 2009. Accessed 26 Sep 2011. http://whqlibdoc.who.int/publications/2009/9789241597906_eng.pdf.

17. World Health Organization. Save Lives: Clean Your Hands: Guide to Implementation. Aug 2009. Accessed 26 Sep 2011. http://whqlibdoc.who.int/hq/2009/WHO_IER_PSP_2009.02_eng.pdf.

18. Allegranzi B, et al. Burden of endemic health-care-associated infection in developing countries: Systematic review and meta-analysis. *Lancet.* 2011 Jan 15;377(9761):228–241.

19. World Health Organization. WHO CleanHandsNet—A Network of Campaigning Countries. Accessed 26 Sep 2011. http://www.who.int/gpsc/national_campaigns/en/.

20. World Health Organization. Save Lives: Clean Your Hands–WHO's Global Annual Campaign. May 2011. Accessed 26 Sep 2011. http://www.who.int/gpsc/5may/en/.

21. World Health Organization. The SIGN Alliance. Accessed 26 Sep 2011. http://www.who.int/injection_safety/sign/en/.

22. World Health Organization. GIPC Network Launch Meeting and Next Steps. 29 Jul 2011. Accessed 26 Sep 2011. http://www.who.int/csr/bioriskreduction/laboratorynetwork/gipc_next_steps/en/index.html.

23. Jha AK, et al. Patient safety research: An overview of the global evidence. *Qual Saf Health Care.* 2010 Feb;19(1):42–47.

Table 2-1. Main WHO Programs Focused on Health Care–Associated Infection (HAI) Prevention and Control

Blood Transfusion Safety (http://www.who.int/bloodsafety/en/)

Prevention of transfusion-transmissible infections (including HIV, hepatitis B, hepatitis C, and syphilis, and bacterial contamination of blood and blood products)

Relation to HAI prevention and control	Main guidelines and documents*
<ul><li>To develop norms, standards, best-practice guidelines, tools, and materials relating to the entire blood-transfusion process from donor to patient to ensure blood safety</li><li>To support the establishment of sustainable national blood programs, ensuring the provision of safe, high-quality blood and blood products to all patients requiring transfusion and their safe and appropriate use</li><li>To build capacity in countries through structured training activities, voluntary unpaid blood donation, donor selection, donation testing, risk assessment and management, data and quality management, external quality assessment, blood cold chain, hemovigilance, and the clinical use of blood</li><li>To support the implementation of a quality system in all aspects of blood collection, processing, testing, and clinical use, including setting up the system for surveillance, vigilance, and monitoring</li><li>To support the development of education and training programs and to incorporate transfusion medicine into medical and nursing school curricula</li><li>To establish a global monitoring mechanism on safe blood and blood products and to collect, to analyze, and to disseminate reliable information on blood safety and availability</li><li>To promote harmonization and collaboration of international efforts to ensure sufficient quantities of safe blood and blood products</li><li>To promote research and development in the provision and appropriate use of safe blood and blood products</li></ul>	<ul><li>Information sheet</li><li>Prevention of health care–associated HIV infection: Flyer</li><li>*Aide-mémoire* for good policy process for blood safety and availability</li><li>*Aide-mémoire* for national health authorities: Developing a national blood system</li><li>Universal access to safe blood transfusion</li><li>Guidelines: Maintaining a safe and adequate blood supply during pandemic influenza</li><li>WHO resource materials on blood safety: CD-ROM</li><li>The Melbourne declaration on 100% voluntary nonremunerated donation of blood and blood components</li><li>Toward 100% voluntary blood donation: A global framework for action</li><li>Developing a voluntary blood donor program (DONOR): Facilitator's toolkit (6 modules): CD-ROM</li><li>Blood-donor selection: Recommendations on assessing suitability for blood donation</li><li>Screening donated blood for transfusion-transmissible infections: Recommendations for blood transfusion services</li><li>*Aide-mémoire*: The blood cold chain</li><li>The blood cold chain: Guide to the selection and procurement of equipment and accessories</li><li>Manual on the management, maintenance, and use of blood cold chain equipment</li><li>*Aide-mémoire*: The clinical use of blood</li><li>*Aide-mémoire*: Clinical transfusion process and patient safety</li><li>Developing a national policy and guidelines on the clinical use of blood recommendations</li><li>The clinical use of blood: Information sheet for clinicians</li><li>The clinical use of blood: Handbook</li><li>The clinical use of blood in general medicine, obstetrics, pediatrics, surgery and anesthesia, trauma, and burns: Module</li><li>The clinical use of blood: CD-ROM</li><li>*Aide-mémoire*: Quality systems for blood safety</li><li>Quality management training for blood transfusion services: Facilitator's toolkit (5 books, 15 modules, CD ROM)</li><li>Distance learning in blood safety: Flyer</li><li>Establishing a distance-learning program in blood safety: A guide for program coordinators</li><li>Safe blood and blood products: Distance-learning materials (five modules)<ul><li>– Safe blood and blood products: Trainer's guide</li><li>– Introductory module: Guidelines and principles for safe blood-transfusion practice</li><li>– Module 1: Safe blood donation</li><li>– Module 2: Screening for HIV and other infectious agents</li><li>– Module 3: Blood-group serology</li></ul></li></ul>

Continued

Table 2-1. Main WHO Programs Focused on Health Care–Associated Infection (HAI) Prevention and Control *(continued)*

Relation to HAI prevention and control	Main guidelines and documents*
Clean Care Is Safer Care (http://www.who.int/gpsc/en/) HAI prevention control, and in particular, surveillance and prevention of the endemic burden of HAIs, with special focus on hand	

• To raise awareness of the burden of HAIs worldwide and the importance of hand hygiene in health care
• To catalyze political and stakeholders' commitment to reducing HAIs
• To develop technical guidance and recommendations on hand hygiene and infection control measures and to support their implementation in Member States
• To promote and to sustain hand-hygiene improvement at the point of care, through the *SAVE LIVES: Clean Your Hands* initiative and through a network of hand-hygiene campaigning countries—the *CleanHandsNet*
• To undertake reviews and to report updates related to the endemic burden of HAIs and to promote HAI surveillance and data reporting
• To evaluate the impact of infection control interventions to reducing the HAI burden, with particular focus on settings with limited resources
• To coordinate the development of new approaches for the prevention of surgical site infections
• To integrate infection control and hand hygiene in the approach to preventing bloodstream infection
• To support development and strengthening of infection control capacity and knowledge, skills, and behaviors at regional, subregional, and country levels through the provision of tools and materials
• To develop and to coordinate educational, training, and research activities
• To advise WHO on infection control measures and priorities and their integration with patient-safety strategies
	• Guidelines on hand hygiene in health care
	• Guide to implementation of the WHO multimodal hand-hygiene improvement strategy
	• Hand Hygiene Implementation Toolkit (32 tools):
	  – Tools for system change
	  – Tools for training and education
	  – Tools for evaluation and feedback
	  – Tools as reminders in the workplace
	  – Tools for institutional safety climate
	• Hand-hygiene self-assessment framework
	• "Hand Hygiene Moment 1—Global Observation Survey": Summary report
	• *SAVE LIVES: Clean Your Hands* promotional video
	• Outline action plan and top 10 tips for country/area campaigns
	• Using hand-hygiene improvement tools to implement country/area campaigns
	• Report on the endemic burden of HAIs worldwide
	• HAIs fact sheet
	• Scientific publications in peer-reviewed journals

Infection Prevention and Control in Health Care (http://www.who.int/csr/bioriskreduction/infection_control/en/index.html) HAI prevention and control; in particular, prevention, preparedness, and response to epidemics that can be associated with or amplified by health care	
• To support IPC capacity building in Member States through technical assistance and development of guidance on core elements for national and local IPC programs • To provide support to help prevent spread of infectious diseases through development and dissemination of evidence-based infection control measures in health care settings • To provide IPC tools for health care facility preparedness to respond to pandemics and epidemics • To coordinate the Global Infection Prevention and Control (GIPC) Network to foster alignment of policies and to enhance IPC practices worldwide • To support Member States in responding to outbreaks through the WHO Global Outbreak Alert and Response Network (GOARN) • To develop evidenced-based norms and standards for antimicrobial-resistance containment strategies in health care settings • To support infection control preparedness to cope with public health emergencies	• Prevention of hospital-acquired infections • Practical guidelines for infection control in health care facilities • Infection prevention and control of epidemic- and pandemic-prone acute respiratory diseases in health care WHO interim guidelines and an accompanying set of implementation tools for community and hospital health care facilities • Interim infection control recommendations for care of patients with suspected or confirmed filovirus (Ebola, Marburg) or hemorrhagic fever • Core components for IPC programs and an accompanying set of implementation tools for national and local programs • WHO policy on tuberculosis (TB) infection control in health care facilities, congregate settings, and households • Natural ventilation for infection control in health care settings • Advice on the use of masks in the community setting in Influenza A (H1N1) outbreaks • IPC during health care for confirmed, probable, or suspected cases of pandemic (H1N1) 2009 virus infection and influenza-like illnesses

Continued

Table 2-1. Main WHO Programs Focused on Health Care–Associated Infection (HAI) Prevention and Control *(continued)*

Relation to HAI prevention and control	Main guidelines and documents*
Injection Safety (http://www.who.int/injection_safety/en/) Prevention of blood-borne pathogens transmission through unsafe injection practices	
• To promote the rational use of injections and safe practices for injections and related procedures, including phlebotomy, intravenous, and fingerpick procedures • To produce policies on the prevention of needlestick injuries in HCWs and the use of personal protective equipment (PPE) following accidental stick injuries • To support the implementation of the recommendation for providing hepatitis B vaccine for all HCWs • To improve access to safety-engineered injection devices and sharps containers • To promote safe sharps waste management • To provide the secretariat for the "Safe Injection Global Network" (SIGN), which aims to achieve safe and appropriate use of injections throughout the world	• First, do no harm: Introducing auto-disable syringes and ensuring injection safety in immunization systems of developing countries • WHO best practices for injections and related procedures toolkit • WHO guidelines on drawing blood: Best practices in phlebotomy • Revised injection-safety assessment tool • Communication strategy for the safe and appropriate use of injections • The injection-safety policy planner • Guiding principles to ensure injection-device security • Guide to supervising injection providers • SIGN 2010 meeting report
Occupational Health (http://www.who.int/occupational_health/topics/hcworkers/en/index.html) Prevention of HAIs among HCWs	
• To promote the protection of occupational health of HCWs and the greening of the health sector (for example, less toxic disinfectants, natural ventilation) • To support the hepatitis B immunization campaign for HCWs (linked in regions to vaccination week and other vaccine-preventable diseases) • To reduce the exposure to HIV and other sharps-related infections (hepatitis B and C) associated with injections in HCWs • To review and to report data on the global burden of disease from sharps injuries to HCWs	• Joint WHO-ILO-UNAIDS policy guidelines for improving HCW access to HIV and TB prevention, treatment, care, and support services • Occupational health: A manual for primary HCWs • Role of the occupational health nurse in the workplace • Protecting HCWs—preventing needlestick injuries tool kit • Joint WHO/ILO guidelines on postexposure prophylaxis (PEP) to prevent HIV infection
Safe Surgery Saves Lives (http://www.who.int/patientsafety/safesurgery/en/index.html) Reduction of complications due to surgery, including surgical site infections (SSIs)	
• To improve the safety of surgical care around the world by ensuring adherence to proven standards of care in all countries • To contribute to the prevention of SSIs through the use of the WHO surgical-safety checklist	• WHO surgical-safety checklist • Checklist implementation manual
Water Supply, Sanitation, and Hygiene Development (http://www.who.int/water_sanitation_health/hygiene/en/) Promotion of environmental health in health care settings; in particular, safe health care waste management	
• To support the development and implementation of national policies, guidelines on safe practices, and training and promotion of effective messages in a context of healthy settings • To develop technical guidance on environmental health standards in health care • To develop technical guidance materials for assessing the quantities and types of waste produced in different facilities • To develop national health care waste-management guidelines • To build capacity at national level to enhance the way health care waste management is dealt with in low-income countries	• Safe health care waste management: Policy paper • WHO core principles for achieving safe and sustainable management of health care waste • Management of solid health care waste at primary health care centers: A decision-making guide • Essential environmental health standards in health care • Natural ventilation for infection control in health care settings • Mercury in health care: Policy paper

* These documents are all available in PDF format on the cited website pages related to the corresponding WHO program.

Joint Commission International's Infection Prevention and Control Standards and Requirements

A Detailed Study

The prevention and control of infections represent one of the most significant safety initiatives for a health care organization. Infections can be acquired in any health care setting, transferred between organizations, or brought in from the community. Because infections are a significant safety risk for patients, other care recipients, and health care workers (HCWs), infection prevention and control (IPC) must be high on every organization's list of priorities.

To help organizations focus on IPC issues and address related challenges, Joint Commission International (JCI) has developed IPC and related standards in all of its accreditation and certification programs as follows:

- Ambulatory Care: Infection Control and Facility Safety (IFS; partial chapter)
- Clinical Laboratories: Resource Management and Laboratory Environment (RSM; 1 standard)
- Home Care: Infection Prevention and Control (IPC; entire chapter)*
- Hospitals: Prevention and Control of Infections (PCI; entire chapter)
- Long Term Care: Infection Prevention and Control (IPC; entire chapter)*
- Medical Transport: Exposure to and Transmission of Biologic and Chemical Agents (BCA; entire chapter)
- Primary Care: Organization and Delivery of Services (ODS; chapter portion on IPC)
- International Patient Safety Goal 5 (IPSG.5)—Reduce the Risk of Health Care–Associated Infections (goal applicable for all accreditation and certification programs except Medical Transport)

The purpose of this chapter is to provide an in-depth look at JCI IPC requirements. A complete list of all JCI IPC requirements at the time of this publication is provided in Appendix 1. For the current IPC requirements regarding any JCI accreditation or certification program, please consult the applicable JCI comprehensive accreditation or certification manual or access JCI's accreditation and certification Web pages at http://www.jointcommissioninternational.org /Accreditation-and-Certification-Process/.

Please note: The majority of organizations surveyed by JCI are hospitals—three out of four organizations, as of the publication of this book—and as a result, the JCI hospital

standards are used as the foundation of much of this chapter and of Chapter 4. However, it is important to note that JCI accreditation standards are similar in theme, tone, and detail across accreditation and certification programs, and, therefore, JCI requirements are similar no matter the accreditation or certification program.

It is also important to note that for the sake of the following discussion, only JCI requirements with direct application to IPC are noted. Many JCI standards could and do apply indirectly to the concepts discussed below, but only those requirements specific to prevention and control of infections are noted.

JCI Requirements

Most JCI requirements are in the form of standards, which were created to respond to requests from the international community for external, objective, standards-based ways to evaluate health care practices and organizations. The goal of the accreditation program is to stimulate demonstration of continuous, sustained improvement in health care organizations by applying international consensus standards and indicators. JCI standards require a focused look at IPC across an organization and have an underlying philosophy of quality management, continuous quality improvement, and patient safety. These standards guide the organization leadership to establish and to maintain a comprehensive, integrated IPC program that is adequately supported and well managed.

JCI standards discuss the components of a comprehensive IPC program and the resources and support systems necessary to successfully implement such a program. There are three parts to the JCI standards: the standards, intent statements, and measurable elements.

Standards

JCI standards define the performance expectation, structures, or functions that must be in place for IPC. These standards were developed using a consensus process with a task force of international experts. The standards are based on accreditation experiences during recent years in more than 40 countries. The standards are validated through accreditation surveys and are designed to incorporate local or national laws and regulations. JCI has determined that organizations being surveyed must satisfactorily meet the requirements of all standards for the prevention and control of infection to achieve accreditation. These standards are designed to create a culture of patient safety and to lead organizations to best-practice levels to protect fundamental patient and family rights, to reduce risks during patient

* At the time of publication, the first edition of the JCI Home Care and Long Term Care manuals were being developed for publication in January 2012. Standards for both programs were derived from JCI's Care Continuum standards and will be in effect starting 1 July 2012. For the current status of these initiatives, visit the JCI Accreditation website (http://www.jointcommissioninternational.org /Accreditation-and-Certification-Process) or e-mail JCI Accreditation at JCIAccreditation@jcrinc.com.

care processes, and to enhance a safe environment where care is provided.

A 12-member International Standards Subcommittee, composed of experienced physicians, nurses, administrators, and public-policy experts, guides the development and revision process of the JCI standards. The subcommittee consists of members from six major world regions: Latin America and the Caribbean, Asia and the Pacific Rim, the Middle East, Central and Eastern Europe, Western Europe, and Africa. The work of the subcommittee is refined based on an international field review of the standards and the input from experts and others with unique content knowledge.

Intent Statements

A standard's intent statement helps explain the full meaning of the standard. The intent describes the purpose and rationale of the standard, providing an explanation of how the standard fits into the overall program, sets parameters for the requirement(s), and otherwise "paints a picture" of the requirements and goals.

Measurable Elements

Measurable elements of a standard indicate what is reviewed and assigned a score during the survey process. The measurable element(s) for each standard identify the requirements for full compliance with the standard. The measurable elements are intended to bring clarity to the standards and to help the organization fully understand the requirements, to help educate leaders and HCWs about the standards, and to guide the organization in accreditation preparation.

Examples of the standards, intent statements, and measurable elements are found throughout this book (*see*, for example, Box 3-1). The standards are updated approximately every three years based on the ongoing assessment of science, contemporary health care practice, available technology, quality and patient-safety practices, and other information.

Components of a Comprehensive IPC Program

The goal of an organization's infection surveillance, prevention, and control program is to identify and to reduce the risks of acquiring and transmitting infections among patients, HCWs, contract workers, volunteers, students, and visitors.

IPC programs differ from one organization to another, depending on the organization's geographic location, community, socioeconomic and physical environment, patient volume, populations served, types of clinical activities, and

---

Box 3-1. Example of JCI Standard, Intent, and Measurable Elements

Standard PCI.1

One or more individuals oversee all infection prevention and control activities. This individual(s) is qualified in infection prevention and control practices through education, training, experience, or certification.

Intent of PCI.1

The infection prevention and control program has oversight appropriate to the organization's size, level of risks, complexity of activities, and the program's scope. One or more individuals, acting on a full-time or part-time basis, provide that oversight as part of their assigned responsibilities or job descriptions. Their qualification depends on the activities they will carry out and may be met through
- education;
- training;
- experience; and
- certification or licensure.

Measurable Elements of PCI.1

❏ 1. One or more individuals oversee the infection prevention and control program.

❏ 2. The individual(s) is qualified for the organization's size, level of risks, and program scope and complexity.

❏ 3. The individual(s) fulfills program oversight responsibilities as assigned or described in a job description.

---

number and education of employees. Effective programs include identified leaders, appropriate policies and procedures, HCW education, coordination throughout the organizations, and systems to identify risks and to intervene to minimize or to eliminate infections.

The JCI hospital IPC standards are organized into the following six major sections:
1. Program Leadership and Coordination
2. Focus of the Program
3. Isolation Procedures
4. Barrier Techniques and Hand Hygiene
5. Integration of the Program with Quality Improvement and Patient Safety
6. Education of Staff About the Program

As mentioned earlier in this chapter, other JCI accreditation programs also have IPC requirements listed. Where those requirements overlap with JCI hospital standards is noted below.

Program Leadership and Coordination

Applicable JCI Standards	
The following JCI standards are directly applicable to this section of text. For complete standard text and further compliance information, *see* Appendix 1.	
Ambulatory Care	IFS.1 through IFS.4
Clinical Care Program (Certification)	
Clinical Laboratories	
Home Care	IPC.1 through IPC.3
Hospitals	PCI.1 through PCI.4
Long Term Care	IPC.1 though IPC.3
Medical Transport	BCA.1 through BCA.3
Primary Care	ODS.27 through ODS.29

JCI's program leadership and coordination requirements describe the organization's responsibilities for determining the focus of the IPC program. These requirements indicate that one or more full- or part-time HCWs—as part of their assigned responsibilities or job description(s)—oversee all IPC activities and that the individual(s) be qualified in IPC practices through education, training, experience, or certification. The designation of a particular individual(s) helps in the coordination of the multiple facets of the program. The IPC program's oversight should be appropriate to the organization's size and risk levels, and the program's scope and complexity. Although decentralization of IPC leadership can be effective, it sometimes leads to gaps in performance and less accountability. The person(s) designated for the oversight role coordinates the dynamics of program management, including addressing changing infection risks and implementing intervention strategies; ensures inclusion of all programs and services; and generates policies and procedures to guide compliance with best IPC practices. Therefore, it is important for this person(s) to have clinical expertise and program management skills to oversee all the IPC activities.

These requirements also call for program management by designating those persons or group that monitors and coordinates IPC activities in the organization and directs the coordination of IPC activities. This group must include representatives from at least medicine, nursing, IPC (for example, health care epidemiologist, infection control physician, IPC officer, and infection control nurse), and housekeeping. Others may be included as appropriate to the organization. IPC activities involve individuals in every department or service who perform nearly every function within a health care organization.

When the program oversight activities reside with a committee, it is incumbent on the organization to provide each member with education and training as well as clearly defined roles and responsibilities. *See* Chapter 5 for more discussion of the multidisciplinary oversight team.

These JCI standards are also focused on grounding the IPC program in science, practice guidelines, regulation, and technology and on providing sufficient resources to establish that scientific and technological foundation. JCI requires that the IPC program be based on current scientific knowledge, accepted practice guidelines, and applicable laws and regulations. Current scientific information is required to understand and to implement effective surveillance and control activities; practice guidelines provide information on preventive practices and infections associated with clinical services; and applicable laws and regulations define elements of the basic program and reporting requirements. Many of these guidelines are available online from government agencies and from professional societies. *See* Appendix 2 for selected websites and organizations providing practice guidelines. JCI requirements also state that leaders provide adequate resources to support the IPC program, particularly via information-management systems. Such systems are key resources to support the tracking of risks, rates, and trends in health care–associated infections (HAIs). Leadership roles and responsibilities are discussed in Chapter 5. Functions covered in these standards include data analysis, interpretation, and presentation of findings.

Focus of the Program

Applicable JCI Standards	
The following JCI standards are directly applicable to this section of text. For complete standard text and further compliance information, *see* Appendix 1.	
Ambulatory Care	IFS.5
Clinical Care Program (Certification)	
Clinical Laboratories	RSM.6.1*
Home Care	IPC.4 through IPC.5
Hospitals	PCI.5 through PCI.7.5
Long Term Care	IPC.4 through IPC.5.5
Medical Transport	BCA.1 through BCA.3
Primary Care	ODS.27 through ODS.29
* RSM.6.1 deals with a laboratory using a coordinated process to reduce the risks of infection as a result of exposure to biohazardous materials and waste only.	

Program-focus standards describe the organization's responsibilities for determining the focus of the IPC program. These requirements emphasize that the organization design and implement a coordinated and comprehensive program and plan to reduce the risks of HAIs for patients and HCWs. Safe, high-quality care for patients and a safe work environment for employees are intertwined because employees and patients who become infected can transmit the infection to other patients or HCWs. These standards imply a close working relationship between the IPC and employee health services.

Under these standards, the IPC program is guided by a plan that addresses infection issues that are epidemiologically important to the organization. This requires assessing risks and key issues that pertain to the particular infections, populations, environment, and other factors that are specific to the organization. In addition, the standard requires that the IPC program be designed to be appropriate to the organization's size, geographic location, services, and patients. A facility that treats primarily trauma patients rather than pediatric or cancer patients or is an ambulatory care center rather than an acute inpatient facility must address the issues most relevant to its patients, services, and setting. Organizations in very rural settings may have challenges that differ from those of facilities in urban settings. Conditions that should be considered in assessing geographic and environmental influence on infections include the following:

- Natural environmental disruptions—floods, hurricanes, earthquakes, and other events
- Temperature variations—tropical versus cold
- Vector density—mosquitoes, rodents
- Contaminated water sources or lack of water
- Ecological changes—deforestation, global warming, air pollution, and so forth
- War, migrations, displaced persons
- Urban versus rural—congested housing versus agricultural environments
- Availability, lack of, or disruption of services

Another key element of these requirements is that the IPC program include surveillance activities that are proactive and systematic. Surveillance (*see* Box 3-2), or the observing of practice and collecting of infection data, is essential to identify endemic (usual) infections and outbreaks (unusual infections or numbers of infections above the usual endemic rates). Not only must the surveillance activities help the IPC professionals identify ongoing or unusual infections, but the IPC program must have the capability to investigate infection clusters or outbreaks to identify which infections are occurring and why, the source, the mode of transmission, processes contributing to the infections, and potential solutions to resolve the outbreak and to stop the infections. Once this information is clear, it should be used to implement prevention strategies that will prevent the recurrence of the infections in the future.

JCI standards require that the ICP program be informed by a periodic assessment of the organizational risks for infections and guided by policies and procedures to prevent or to

---

Box 3-2. Surveillance

According to the US Centers for Disease Control and Prevention (US CDC), *surveillance* "is the ongoing systematic collection, analysis, and interpretation of health data for purposes of improving health and safety."[1]

Surveillance allows hospital personnel to identify risks and areas for improvement, to target infection-reducing initiatives, and to monitor progress toward reducing the number and spread of infections within a facility, as well as allowing ICP and other HCWs to do the following[2–5]:

- Establish endemic rates of HAIs.
- Identify outbreaks.
- Search out cases of a specific disease.
- Determine whether processes used to prevent and to control infections are functioning properly.
- Check the success of any changes made to a system or process.
- Monitor the occurrence of adverse outcomes to identify potential risk factors.
- Ensure compliance with federal and state regulations and accreditation requirements.
- Monitor injuries and identify risk factors for occupational injuries in HCWs.
- Help with health care and support HCW education efforts.

References

1. US Centers for Disease Control and Prevention. Surveillance. (Updated 8 Oct 2010) Accessed 18 Apr 2011. http://www.cdc.gov/niosh/topics/surveillance.
2. The Joint Commission. *The Joint Commission Infection Prevention and Control Handbook for Hospitals*. Oak Brook, IL: Joint Commission Resources, 2009.
3. Lautenbach E, Woeltje KF, Malani PN. Society for Healthcare Epidemiology of America. *Practical Healthcare Epidemiology*, 3rd ed. Chicago: University of Chicago Press, 2010.
4. Yokoe DS, et al. A compendium of strategies to prevent healthcare-associated infections in acute care hospitals. *Infect Control Hosp Epidemiol.* 2008 Oct;29 Suppl 1:S12–21.
5. Association for Professionals in Infection Control and Epidemiology (APIC). *APIC Text of Infection Control and Epidemiology*, 3rd ed. Washington, DC: APIC, 2009.

---

mitigate those risks. IPC policies should be based on the best available evidence and science, which requires infection professionals to continually review the literature, new guidelines, and laws and to incorporate them into organizational policies and procedures. The organization sets risk-reduction goals and measurable objectives that help formulate the IPC plan, provide focus for the program, and permit objective evaluation of progress toward risk reduction.

JCI standards also indicate that the IPC program involve all patient, HCW, and visitor areas of the organization.

Because infection can potentially be transmitted by any of the above persons as well as by vendors, volunteers, and students, any of the areas where these persons work should have IPC policies and procedures and should be considered an integral part of the organization's IPC program.

JCI directs the organization to use a risk-based approach to establish the focus of the HAI prevention and reduction program. Each organization must determine those epidemiologically important infections, infection sites, and associated devices and procedures that will provide the focus of efforts to prevent and to reduce the incidence of HAIs. Organizations consider, as appropriate, infections that involve the following:

- Respiratory tract—such as the procedures and equipment associated with respiratory therapy, intubation, mechanical ventilatory support, tracheostomy, and so on
- Urinary tract—such as the invasive procedures and equipment associated with indwelling urinary catheters, urinary drainage systems, and so on, along with associated care
- Intravascular invasive devices—such as the insertion and care of central venous catheters and peripheral venous lines
- Surgical sites—such as their care, type of dressing, and aseptic procedures
- Epidemiologically significant diseases and organisms—including multidrug-resistant organisms and highly virulent infections
- Emerging or reemerging infections in the community

In addition to specific infections, such issues as employee exposures or environmental hazards may be selected as areas that are considered epidemiologically important and should be addressed in planning the focus of the IPC program. When the evaluation or analysis of the data of any of these infections indicates the need for action, the organization refocuses its attention to these areas. The organization assesses these risks at least annually, or more often if desired, and documents its findings. In addition, when the risk analysis identifies direct-care or support processes that may be contributing to infection, the organization addresses these processes through policies and procedures, education, changes in practice, or other activities to work toward the reduction or elimination of risk.

JCI standards on program focus also address risk inherent with particular equipment, departments, and other scenarios. JCI requires organizations to ensure that their medical equipment, laundry, and linen are cleaned, disinfected, or sterilized to minimize infection risk and that processes for doing so are consistent throughout the organizations. For example, if more than one area performs sterilization procedures, such as a central sterilizing department and satellite areas, each of the areas

performing these functions must meet the same organizational and best-practice standards. Ensuring this quality requires oversight and coordination. Areas affected by this standard include the following:

- Equipment cleaning and sterilization—in particular, invasive equipment, such as endoscopes and surgical instruments
- Laundry and linen management

JCI requirements state that a policy and procedure identify the process for managing expired supplies and define the conditions for reusing single-use devices (SUDs) when laws and regulations permit and an organization decides to take this approach. SUDs are permissible when permitted by local laws and regulations, as long as carefully designed policies are in place that identify at least the following:

- Devices and materials that can never be reused
- Maximum number of reuses specific for each device and material that is reused
- Types of wear and cracking, among other concerns, that indicate the device cannot be reused
- Cleaning process for each device that starts immediately after use and follows a clear protocol
- Process for the collection, analysis, and use of IPC data related to reused devices and materials

One organization's process to develop its SUD policy is described in Case Study 3-1.

CASE STUDY 3-1
Reprocessing Single-Use Devices (Canada)

Sandra Callery, RN, MHSc, CIC

Introduction

The finance department at Sunnybrook Health Sciences Centre (SHSC) asked for cost-saving measures throughout the hospital. The operations director for the operating room (OR) and outpatient procedures requested that the Reprocessing Steering Committee (the Committee) consider approving the reuse of some high-cost single-use devices (SUDs) that are used in the cardiac catheterization unit and the OR. Currently the hospital's policy on reuse states that it would not consider reprocessing any critical or semicritical SUD within the institution. However, if an area or user chooses to have an SUD reprocessed by a third party, the third party must provide documentation to the Committee that it follows the methodology and validation processes as outlined by an established regulatory body, such as the US Food and Drug Administration (US FDA).

Methods

The Committee reviewed government regulations regarding reprocessing SUDs, including liability. The Committee established the hospital's weighted criteria at the time of submission of request for purchase (RFP). The responses to the RFPs were assessed by the Committee. Reference checks were conducted. Prior to selection, a site tour of the licensed reprocessor's facility was conducted by the Committee to review practices and procedures and to ensure that it had been certified by a regulatory authority or an accredited quality system auditor to ensure the cleanliness, sterility, safety, and functionality of the reprocessed equipment/devices. In addition, the Committee verified its ability to

a) track and label equipment/devices;
b) recall improperly reprocessed medical equipment/devices;
c) test for pyrogens;
d) report adverse events;
e) provide good manufacturing procedures; and
f) establish the maximum number of reuses specific for each device.

The Committee collaborated with the prospective third-party reprocessors to determine eligible instruments and to perform a cost-benefit analysis.

Staff and departments involved included representation from senior leadership and the following teams and departments: IPC, OR, ambulatory care, central reprocessing, and materials management. The Committee has a reporting structure to the IPC Committee and the Medical Advisory Committee of the hospital.

Results

Canadian regulations do not recommend the reprocessing of SUDs by health care institutions unless the reprocessing is done by a licensed reprocessor. Submissions were reviewed by a hospital committee, site tours were conducted, and SHSC selected a licensed reprocessor to reprocess 100 different critical SUD items, with annual savings of more than $300,000.

Lessons Learned

Careful consideration and execution must be used when entering into reprocessing of SUDs, including the following tips:

• Provide adequate time for discussion with the Committee members and to the reporting committees.
• Ensure adequate representation of affected hospital services/programs during preliminary discussions.
• Do homework by reviewing hospital policies regarding hospital liability.
• Develop exclusion and inclusion criteria.
• Keep physicians and surgeons informed of the decisions throughout the process.
• Ensure that hospital policies and procedures give clear direction on the hospital's position and ongoing monitoring of compliance with the reprocessing protocols.

A policy that identifies the process for ensuring proper handling of expired supplies, including IV fluids, catheters, sutures, and others, must be in place and enforced. This policy may include the frequency of examining supplies to determine whether they are near expiration or have expired; a process, such as "first in–first out," to reduce the amount of expired supplies; and the way expired supplies are removed from general stores or shelves and supply rooms on patient units.

JCI standards also call for risk reduction in the processes of disposing of blood and blood components as wells as infectious waste and body fluids from any organization area, including the mortuary and postmortem areas. These wastes must be handled and disposed in a manner that protects the employees who are disposing of the wastes and the environment where the wastes reside or are disposed (eliminated) to prevent the transmission of infectious agents in the wastes and fluids. Similar requirements are in place regarding sharps and needles, with particular focus on the containers that are used to hold used sharps, the method of disposal of the containers, and the surveillance of the disposal process. The sharps disposal process should be consistent with safe practices; local, regional, or national laws; and other regulations. The organization may manage this process or contract with an outside agency to dispose of sharps and needles.

Kitchen sanitation, food preparation and handling, and mechanical and engineering controls (such as system ventilation, biological hoods, and others) should be managed to minimize or to eliminate infection risk.

JCI standards require organizations to reduce the risk of infection in the facility during demolition, construction, and renovation and to consider, among other factors, air quality, dust, and other risks to patients or HCWs. It is essential that infection control HCWs be involved in construction and renovation from the beginning to the end of the process to ensure that infection prevention risks are addressed. This and other related content are discussed further in Chapters 5 and 6.

Isolation Procedures

Applicable JCI Standards
The following JCI standards are directly applicable to this section of text. For complete standard text and further compliance information, *see* Appendix 1.

Ambulatory Care	
Clinical Care Program (Certification)	
Clinical Laboratories	
Home Care	
Hospitals	PCI.8
Long Term Care	IPC.6
Medical Transport	BCA.6
Primary Care	

Isolation standards require that patients—especially when immunosuppressed—as well as visitors and HCWs be protected from infections via barriers and isolation. Precautions regarding airborne transmission are especially important components of this requirement, including JCI's preference that patients with airborne infections be isolated in negative-pressure rooms until the infections are no longer communicable. For organizations unable to construct negative-pressure rooms, an acceptable alternative is a high-efficiency particulate air (HEPA) filtration system that functions at the rate of at least 12 air exchanges per hour. When neither a negative-pressure room nor HEPA filtration is available, organizations must have a policy and a procedure for how to manage for short periods of time patients who may spread infection by the airborne route.

In addition, these JCI requirements indicate that the organization must have a strategy to deal with an influx of patients with contagious infectious diseases. This will require advance planning and forethought, including the careful education of HCWs in the management of such patients.

Barrier Techniques and Hand Hygiene

Applicable JCI Standards
The following JCI standards are directly applicable to this section of text. For complete standard text and further compliance information, *see* Appendix 1.

Ambulatory Care	IFS.7
Clinical Care Program (Certification)	
Clinical Laboratories	
Home Care	IPC.6
Hospitals	PCI.8 and PCI.9
Long Term Care	IPC.7
Medical Transport	BCA.4
Primary Care	ODS.16 and ODS.24.3

JCI's barrier-technique and hand-hygiene requirements indicate that gloves, masks, soap, and disinfectants be available and used correctly when required. Hand-hygiene materials, barrier techniques, antiseptics, and disinfecting agents are fundamental to IPC. The organization must identify those situations in which masks and gloves are required and ensure that the products are available and accessible. For example, soap, alcohol hand preparations, and disinfectants should be located in those areas where hand hygiene and disinfecting procedures are required. Organizations should also adopt and post hand-hygiene guidelines in appropriate areas throughout the organization. (The use of guidelines is scored at IPSG.5, ME 2; *see* "Infection Prevention and Control and the International Patient Safety Goals," beginning on page 27, for more details.) HCWs must be educated in proper hand-washing and disinfecting procedures.

Integration with Quality Improvement and Patient Safety

Applicable JCI Standards
The following JCI standards are directly applicable to this section of text. For complete standard text and further compliance information, *see* Appendix 1.

Ambulatory Care	
Clinical Care Program (Certification)	
Clinical Laboratories	MGT.4.2.1 and MGT.4.6
Home Care	IPC.1
Hospitals	PCI.10 through PCI.10.6
Long Term Care	IPC.1
Medical Transport	QMI.3.7
Primary Care	ODS.27 and ODS.29

JCI requires organizations to make certain that IPC measures are given equal weight with other quality-improvement measures. These standards require that the IPC process be integrated with the organization's overall quality-improvement and patient-safety program. It is important to have IPC representation on the quality and patient-safety oversight group and to ensure that IPC data and issues are discussed in this setting.

The IPC process is designed to lower the risk of infection for patients, HCWs, and others. To reach this goal, the organization must proactively monitor and track risks, rates, and trends in HAIs. This tracking is the core of the surveillance program and is discussed further in Chapters 5 and 6.

JCI standards state that the organization should also use indicators to monitor infections that are epidemiologically important to the organization. If an organization has a large cardiac or neurosurgical surgery service, an extensive neonatal intensive care unit(s), or rehabilitation patients, it should select infection indicators specific for these patient populations. If the organization has a challenging problem with ventilator-associated pneumonia (VAP) in critical care patients, it may choose outcome indicators of infection in populations at risk for VAP for the monitoring or auditing process.

JCI requires that risk, rate, and trend information from surveillance, monitoring, or auditing processes be used to design or to modify processes to reduce infections to the lowest possible levels. As the information and the associated risks change, the organization must review and modify existing procedures, such as those associated with care of the ventilated patient or designed to decrease risk in a surgical patient. The organization uses its performance-improvement model to guide these improvement efforts.

JCI also requires that organizations evaluate their IPC data and information by comparing their IPC rates and trends against those of similar organizations through comparative databases and against best practices and scientific evidence. This process must be carefully designed to ensure that common definitions are used to classify infections as health care associated and that the frequency, intensity, and methods of surveillance are consistent for the comparative organizations. It is important for the IPC program to regularly communicate the results of IPC monitoring to the appropriate HCWs, physicians, and management. The leaders of the organization will use this information to provide guidance to the IPC program staff and to determine priorities and resources allocated to the IPC program. In addition to internal reporting, these standards require the organization to disseminate information on infections to the appropriate external public health agencies to comply with any regulations. The recipients of IPC data will vary among countries. Some countries have a nationwide database on infections; in other countries, all information is collected by the ministry of health or other governmental organization. When the organization receives information and reports from its public health agencies, it must take appropriate action to respond to these reports.

Staff Education

Applicable JCI Standards	
The following JCI standards are directly applicable to this section of text. For complete standard text and further compliance information, *see* Appendix 1.	

Ambulatory Care	
Clinical Care Program (Certification)	
Clinical Laboratories	
Home Care	IPC.7
Hospitals	PCI.11
Long Term Care	IPC.8
Medical Transport	BCA.10 through BCA.10.2
Primary Care	

The last section of the JCI requirements calls for maintaining knowledgeable HCWs. JCI standards state that organizations will provide IPC education to HCWs, patients, and, as appropriate or applicable, family and other caregivers. For an organization to have an effective IPC program, it must educate HCWs about the program when they begin working in the organization and regularly thereafter. The education program includes professional physicians and nurses, clinical and nonclinical support staff, and even patients and families, if appropriate. The program may also include tradespeople and other visitors. The education focuses on the policies, procedures, and practices that guide the organization's IPC program. The education also includes the findings and significant trends from monitoring or auditing activities, new services, or changes in IPC practices.

All JCI standards with direct and indirect IPC applicability are listed in Appendix 1.

Infection Prevention and Control and the International Patient Safety Goals

Applicable JCI Programs
International Patient Safety Goal 5 (IPSG.5) is applicable to the following JCI accreditation and certification programs:
• Ambulatory Care
• Clinical Care Program (Certification)
• Clinical Laboratories
• Home Care
• Hospitals
• Long Term Care
• Primary Care

JCI presented its first set of six International Patient Safety Goals in 2006, with requirements that organizations directly address frequently problematic health care issues. Among those goals is International Patient Safety Goal 5 (IPSG.5), the full text of which is in Box 3-3. Case Study 3-2 shows how one organization complied with the requirements of IPSG.5.

Box 3-3. International Patient Safety Goal 5 (IPSG.5)

Goal 5: Reduce the Risk of Health Care–Associated Infections

Standard IPSG.5

The organization develops an approach to reduce the risk of health care–associated infections.

Intent of IPSG.5

Infection prevention and control are challenging in most health care settings, and rising rates of health care–associated infections are a major concern for patients and health care practitioners. Infections common to all health care settings include catheter-associated urinary tract infections, blood stream infections, and pneumonia (often associated with mechanical ventilation).

Central to the elimination of these and other infections is proper hand hygiene. Internationally acceptable hand-hygiene guidelines are available from the World Health Organization (WHO), the US Centers for Disease Control and Prevention (US CDC), and various other national and international organizations.

The organization has a collaborative process to develop policies and/or procedures that adapt or adopt currently published and generally accepted hand-hygiene guidelines and for the implementation of those guidelines with the organization.

Measurable Elements of IPSG.5

❏ 1. The organization has adopted or adapted currently published and generally accepted hand-hygiene guidelines.

❏ 2. The organization implements an effective hand-hygiene program.

❏ 3. Policies and/or procedures are developed that support continued reduction of health care–associated infections.

CASE STUDY 3-2

Increasing Compliance with Hand-Hygiene Protocol (Turkey)

Özlem Yıldırım, PhD, MSEM, BSIE; Birsen Cetin, MD; Fatma Kucukerenkoy, MM, RN; Rahsan Boyoglu, MSN, RN; Nilufer Dogan, RN

Introduction

Citing published data indicating that increased hand-hygiene compliance leads to fewer HAIs, leaders at American Hospi-tal, Istanbul, Turkey, made a priority of increasing its baseline rate of 56% compliance.

Methods

A multidisciplinary improvement team was formed to address hand-hygiene compliance. The team included leaders and support staff from the American Hospital's Infection Control Committee (ICC) as well as staff from nursing, continuous quality improvement, and selected clinical departments. The team's first task was to develop and to design a Hand-Wash Observation Form and to supply the form to a group of "observers." Observers were trained on the hospital's policy for effective hand hygiene and were strategically stationed to observe HCWs' compliance. Observation methodology was discussed, including the following:

- Criteria for appropriate hand washing, including opportunity, method, and duration
- Opportunities to observe, such as before and after patient contact, medication preparation, or collection of dirty linens
- Identification of physicians, nurses, respiratory therapists, physiotherapists, and technicians as the persons to be observed

Through this surveillance, the observers identified incidents of noncompliance. The compliance rate was calculated based on the number of observations of HCWs in compliance with the hand-hygiene protocol divided by the total number of observations (opportunities). Following the aggregation of collected data, data were stratified by profession, clinical service, and unit. This information was sent to the units monthly, and hand-hygiene compliance indicators were monitored as one of the key performance indicators for the hospital. The trends were monitored monthly by the ICC and quarterly by the Quality Improvement and Management Committee and disseminated at regular departmental meetings. An improvement plan was developed and implemented.

Actions, Strategies, and Interventions

Because hand-hygiene compliance data had not been previously quantified, most departments were not aware of their actual hand-hygiene performance levels. Prior to this initiative, many HCWs were not fully aware of their hand-hygiene responsibilities, because practical knowledge and communication of that knowledge were lacking.

Strategies for improving compliance were identified, including the following:

- Infection control nurses formally educated HCWs about the theory underlying hand hygiene before and after patient care and trained the HCWs on proper hand-hygiene technique.

- To increase HCW awareness and to make the process more practical, mirrors were installed above sinks, and walls containing sinks were painted green to further identify the areas and to draw HCWs' attention. Sensor-based faucets were installed.
- With the support of the top management, the ICC increased the number of alcohol-based hand-rub dispensers. The hand rub was made available in specific locations, such as the entrance to key locations, including patients' rooms, blood-draw rooms, pharmacy, and near sinks. In addition, a practical document explaining the use of the hand rub was prepared and displayed on each dispenser.
- Laboratory technicians were provided with pocket-sized containers of alcohol-based hand rub.
- The organization's Communications Department shared the hand-hygiene protocol with HCWs via the hospital's intranet site and "Clean Hands Save Lives" coasters.
- An observational "hand-hygiene rate" was established as a key performance measure, and results were shared monthly.
- Based on the results, discipline- and department-specific training programs were organized.

Results

At the end of the measurement period, hand-hygiene compliance had increased to 72%, exceeding the targeted compliance rate of 65%.

During the first year of implementation, the hand-hygiene compliance rate was monitored at the following times:

- Hand hygiene prior to patient contact
- Hand hygiene following patient contact
- Compliance with all the steps for proper hand-hygiene technique

The compliance rate was calculated as the average of these three steps. Because HCW compliance was lowest in "hand hygiene prior to patient contact," greater emphasis was placed on increasing compliance in that area, including education for reasons for hand washing during each step. The data analysis was done by discipline (physicians, nurses, nurse aides, physiotherapists, radiology technicians, and laboratory technicians). Starting in 2009 respiratory therapists, cardiology technicians, and anesthesia technicians also were included. In 2010 the hospital's dental clinic opened, and dental technicians were added to the monitoring process.

During those three years (2007–2010), data show that nurses had the best compliance rate with 89%, followed by dental technicians (2010 only) with 87%, and respiratory

therapists with 84%. Most-improved categories were nurse aides and physiotherapists with an 86% increase during that time frame, and anesthesia technicians, who achieved an 81% increase.

Compliance measurement is ongoing, and the results are aggregated and reported to the related department managers monthly. Likewise, compliance data are being shared with the ICC. The organization's target compliance rate is also discussed by the ICC in an ongoing manner. Due to the success of this initiative, leadership implemented a new strategy to create a more effective hand-hygiene program, instructing the ICC to also monitor alcohol-based hand-rub usage rates and the quantity of hand rub used per 1,000 patient census days per month.

The committee monitored the hand-hygiene rates as an indicator of compliance with JCI's International Patient Safety Goal 5 (*see* Box 3-3). Compliance with hand-rub use per 1,000 patient census days increased from an initial rate of 18% in January 2009 to 41% in June 2011.

Lessons Learned

- Leadership was essential to facilitating change in hand-hygiene compliance. Without leadership buy-in, HCWs would have been less motivated to change their behavior.
- The power and effectiveness of data collection were evident to team members, as they learned to quantify the performance of a practice through observation.
- Culture change required time, and sustaining the improvement took frequent, repeated performance measurements.
- On-the-job training was essential for changing HCWs' behavior. HCWs need to understand their responsibilities and receive ongoing feedback to ensure continuous performance improvement.

IPSG.5 addresses the issue of IPC by suggesting that organizations comply with the World Health Organization's (WHO's) or US CDC's guidelines on hand hygiene, depending on local regulations or preferences. (Although WHO and US CDC guidelines are suggested as ways to meet this safety goal, an international organization can use another set of guidelines that is "published and generally accepted." This will usually mean guidelines that are evidence based.) According to WHO, low hand-hygiene compliance rates are reported from developed and developing countries. Despite worldwide attention to the issue of hand hygiene and its relationship with the spread of infection to patients and others, WHO places hand-hygiene compliance rates from 5% to 89% and an overall average of 38.7%.[1]

Chief reasons for this shortfall, according to WHO,[1] include the following:

- Hand-washing agents that cause irritations and dryness
- Sinks inconveniently located/shortage of sinks
- Lack of soap, paper, or towel
- Insufficient time
- Prioritizing patient needs
- Interference with HCW–patient relationship
- Low risk of acquiring infection from patients
- Belief that glove use eliminates the need for hand hygiene
- Lack of knowledge of guidelines/protocols, experience, and education
- Lack of rewards/encouragement
- Lack of role model from colleagues or superiors
- Forgetfulness
- Skepticism about the value of hand hygiene
- Disagreement with the recommendations
- Lack of scientific information of definitive impact of improved hand hygiene on HAIs

WHO (in 2009) and the US CDC (in 2002) have released guidelines for hand hygiene in health care settings based on extensive review of the scientific literature and the consensus of world experts. The guidelines advise, among other things, the preferential use of alcohol-based hand rubs for routine hand hygiene as well as traditional soap and water when hands are visibly soiled and sterile gloves when appropriate to protect patients in health care settings. Also included are recommendations for care of the hands, advice against use of artificial nails, proper use of gloves, and leadership guidelines. WHO's recommended hand-washing techniques using either soap and water or alcohol-based formulations can be found in Figure 3-1. The full text of WHO and US CDC guidelines are available via the Web in the following places:

- WHO Hand Hygiene Guidelines
  http://whqlibdoc.who.int/publications/2009/9789241597 906_eng.pdf
- CDC Hand Hygiene Guidelines
  http://www.cdc.gov/handhygiene/Guidelines.html

Although WHO guidelines outline the appropriate use of alcohol-based hand rubs (if hands are not visibly soiled, the use of hand rubs is appropriate and preferred), individuals are not required to use them. However, if an individual chooses not to use them, then he or she should use soap and water instead. Towelettes (that is, paper towels embedded with an antiseptic product, such as alcohol) are not a substitute for hand washing, and non-alcohol-based rubs are not recommended.

The guidelines offer appropriate techniques for hand hygiene, including using soap and water for 15 seconds and rubbing the hands together with an alcohol-based hand rub until the hands are dry. The guidelines also cover the appropriate selection of hand-hygiene agents, formulas for preparing alcohol-based hand-hygiene agents in the organization, and recommendations for appropriate skin care.

For updates on this or any WHO initiative, *see* Chapter 2 and the WHO website at http://www.who.int.

Some organizations have expressed concern that alcohol-based hand rubs are flammable. While acknowledging this concern, JCI believes that the typical alcohol gel and foam dispensers in the health care setting are of such limited size and volume that the alcohol gel's contribution to the acceleration of fire development or fire spread is "negligible." In all cases, organizations are advised to consult with and to follow the advice of their local fire authorities.

The Joint Commission Center for Transforming Healthcare's Hand-Hygiene Solutions

Established in 2009, the US-based Joint Commission Center for Transforming Healthcare strives to solve health care's most critical safety and quality problems. The Center participants—some of the leading hospitals and health systems in the United States—use a systematic approach to analyze specific breakdowns in care and to discover their underlying causes to develop targeted solutions that solve these complex problems. The first set of targeted solutions was created by eight leading health care organizations in the United States that worked with the Center to tackle hand hygiene. (Targeted solutions for surgical site infections [SSIs]—particularly in the area of colorectal procedures—were scheduled for publication in late 2011 at the same time of this publication; *see* http://www.centerfor transforminghealthcare.org/projects/detail.aspx?Project=4 for updated information on this initiative.)

The Center's Targeted Solutions Tool™ (TST)—provided free of charge to Joint Commission–accredited organizations in the United States—guides health care organizations through a step-by-step process to accurately measure their actual performance, to identify their barriers to excellent performance, and to direct them to proven solutions that are customized to address their particular barriers. As of October 2011, the TST is being used by more than 1,100 distinct health care organizations in the United States.

The TST provides the foundation and framework of an improvement method that, if implemented correctly, will improve an organization's hand-hygiene compliance and contribute substantially to its efforts to reduce the frequency of HAIs. Participating hospitals that developed the hand-hygiene solutions have achieved and continue to show major and sustained gains in hand-hygiene compliance. At the time of this

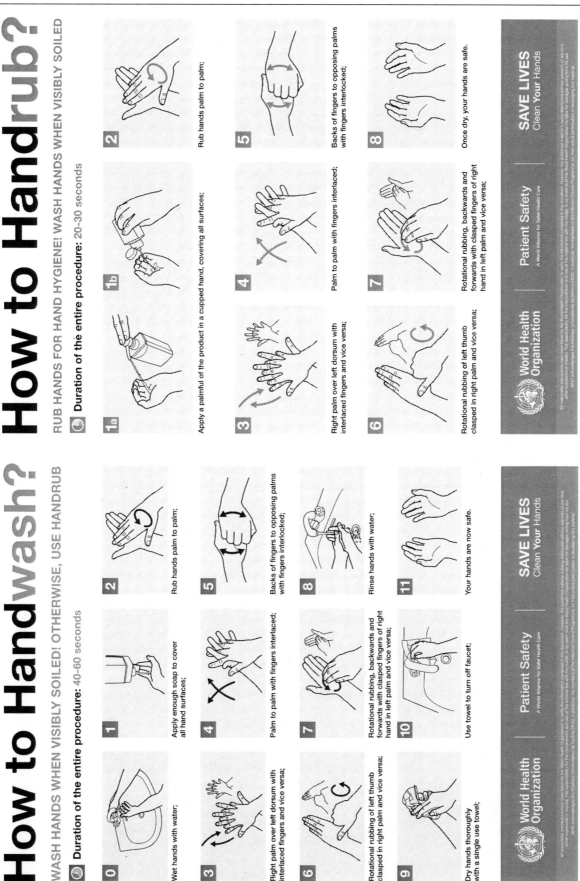

Figure 3-1. WHO Hand-Wash and Hand-Rub Technique

Source: © 2009 World Health Organization. Used with permission.

publication, compliance in participating hospitals had climbed from its baseline of 49% to an average of 81%. Some of the participating hospitals have also been tracking the correlation between hand-hygiene compliance and the occurrence of HAIs. The hospitals started to notice that as the hand-hygiene compliance rate increased, the HAIs rate started to decrease.

Although the Center's efforts thus far have been focused in the United States, its intent is to expand the Center's scope to non–US organizations, possibly as soon as 2012. More important, the issues the Center addresses are important to health care organizations throughout the world, and the

processes used by the TST and other solutions can be considered by all organizations.

Further and updated information on the Center is available at its website, http://www.centerfortransforming healthcare.org/.

Evaluating compliance with the JCI requirements is examined in depth in Chapter 4.

Reference

1. World Health Organization. WHO Guidelines on Hand Hygiene in Health Care. 2009. Accessed 19 Apr 2011. http://whqlibdoc.who.int /publications/2009/9789241597906_eng.pdf.

Surveying Infection Prevention and Control

*The Role of Infection Prevention and Control
in the Accreditation Survey Process*

Chapter Four

The surveillance, prevention, and control of infections affect every part of an organization and every aspect of patient care and employee safety. Lack of attention in this area can lead to decreased patient safety, adverse events, tremendous organizational expense, and ultimately an unsafe organization. Because it has a significant impact on an organization's provision of safe and high-quality care, it is not surprising that infection prevention and control (IPC) is evaluated in multiple ways during the accreditation process. This chapter offers a brief look at the Joint Commission International (JCI) accreditation process specifically for IPC and offers examples for compliance readiness. The IPC portion of the JCI survey consists of the following main activities:

- Surveyor planning session
- Document review
- Facility tour
- Tracer methodology, which includes the following:
  - Individual patient tracer
  - Infection control system tracer

The surveyor planning session, document review, facility tour, and tracer methodology are described in more detail in subsequent chapter sections. Two programs—Medical Transport and Clinical Laboratories—also have a formal Infection Control interview as part of the on-site survey. That portion of the on-site survey is also examined briefly later in the chapter.

Please note: JCI standards and on-site survey processes for each accreditation and certification program have unique, differentiating characteristics. Also, some programs' standards and survey processes have been updated more recently than others. This chapter deals generally with standards and survey processes and indicates program-specific differences as necessary.

It is also important to note that the JCI on-site survey is only a part of the overall JCI accreditation and certification process. Although the on-site survey takes place over three to five days every three years, JCI accreditation is intended to help organizations—to improve the safety and quality of patient care, to ensure a safe care environment, and to continually work to reduce risks to patients and health care workers (HCWs). The on-site survey should not measure results that are produced when HCWs know they're being tested; the survey is meant to determine the quality of care provided all day, any day.

Surveyor Planning Session

The surveyor planning session is held the first day of the on-site survey, normally following the Opening Conference and Orientation to the Organization's Services and the Quality Improvement Plan. During this session, surveyors review data and information about the organization and plan the survey agenda, including selecting initial tracer patients.

Please note: Although much of this information may not seem applicable to IPC, the nature of the tracer activities later in the on-site survey process makes collecting and analyzing these types of data essential during this session. For more on tracers, read the section later in this chapter, "Tracer Methodology and the On-Site Survey."

The organization should provide space for this session, usually in a room designated as the "surveyor headquarters" during the course of the entire on-site survey. This space should have the following items:

- Conference table
- Power outlets
- Telephone
- High-speed Internet connection or access for each surveyor
- Printer

Participants in the surveyor planning session should include at least the following:

- Organization's survey coordinator (as needed by surveyor team)
- Translators (as needed by surveyor team)
- All surveyors

Surveyors will inform the organization if any other personnel should attend this session, but the organization should plan to have at least the people noted above available.

The session's purpose is to allow the surveyors to review and to discuss pertinent data and to plan the survey agenda. The surveyors review the following items (as applicable to the setting), and these materials should remain available to surveyors for the entire duration of the survey:

- IPC surveillance data, including committee meeting minutes, for 12 months prior to the triennial survey and 4 months prior to an initial survey
- Performance improvement data, including committee meeting minutes, for 12 months prior to the survey and 4 months prior to an initial survey
- Facility management and safety-plan annual reviews. Surveyors will review these documents to prepare for the facility tour session.
- Facility management and safety multidisciplinary team meeting minutes for the 12 months prior to the survey and 4 months prior to an initial survey. Surveyors will review these documents to prepare for the facility tour session.
- A list of departments/units/areas/programs/services within the organization (if applicable)
- An organization chart and map
- A current list of inpatients, including their names, diagnoses, ages, admission dates, physicians, and units/services

- A list of the operative and other invasive procedures scheduled for the day, including surgeries in the operating theatre(s), day surgeries, cardiac catheterizations, endoscopies/colonoscopies, and in vitro fertilizations
- A list of the scheduled home visits for the duration of the survey, including types of service, disciplines, dates of admission, and locations. The list should include branch locations (if applicable).
- Name of key contact person (such as a supervisor or scheduler) who can assist surveyors in planning tracer selection
- A list of contact telephone numbers in case surveyors need to reach key staff

Document Review

The document review session, normally conducted the first day of the survey, provides surveyors the opportunity to evaluate standards that require some written evidence of compliance. In addition, this session orients the survey team to the structure of the organization and management. This session is also usually done the first day of the on-site survey and in the same room provided for the surveyors for the duration of the survey.

Participants should include organization staff members who are familiar with the documents that will be reviewed, can translate these, and are able respond to questions the surveyors may have during the session. At the discretion of the team, surveyors may designate a limited number of staff members to attend and to participate in the document review session. The session may be conducted as an interview of staff about the documents.

The documents that should be available to the survey team for their review or reference during the survey process for IPC include the following:

- Required policies and procedures, written documents, or bylaws, including the risk-assessment and IPC plan(s)
- Minutes of the key committees for the past year, such as IPC committee minutes, preferably with attachments and any other minutes that would indicate IPC participation or contribution, such as those from Performance Improvement, Safety, Leadership/Management Team Meetings, and Pharmacy and Therapeutics
- An accurate list of the patients currently receiving care in the organization
- A list of the operative and other invasive procedures scheduled for the day, including surgeries in the operating theatre(s), day surgeries, cardiac catheterizations, endoscopies/colonoscopies, and in vitro fertilizations
- A sample action plan for a root cause analysis for a sentinel event or a near miss that involves some aspect of IPC

- An example of a measure from the International Library of Measures on which a validation was performed, such as hand hygiene

In addition, the organization should complete and have available for the survey teams the worksheet related to relevant national or local health care–related laws and regulations that may affect infection control activities.

Documents Available in English

JCI organizes a team of surveyors to match the organization's needs and unique characteristics. JCI will make every effort to provide surveyors who are fluent in the language(s) used at the organization. If JCI surveyors with the appropriate language capabilities are not available, it is the organization's responsibility to provide interpreter services throughout the survey. The interpreter(s) must be fluent in English and the language(s) used at the organization, be experienced in verbal and written translation, be able to follow recognized Medical Interpreting Standards of Practice, and abide by the confidentiality policies and regulations set up by the organization.

No matter who is responsible for translations, documents showing evidence of compliance with some standards must be provided to the surveyors in English. Those standards with direct application to IPC are the following:

- Policies and/or procedures are developed that support continued reduction of health care–associated infections. (IPSG.5, ME 3)
- The program is guided by appropriate policies and procedures [to reduce risks of health care–associated infections]. (PCI.5, ME 5)
- When single-use devices and materials are reused, the policy includes items (a) through (e) in the intent statement. (PCI.7.1.1, ME 2)
- The organization develops an IPC program that includes all staff and other professionals and patients and families. (PCI.11, ME 1)

For a full listing of documents related to IPC that must be provided to JCI surveyors—in English or otherwise—*see* Appendix 1.

The documents should be made available to the survey team in the meeting room that has been designated for its use throughout the duration of the survey. At the beginning of the session, one staff person should briefly orient the survey team to the organization of the documents. During the remainder of the session, a staff member who can respond to any questions the surveyor(s) may have should be readily available (in person or by telephone). The materials should remain available to the survey team throughout the survey for reference purposes. However, if documents are required for use by organization staff, they can be removed.

It is highly probable that many of the required documents will be part of larger documents. Organizations do not need to remove or to photocopy pertinent sections of these documents. Instead, organizations can identify these sections using bookmarks or tabs. Guidelines for cross-referencing this information are provided in the next section. Other documents, such as minutes and reports, may be freestanding or individual documents. Organizations should decide whether to provide the original documents or photocopies. It is always beneficial to have several examples of these documents, such as committee minutes from the last few meetings.

Because the issues identified in the document review list may be addressed in different documents, depending on the organization, the following guidelines for organizing the documents to be used by the surveyors are provided.

Group the freestanding or individual documents according to the following three lists provided in this guide:
1. Required quality monitors
2. Required organization plans
3. Required policies and procedures, written documents, or bylaws

The documents reviewed by the survey team provide an overview of what they expect to see in actual practice during the survey process. For example, they would expect to find the following when a new procedure on the disposal of infectious waste is developed:

- That appropriate HCWs have been educated about the new procedure
- That any special skills or other needed training has taken place
- That waste is actually being disposed of according to the new procedure
- That any documentation required by the procedure is available for review

The presence of a policy or procedure alone usually does not determine the score of the standard. Rather, the score is determined by the daily practice (implementation) of the policy or procedure. The survey team will look for evidence that the practice related to the policy or procedure is well implemented, as appropriate, throughout the organization and thus is sustainable. In the event the implementation appears incomplete to the survey team, or the implementation occurred in a manner that is not sustainable or was implemented too recently to determine sustainability, the survey team will make a recommendation that more time be allowed to collect better evidence of sustainable implementation and to incorporate the recommendation into the survey follow-up

requirements. For example, JCI hospital standard PCI.7.1.1 requires organizations to establish a policy and procedure that identifies the process for managing expired supplies and defines the conditions for reuse of single-use devices (SUDs) when laws and regulations permit. Part of the process for establishing a policy and procedure includes identifying which SUDs the organization will reuse, how those items will be cleaned and sterilized, and how to monitor the process and progress of the initiative. If the policy to reuse SUDs was developed over a one-year period but was implemented only two months before the on-site survey, surveyors will note that the effectiveness of the policy and procedure cannot yet be fully evaluated.

In general, the length of time a policy has been implemented is referred to as a "track record." The survey team will look for a 4-month track record for policy-related standards during an initial survey and for a 12-month track record during a triennial survey. For policy-related standards to be scored "fully met," the track-record requirement must be met. When the track-record period has not been met, but the survey team finds that the policy has been implemented in a sustainable manner, the team has the prerogative to score the standard as "fully met."

For example, if the organization instituted a new program for sharps disposal (as required by JCI hospital standard PCI.7.3) 8 months before its triennial survey, the organization must present data to JCI surveyors that indicate it has developed and communicated (PCI.2), educated (PCI.11), and enforced (PCI.5) sharps-disposal policies as follows:

- Sharps and needles are collected in dedicated, puncture-proof containers that are not reused.
- The hospital disposes of sharps and needles safely or contracts with sources that ensure the sharps containers are disposed of in dedicated hazardous waste sites or as determined by national laws and regulations.
- The disposal of sharps and needles is consistent with IPC policies of the organization.

If any portion of that process has not been properly implemented for the previous 5 months, the organization will be found not compliant, partially met, or not met, depending on the level of compliance demonstrated, according to the JCI scoring guidelines.

Facility Tour

The facility tour consists of in-person visits to selected patient-care settings, inpatient and ambulatory units, treatment areas, and other areas, including, but not limited to, admitting, kitchen, pharmacy, central storage, laundry, morgue, and power plant (if applicable), to examine high-risk areas for safety and security. (Note: JCI distinguishes between the terms *safety* and *security* as follows: *Safety* is the degree to which the organization's buildings, grounds, and equipment do not pose hazards or risks to patients, staff, or visitors; *security* is protection from loss, destruction, tampering, or unauthorized access or use.) Surveyors also use the facility tour to see whether the corridors and exit paths of travel are free for the safe exit of the facility in an emergency. The tour is designed to address IPC practices in addition to other issues, such as medical and other equipment, hazardous materials and waste, HCW education, and the physical facility, many of which may have IPC aspects.

Participants in the facility tour include the following:

- Administrator surveyor (physician and/or nurse surveyors when team does not include an administrator)
- Infection control practitioner (also known as infection preventionist)
- Chief engineer
- Safety officer and/or facility manager
- Directors of admitting, pharmacy, and dietary (when surveyors are present in their areas)

In addition to Prevention and Control of Infections (PCI) requirements, standards from the following chapters are surveyed during the facility tour:

- Facility Management and Safety (FMS)—covering the physical facility, medical and other equipment, and people (HCWs, patients, and visitors); for example, the effectiveness of disinfecting medical equipment
- Staff Qualifications and Education (SQE)—covering the skills and qualifications of HCWs and the quality and frequency of the education provided and received; for example, ensuring that caregivers receive ongoing training on proper insertion, maintenance, and removal of central lines
- Assessment of Patients (AOP)—an ongoing, dynamic process that includes collecting information and data on the patient's physical, psychological, social status, and health history; analyzing the data and information, including the results of laboratory and imaging diagnostic tests, to identify the patient's health care needs; and developing a plan of care to meet the patient's identified needs; for example, a proper health history can reveal that a patient has spent significant time in hospitals recently, has been treated with a variety of antibiotics, and therefore could be at increased risk of acquiring multidrug-resistant organism (MDRO) infections.
- Management of Communication and Information (MCI)—communication to and with the community, patients and their families, and other health professionals; for example, aggregate data from IPC measurements and

utilization review can help the organization understand its current IPC performance and identify opportunities for improvement.

The surveyors visit patient-care areas as well as non-patient-care areas of the facility. In all areas, the surveyor(s) will observe the facility and interview staff to learn how the organization manages the facility to minimize infections, to maintain safe conditions for patients and staff, and to implement emergency response plans, such as when there is an influx of infectious patients.

Please note: In some survey agendas, two surveyors will visit separate sections of the facility at the same time. The organization should be prepared to have staff available to guide and to assist each surveyor on the tour of the facility.

The non-patient-care areas visited by the surveyor(s) that often involve infection risks include the central storage areas or warehouse, central sterile supply department, laboratory, laundry (if applicable), food service/kitchen, hazardous-materials storerooms, clean and soiled linen rooms, the bottoms of laundry and garbage chutes, the morgue, heating and air-conditioning equipment, and rooms to evaluate storage practices and utility-systems maintenance.

Preparing for the facility tour should include the following steps for infection control professionals:

- Prior to survey, the organization's leaders and facility manager(s) should carefully read the relevant infection prevention standards.
- The facility manager(s) should tour the facility, conduct an inspection according to the standards, and attempt to address any infection deficiencies prior to survey.
- Prior to survey, the organization should ensure that all medical equipment has been inspected, tested, and maintained and that these activities are documented.
- Representatives of the organization should be prepared to explain or to demonstrate how potable water and electrical power are available 24 hours a day and alternate plans.

Tracer Methodology and the On-Site Survey

JCI's on-site survey uses tracer methodology to follow—or "trace"—a sample of active patients through their experiences of care in the organization and to evaluate individual components and systems of care.

Tracer methodology accomplishes the following:

- Incorporates the use of information provided in the accreditation survey application and previous survey and monitoring reports
- Follows the experience of care for a number of patients through the organization's entire health care process

- Allows surveyors to identify issues in one or more steps of the patient-care process or the interfaces between processes

Two types of tracers are used for JCI's on-site surveys: individual patient tracers and infection control system tracer, the latter of which includes individual-based system tracers.

Individual Patient Tracers

The individual patient tracer activity measures the care experiences that a single patient had while in an organization's care. From that exercise, JCI can analyze an organization's system of providing care, treatment, and services for any patient at any time. All aspects of an organization's caregiving—including IPC—are measured as part of any individual patient tracer.

During an individual tracer, surveyors will perform the following tasks:

- Follow the course of care, treatment, and services provided to the patient by and within the organization, using current records whenever possible
- Assess the interrelationships between and among disciplines and departments, programs, services, or units, and the important functions in the care and services being provided
- Evaluate the performance of relevant processes, with particular focus on the integration and coordination of distinct but related processes
- Identify potential concerns in the relevant processes

Using the information from the application, the surveyors will select patients from an active patient list to "trace" their experiences throughout the organization. Patients typically selected are those who have received multiple or complex services and therefore have experienced more contact with various parts of the organization. Often a patient is selected who is on isolation precautions, was admitted with a communicable disease, or has an infection caused by an MDRO or other infection. This interaction will provide the opportunity to assess continuity-of-care issues. To the extent possible, surveyors will make every effort to avoid selecting tracers that occur at the same time and that may overlap in terms of sites within the organization.

Patient tracer selection may be based on, but not limited to, the following criteria:

- Patients in the top five diagnoses groups for that organization
- Patients related to system tracers, such as IPC and medication management
- Patients who cross programs, such as the following:
  - Patients scheduled for a follow-up in outpatient care or patients transitioning from the organization to home

care, such as a post–orthopedic surgery patient having a hip replacement
  - Patients entering or leaving the organization from or to the care continuum—for example, long term care and home care—such as an elderly patient with pneumonia who is being transferred from a hospital to a long term care facility, is fragile, and is at risk for reinfection if not properly cared for in the long term care facility.

Surveyors will follow the patient's experiences, looking at services provided by various individuals and departments within the organization as well as "handoffs" between them. The communication from one care setting to another is critical for patients with infections to ensure that they receive any needed monitoring, isolation, or treatments.

This type of review is designed to uncover systems issues, to look at the individual components of an organization, and to examine how the components interact to provide safe, high-quality patient care.

Surveyors may start a tracer where the patient is currently located. He or she can then move to where the patient first entered the organization's systems; to an area of care provided to the patient that may be a priority for the organization; or to any of the areas in which the patient received care, treatment, and services. The order will vary. For example, a tracer may start in the surgery department, where a patient is identified, and the surveyor may then go to the admitting department, preanesthesia care unit, the patient's clinical unit, and the laboratory or radiology to discuss the care before the patient arrived in surgery. The surveyor may then discuss the patient's care with rehabilitation services and others who will interact with the patient after the surgical procedure.

The number of patients followed under tracer methodology will depend on the size and complexity of the organization and the length of the on-site survey. As appropriate to the provision of care being reviewed, the tracer will include the following elements:

- Review of the patient record with the HCW responsible for the patient's care, treatment, or service provided. If the responsible HCW is not available, surveyors may speak with other HCWs. Supervisor participation in this part of the tracer should be limited. Additional HCWs involved in the patient's care will meet with surveyors as the tracer proceeds. For example, surveyors will speak to a dietitian if the patient being traced has nutritional issues. The following observations and discussions are part of the IPC tracer methodology:
  - Observation of direct patient care
  - Observation of medication processes
  - Observation of IPC practices

– Observation of care-planning processes
- Discussion of IPC data use in the organization. This includes measures being used, information that has been learned, improvements made using data, and data dissemination.
- Observation of the impact of the environment on safety and staff roles in minimizing environmental risks related to infection
- Observation of maintenance of medical equipment and review of qualified personnel responsible for the maintenance of the medical equipment to prevent transmission of pathogens from equipment to patients or to staff
- Interview with the patient and/or family (if it is appropriate, and permission is granted by the patient and/or family). The discussion will focus on the course of care and, as appropriate, will attempt to verify issues identified during the tracer related to IPC.
- Address emergency management and explore patient-flow issues in the emergency department should patients with communicable diseases need care during routine times (tuberculosis) or during a period of influx (H1N1 outbreak).

Surveyors may select and review two to three additional open or closed records to verify issues that may have been identified. For example, the surveyors will review the medical record to determine whether the accepted procedure for inserting a Foley catheter has been followed. Surveyors may ask HCWs in the unit, program, or service to assist with the review of the additional records. The following criteria can be used to guide the selection of additional records, depending on the situation:
- Similar or same diagnosis or tests
- Patient close to discharge
- Same diagnosis but different physician/practitioner
- Same test but different location
- Same age or sex
- Length of stay
- Interview with HCWs
- Review of minutes and procedures as needed

A sample infection control individual patient tracer for an ambulatory surgery center setting is shown in Box 4-1.

Individual-Based System Tracers

Individual-based system tracers look at a specific system or process across the organization. When possible, this activity focuses on the experiences of specific patients or on activities relevant to specific patients. This differs from the individual tracers in that during individual tracers, surveyors follow a patient through his or her course of care, evaluating all aspects

of care rather than a system of care. During an individual-based system tracer, surveyors perform the following tasks:
- Evaluate the performance of relevant processes, with particular focus on the integration and coordination of distinct but related processes
- Analyze communication among disciplines and departments
- Identify potential concerns in relevant processes

An individual-based system tracer includes unit/department visits to evaluate the implementation of the system process, such as IPC, and to review the impact on patient-care services and treatments. The tracer also includes an interactive session that involves surveyors and relevant staff members and that utilizes information from unit/department visits and individual tracers.

Points of discussion in the interactive session include the following:
- The flow of a process across the organization, including identification and management of risk points, integration of key activities, and communication among staff/units involved in the process
- Strengths in the process, weaknesses in the process, and possible actions to take in areas needing improvement
- Issues requiring further exploration in other survey activities
- A baseline assessment of international standards and International Patient Safety Goal (IPSG) compliance
- Education by surveyors, as appropriate

Although individual-based system tracers are used to measure many systems and processes throughout the organization, the infection control system tracer is the only individual-based tracer this text covers in depth.

Infection Control System Tracer

The individual-based infection control system tracer explores an organization's IPC processes. The goals of this session are to assess an organization's compliance with the relevant IPC–related standards and requirements, to identify IPC issues that require further exploration, and to determine actions that may be necessary to address any identified risks and to improve patient safety.

During the discussion of the IPC program, surveyors and organization are able to accomplish the following:
- Identify strengths and potential areas of concern in the IPC program
- Begin determining actions necessary to address any identified risks in IPC processes
- Begin assessing or determining the degree of compliance with relevant standards
- Identify IPC issues requiring further exploration

Box 4-1. Sample Infection Control Individual Patient Tracer, Ambulatory Surgery Center

A surveyor conducted this individual patient tracer in an ambulatory surgical center that provided a variety of surgical services, including ophthalmologic surgery. The surveyor selected a 63-year-old female patient who had undergone cataract surgery the day before.

Registration

The surveyor began her tracer in the reception/check-in/registration area by asking the registration staff members what process they followed when a new patient came to the center for surgery. She also asked what kinds of consent, education, and information are shared with the patient. The receptionist in the registration area explained that the center contacts patients in advance of their surgery to go over any questions they might have and instructs them to bring in some documents they will receive in the mail in advance of their surgery.

The surveyor asked to see how the registration staff documented this advance contact, and the receptionist showed her the electronic medical record and where on the record this information was documented. She also asked the receptionist what steps were taken to ensure privacy for patients when they were checking in. The receptionist showed the surveyor the sitting area in front of the check-in computer desk, which was positioned a short distance away from the waiting room and provided a quieter spot for the receptionist to check in the patient. The surveyor then asked the receptionist what kind of orientation she received to do her job and what ongoing training was provided. The receptionist responded that because the ambulatory surgical center's record software was recently installed, all reception staff members had undergone several in-service training sessions to learn how to use it. The receptionist added that she attended bimonthly staff meetings at which she received in-service training relating to patient safety and anything else the center's quality-improvement specialist wanted staff to know.

Ophthalmology Service Nurse

The surveyor then visited the ophthalmology service, where the tracer patient had undergone surgery. She first met with the nurse to ask how the service received and assessed surgical patients. The nurse indicated that the patient had come for a presurgical assessment a week earlier. The surveyor asked to see the assessment form and for the nurse to indicate what kind of documentation was included for the patient. The nurse showed the surveyor the physical assessment and medication forms as well as the surgical informed consent form. The surveyor asked how anyone looking at the presurgical information forms would know which information must be included for the form to be complete, whether the nurse had to fill in answers for every question or whether only certain questions were required for

a minimum physical assessment, and whether there is a policy regarding completing the forms. The nurse pointed out instructions on the back side of the form and spoke about training sessions provided to staff when they were first employed by the organization as well as periodic training sessions when the forms were first instituted or modified or when leadership believed compliance with policy needed improvement.

The surveyor then checked the record to verify inclusion of the documentation. Because the patient had been designated as diabetic, the surveyor asked the nurse to describe what kind of, if any, additional assessments or documentation would have needed to be collected for the patient. The nurse said that the patient's diabetes was flagged for Anesthesia Services' attention, and the patient had had to undergo an additional blood screening prior to surgery. The surveyor verified the orders and documentation on the record.

The surveyor then asked what type of presurgical education was provided to the patient, and the nurse showed the educational material and the education checklist that the nurse completed and asked the patient to sign in to acknowledge receiving the information. The surveyor also asked the nurse to describe what kinds of competencies and ongoing training she received for her job.

Anesthesiologist

The surveyor then met with the surgical center's anesthesiologist to discuss preoperative surgical preparation, including his understanding of the Universal Protocol for Preventing Wrong Site, Wrong Procedure, Wrong Person Surgery™—a protocol developed by the US–based Joint Commission featuring three principal components: preprocedure verification, site marking, and a time-out (a final review of pertinent facts on the patient and procedure just before the procedure begins)[1]—and when it is conducted, the presedation assessment and the sedation consent form. The surveyor also asked what the process was to mark the site and who did it. The anesthesiologist explained that he was very familiar with the Universal Protocol and that the entire team followed the Universal Protocol after the patient had been prepared and before she underwent sedation. While he did his presedation check, the anesthesiologist explained, he also had the patient verify the correct eye for the procedure and complete the sedation-consent form. The surgeon, he explained, would usually mark the site after the correct site was verified, although sometimes the anesthesiologist had done it if the surgeon was unavailable. These steps were documented on the presurgical checklist, which the surveyor was able to verify in the record.

Surgical Nurse

The surveyor then visited the postsurgery recovery area where the patients recovered before being discharged. She

Box 4-1. Sample Infection Control Individual Patient Tracer, Ambulatory Surgery Center *(continued)*

met with one of the surgical nurses there to ask her about her postsurgical assessment process and in what kind of discharge planning she is involved. The surveyor noted that several patients were recovering in the area, with family or companions sitting in chairs near the patients' beds. The nurse explained that patients recovered here with family or other designated companions at their bedsides until the surgeon came to check on them, and they were discharged after they had been provided with education and had fully recovered from sedation or anesthesia. She explained that she conducted regular assessments of patients by checking on their postsedation conditions and their pain levels. She also explained her involvement in discharge planning and education, which was provided to the patients and family members throughout their stay in recovery.

The surveyor also asked the nurse whether the organization had a policy about reusing SUDs. The nurse said the policy stated that no SUDs were to be reused. The surveyor asked where used equipment and other waste were taken after the surgery was completed; the nurse pointed out the waste receptacle adjoining the surgical suite and the posted schedule for waste disposal next to the receptacle's opening.

The surveyor asked what specific education was included and what patient follow-up the surgical center undertook. The nurse said that staff members provided education to patients on preventing surgical site infections, postsurgical care instructions, and contact information in case they had any questions. The nurse added that the surgical center did a phone follow-up 24 to 48 hours after the surgery to see how the patient was recovering, and the surgeon also scheduled an office visit to follow up with the patient and to check on recovery.

Based on the tracer, the surveyor may discuss areas of improvement in the daily briefing. The discussion might address the topic of site marking and its documentation.

Sample Tracer Questions

For Registration Staff:

- What is your registration or check-in process?
- How do you document the registration? What education and/or information do you provide to patients upon check-in?
- What consent forms or education about informed consent is shared?
- How do you ensure that the patient is able to complete the registration process with as much privacy as possible? What provision do you have in the event that the patient requires additional privacy?
- What kind of orientation and training do you receive to do your job?

For Ophthalmology Nurse:

- How are new patients checked into the service? Do you perform any presurgical assessments of patients? If so, what are they? What do you assess for infection risk?
- What kind of documentation do you complete for a surgical patient?
- How would anyone looking at the presurgical information forms know which information must be included for the form to be complete? Must you fill in every question, or are only certain questions required for a minimum physical assessment? Is there a policy about that?
- If the patient presents with any high-risk factors, such as diabetes, remote site of infection, current drugs such as antibiotics, what additional assessments or documentation, if any, do you perform?
- What kind of education do you provide to patients in relation to the surgery, infection risk factors, and any postsurgical care? Do you have any documentation to accompany this process?
- What kinds of competency assessments and ongoing training have you received in relation to your job?

For Anesthesiologist:

- What kind of education and process do you follow in relation to the Universal Protocol and infection prevention? What is the surgical center's process?
- Please describe your presedation or preanesthesia assessment. Who performs this assessment?
- What techniques or methods do you use to prevent infections in your patients?
- What is your sedation and operative consent process? Can you show me the form you use?

For Surgical Nurse:

- What type of postsurgical assessment do you perform?
- What would you look for that might indicate infection?
- What is your discharge planning process?
- What is your policy on reusing SUDs?
- Where are used equipment and other waste taken after the surgery is completed?
- How are linens handled that might have blood or body fluids on them?
- What postoperative information, education, and material do you provide to the patient related to infection risk?
- How do you follow up with surgical patients to determine if infection might have developed after the surgery.?

Reference

1. The Joint Commission. Facts About the Universal Protocol. 7 Jan 2011. Accessed 24 Aug 2011. http://www.jointcommission.org /facts_about_the_universal_protocol.

Please note: When a separate infection control system tracer is not noted on the survey agenda (for example, on shorter surveys), surveyors address IPC throughout individual patient tracers and during the improvement in quality and patient safety system tracer.

Individuals from the organization selected for participation should be able to address issues related to the IPC program in all major departments or areas within the organization. This group should include, but not be limited to, representatives from the following departments, as applicable:

- Clinical staff, including all individuals involved in IPC and a sample of individuals involved in the direct provision of care, treatment, and services, including physicians, nurses, and respiratory therapists
- Clinicians and pharmacists who are knowledgeable about the selections of medications available for use and pharmacokinetic monitoring
- Laboratorians who are knowledgeable about microbiology
- Staff responsible for the physical plant
- Organization leadership

Please note: To facilitate a beneficial exchange between surveyors and the organization, the organization should identify a relatively small group of active participants for discussions and interviews. Other staff may attend as observers.

The session opens with introductions and a review of the goals for the infection control system tracer, which include the following:

- Exploration, critical thinking, and potential problem solving about the IPC program
- Identification of potential areas of concern in the IPC program and areas for improvement and actions that could be taken to address these

The tracer process may begin with a short group meeting with individuals responsible for the organization's IPC program or in a patient-care area identified by surveyors for the focused-tracer activity. During the group meeting, surveyors gain a better understanding of the IPC system and identify potential areas that could be explored during the patient-care-area visit and potential areas of concern that require further discussion with staff knowledgeable about the organization's IPC program.

The surveyors may move to other settings as appropriate and applicable to IPC processes across the organization. Surveyors observe staff and engage them in discussion focused on IPC practices in any setting that is visited during this system tracer activity.

Surveyors draw from their tracer activity experience, organizational IPC surveillance data, and other IPC–related data to inspire scenarios for discussion with the organization. Participants are asked to discuss the following aspects of the organization's IPC program as they relate to the scenarios:

- How patients with infections are identified by the organization
- How patients with infections are considered within the context of the IPC program
- Current and past surveillance activity that took place in the previous 12 months or more for re-surveys and 4 months or more for initial surveys
- Type of analysis being conducted on the IPC data, including comparisons
- Reporting of IPC data, including frequency and audience
- Process for handling an influx of infectious patients
- Process used to perform an IPC risk assessment, including the reasons for conducting the assessment and the results of the analysis
- IPC activities (for example, HCW training, education of patient/resident/client population, housekeeping procedures)
- Physical facility changes, either completed or in progress, that have an impact on IPC
- Actions taken as a result of surveillance and the outcomes of those actions
- Effectiveness of implementation of IPSGs 5 and 6 and the hand-hygiene guidelines

Organizations may use IPC data during this part of the activity if the data are relevant to the discussion. Discussion can revolve around patients already included in IPC surveillance and reporting activities or around those not yet confirmed as meeting the definition or criteria for entry into and monitoring through the IPC surveillance system. In addition to surveyor-identified scenarios, the organization is encouraged to present examples of cases that highlight various aspects of the IPC program. Some of the scenarios the surveyors want to discuss, as applicable to the organization, may include, but are not limited to, the following:

- Patients with fever of unknown origin
- Patients with postoperative infections
- Patients admitted to the organization postoperatively
- Patients placed on antibiotics that are new to the list of available medications (preferably ones with corresponding culture and sensitivities, blood levels, and/or other laboratories used for dosing)
- Patients placed in isolation due to infectious diseases. If not easily identifiable, consider patients with any of the following diagnoses (this is not an exhaustive list): varicella, pulmonary tuberculosis, invasive haemophilus influenzae, meningococcal disease, drug-resistant pneumococcal dis-

ease, pertussis, mycoplasma, mumps, rubella, methicillin-resistant *Staphylococcus aureus* (MRSA), vancomycin-resistant *Enterococcus* (VRE), *Clostridium difficile*, respiratory syncytial virus (RSV), enteroviruses, and skin infections (impetigo, lice, scabies).

- IPC practices related to emergency management
- Patients placed in isolation because they are immunocompromised
- Recent changes in physical facilities that have an impact on IPC
- Patients with known cases of active tuberculosis

At the end of the tracer, surveyors and organizational staff summarize identified strengths and potential areas of concern in the IPC program. Surveyors provide education as applicable.

Please note: Usually, a single infection control system tracer session is scheduled. This session is intended to review IPC for all services provided by the organization and therefore should include participants who are able to address IPC in all services.

A sample individual-based system tracer for infection prevention and control in a 250-bed hospital is described in Box 4-2.

The Role of HCWs in Tracer Methodology

HCWs are asked to provide surveyors with a list of patients presently in the organization, including the patients' names, current locations in the organization, and diagnoses, as appropriate. Surveyors may request assistance from organization HCWs for selection of appropriate tracer patients. As surveyors move around the organization, they converse with a wide variety of HCWs involved in the traced patient's care, treatment, and services. These HCWs could include nurses, physicians, therapists, case managers, aides, pharmacy staff, lab personnel (as appropriate), and support staff. If those HCWs are not available, surveyors ask to speak to other HCWs who would perform the same function(s) as the HCWs who have cared for or are caring for the tracer patient. Although it is preferable to speak with the direct caregiver, it is not mandatory, because the questions that are asked are questions that any caregiver should be able to answer in providing care to the patient being traced.

Infection Control Interview

As mentioned earlier in the chapter, the infection control interview is part of some on-site JCI surveys, particularly those in the clinical laboratory programs. (Other programs' on-site surveys elicit similar information via the tracer methodology described above.)

The infection control interview is an approximately 90-minute meeting that helps JCI surveyors assess the processes used to do the following:

- Develop the organization's infection control and surveillance program
- Reduce health care–associated infections
- Ensure that infection control personnel are qualified
- Improve performance in this area, as appropriate to the organization's care continuum priorities
- Collect and monitor meaningful data to evaluate the effectiveness of the infection control program
- Ensure compliance with government and other mandated infection control requirements

The interview is normally conducted in the same meeting room designated for the surveyors' use during the course of the survey. Participants normally include the following people:

- Surveyors, particularly the nurse surveyor
- The organization's medical director
- The individual(s) responsible for the IPC program
- HCWs involved in implementing the IPC program
- Other staff the organization may choose

Issues related to Prevention and Control of Infections, Facility Management and Safety, and Management of Information standards are reviewed and can be found in the Organization and Delivery of Services (ODS) section. In addition, issues related to Improvement in Quality and Safety (IQS) standards will be addressed. Materials necessary for the interview include the following:

- Minutes of any infection control committee meetings
- Surveillance reports
- Quality-improvement reports
- Records of biological testing

These documents can also be included in the document-review session.

To start the interview, the surveyors facilitating the interview explain its purpose. The surveyors may ask participants to explain the components of the infection control program in the organization and to explain how an infectious individual's care is handled from preentry to postdischarge from the primary care organization. A systems tracer may be utilized in which the surveyors may ask about systems issues (for example, information management) that support the infection control program. The surveyors may also ask about how infection control processes are implemented and monitored in alternative settings, such as the individual's home.

Surveyors may ask about specific issues that they have discovered during their visits to individual care units/settings

Box 4-2. Sample Individual-Based System Tracer for Infection Prevention and Control, 250-Bed Hospital

Infection Prevention and Control Director and Committee

The surveyor started the session by meeting with the IPC director and with representative members of the IPC committee. She asked them to explain the committee's mission and focus and asked each to explain his or her role on the committee and in the IPC program.

The IPC director explained that she had coordinated the IPC program in this hospital for about five years. She led the program with a physician who was an epidemiologist. Committee members included representatives from the laboratory, pharmacy, and environmental service; nurses from several areas in the hospital; and an administrator. The committee formally met every other month but was involved in the program on a daily basis.

The surveyor asked the committee representatives to identify the most significant infection control risks that they currently dealt with. She also asked them to identify any studies in which they currently collected data. They explained that they monitored for hand hygiene, which was a focus area for the committee. They also concentrated on potential exposures to needlesticks and other potentially infectious body fluids. In addition, they worked with HCWs regarding compliance with isolation requirements and identification of and interventions for preventing the spread of health care–associated infections, such as *Clostridium difficile* and hospital-acquired vancomycin resistance.

They believed that the incidence of health care–associated methicillin-resistant *Staphylococcus aureus* was actually diminishing, although they saw an increase in community-acquired MRSA infections. The surveyor asked the HCWs to present their studies and to identify how they addressed the identified challenges. The IPC director and medical IPC coordinator described how they accessed national data and information on a daily basis and how they disseminated the relevant information to staff through the hospital's intranet. They also provided periodic education programs for staff.

HCWs

The surveyor asked the HCWs to present data regarding staff compliance with hand-hygiene requirements. She asked how they measured compliance, whether they believed that their measurement strategies were reliable, and whether the interventions were effective.

The surveyor then asked the HCWs to explain the organization's requirements for isolation and when it was used. She also asked how they monitored compliance and whether they collected data to identify the potential risk points in this process.

The Patient's Room

After the formal meeting and review, the surveyor chose a patient with an infection for the tracer. The surveyor observed a nurse entering the tracer patient's room to provide care. She also observed a laboratory technician entering the room to perform a blood draw. She noticed that some family members did not follow the guideline requirements posted outside the patient's room for the use of personal protective equipment (PPE). HCWs said that they educated the family members, but sometimes it was difficult to hold them in compliance, so they generally did not stop them. The laboratory technician fully followed the guidelines. However, the surveyor witnessed that a nurse left the room, went to the medication room, and returned to the patient's room while wearing the same protective garb. Afterward, she was asked whether her conduct was acceptable and safe practice. The nurse responded that she knew she should have removed the garb when leaving the patient's room and put on new protective garb upon reentering, but it was often difficult to follow all the procedures because of her heavy caseload—due to staffing shortages—and the number of times she needed to leave the room for supplies. The surveyor asked her how she prepared for each entry to the patient's room and whether she could plan the visits to include all the equipment and supplies that would be needed. She also asked HCWs how they could assist one another through handoffs of equipment and supplies to ensure full compliance with requirements.

Sample System Tracer Questions

Questions for the Infection Prevention and Control Director and Medical Coordinator of Infection Prevention and Control

- How do you obtain needed and current information regarding IPC?
- How do you disseminate this information to other staff at all levels?
- What are the greatest infection control risks facing your organization?
- What are you doing to diminish the risks and impact on outcomes of care?
- How do you monitor compliance with infection control requirements, such as hand hygiene and contact precautions or isolation-room requirements?
- How do you intervene when you observe noncompliance?
- How do you collect and analyze data regarding risky or problematic trends and patterns?

Questions for Members of the Infection Prevention and Control Committee

- What is your involvement on the committee?
- Why were you selected to be on this committee?
- What data are being studied?

> ### Box 4-2. Sample Individual-Based System Tracer for Infection Prevention and Control, 250-Bed Hospital *(continued)*
>
> - How are the data communicated to you?
> - Do you compare and benchmark your data and outcomes with others? Describe this process. How do you compare?
> - What improvements have you implemented?
>   - Are they effective?
>   - How do you know?
> - How is your staff performing regarding hand-hygiene requirements?
>   - How is hand hygiene monitored?
>   - Have you identified risk areas? If so, how do you address these identified risks?
>   - Has compliance improved?
>   - Is improvement sustained, and is it sustainable?
>   - How do you know?
>
> **Questions for the Nurse and Other HCWs**
>
> - How do you monitor hand-hygiene compliance in staff, visitors, and patients?
> - Do you intervene if you believe the required guidelines for IPC are not being complied with? How?
> - How do you educate patients and families regarding hand hygiene and IPC principles and requirements?
> - How do you document this education?
> - Are you aware of the requirements for the use of PPE for entering the rooms of patients on contact precautions or in isolation?

or home visits or during earlier interviews. Surveyors may ask related questions that they did not have time to ask during their visits to individual care units/settings. They may also ask about how the organization monitors its infection control rates and how it compares to other similar organizations, if this information is available.

Preparation for the infection control interview should include the following steps:

- Becoming familiar with the applicable standards
- Practicing answering questions about the program and how quality management has been able to use infection control monitoring to lower the risk of health care–associated infections in the organization

Conclusion

JCI's accreditation process calls on health care organizations to shift their mind-set from viewing accreditation as a single event in time that provides a somewhat narrow and time-sensitive understanding of how well organizations' systems work together to seeing it more as a continuing dynamic and unfolding process that provides insight into organizations' daily operations. JCI addresses IPC at many points during the survey process to determine how organizations incorporate IPC practices into their daily operations and thus help enhance patient and HCW safety.

With JCI's requirements and means for surveying those requirements now established, Chapters 5 and 6 detail strategies and tools for achieving and maintaining compliance with JCI requirements.

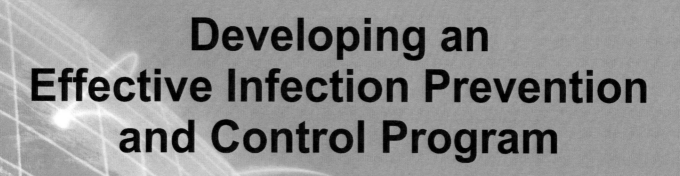

Developing an Effective Infection Prevention and Control Program

Strategies for Success

By
Barbara M. Soule, RN, MPA, CIC, FSHEA
Preeti N. Malani, MD, MSJ
Prof. Ziad A. Memish, MD, FRCPC, FRCPE, FACP, FIDSA

Chapter Five

As discussed in Chapters 3 and 4, the Joint Commission International (JCI) infection prevention and control (IPC) requirements place a strong emphasis on the development, implementation, and evaluation of an integrated and responsive risk-based IPC program. Establishing such a program helps preserve and enhance the quality of care, improve patient, health care worker (HCW), and other staff safety, and prevent adverse events.

The goal of an IPC program is to identify and to reduce or to eliminate the risks of acquiring and transmitting infections among patients, HCWs and other staff, volunteers, students, and visitors. Effective IPC programs have many components that must work together. Several of these components are discussed in this chapter:

- Gaining leadership support for the program
- Establishing an effective infrastructure to support the program
- Involving the whole organization in infection prevention
- Establishing the focus of the program by assessing risk and creating an IPC plan
- Designing strategies to reduce or to eliminate infection risk
- Developing and maintaining a continuous surveillance, data collection, and analysis process
- Evaluating the goals, objectives, and strategies of the IPC program

Successfully achieving these crucial program components requires continual vigilance, persistence, and creativity. This chapter identifies some of the practices and challenges associated with developing and sustaining an effective IPC program and provides strategies, tips, and useful tools to help achieve success. The ideas presented here are fundamental and can be adapted for use in most care settings, depending on program management and available resources. Some of the recommendations are not required by JCI; *see* Chapters 3 and 4 as well as Appendix 1 for all JCI IPC requirements.

Please note: The terms *IPC practitioner* and *IPC professional* are used interchangeably throughout this chapter to identify IPC specialists. In some areas of the world, the preferred term for this same role is *infection preventionist*.

Gaining Leadership Support

In most organizations, the IPC programs that receive visible support from leadership are the ones that HCWs take seriously. Consequently, these programs are typically the ones that are most successful. To have an effective IPC program, it is critical for administrative and clinical leaders to be aware of its functions and goals. Such support ensures the program's effectiveness and contributes to a safer environment for patients. Although most leaders are not directly involved in the day-to-day operations of the IPC program, they should provide oversight and guidance for the development, implementation, and evaluation of the program and provide input to critical initiatives that emerge.[1-6] The decisions that leaders make and the initiatives they support will affect the program and subsequently the quality of care and safety of patients. One of the most effective means to ensure a successful IPC program is for leaders to frame it in the context of an overall culture of patient safety.

Leadership involvement varies in different organizations. Some leaders are actively involved and very knowledgeable about IPC, and others believe that delegating the program to the IPC team is sufficient involvement. A 2008 survey performed in the United States by the Association for Professionals in Infection Control and Epidemiology (APIC) and Premier Inc. Healthcare Alliance identified gaps in how leaders were engaged in IPC programs in their organizations.[7] According to their findings, only about 15% of the survey respondents indicated that the organizational executives and physician leaders were actively engaged or took a leadership role in the efforts to reduce infections in their facility. Yet nearly one third of respondents suggested that the organizational and physician leaders are the most important resources to help address the challenges of health care–associated infections (HAIs).

The leaders' time is valuable, and their support and presence are needed in many areas simultaneously throughout an organization. How do they devote time and energy to IPC in addition to their myriad other priorities? Several ways for leaders to actively and visibly support an IPC program are highlighted in Sidebar 5-1.

An important consideration for the IPC team to gain leadership support is to align the IPC incentives with those of the organization and to stress the similarities when discussing the program or proposing new activities. Increasingly, leaders rely on effectiveness and efficiency when making decisions about how to allocate health care resources. In addition to delivering safe, high-quality care, they are concerned about the "bottom line" or the financial viability of the organization.[8-10] The ability to demonstrate business or financial benefits for implementing best practices in IPC will assist the IPC staff in gaining needed resources (*see* Sidebar 5-2).

Involving Physicians in the IPC Program

Physician leadership is essential for IPC programs. Individual expertise in the pathophysiology, prevention, and treatment of infectious diseases and knowledge of medications and vaccines, diagnostic tests, and treatment modalities are invaluable in guiding policies and procedures pertaining to the clinical aspects of the IPC program. Physicians who partner with the IPC practitioner bring added credibility to recommendations for practice changes for clinical staff. In addition to their clinical specialty, physicians who participate in the IPC program should have special training in health care epidemiology, quality improvement, and patient safety.[11–14] Case Study 5-1 shows how one organization effectively involved physicians in its IPC program.

CASE STUDY 5-1

Reducing Infections in a Medical Intensive Care Unit Using a Proactive Infection Control Program (China)

Zhiyong Zong, PhD, MBBS *(SHEA International Ambassador)*; Dan Pu, MD; Fu Qiao, MBBS

Introduction

Infection control in the intensive care unit (ICU) is challenging, particularly in resource-limited settings. West China Hospital of Sichuan University is an extremely large university hospital with 4,400 beds and serves as the referral center in Chengdu, Republic of China, a region with limited resources. Three ICUs are in this hospital, including a 50-bed medical ICU. This medical ICU is always fully occupied and crowded, has a low nurse-bed ratio (2:1), and is associated with a high prevalence of HAIs, such as ventilator-associated pneumonia (VAP) and catheter-related bloodstream infections (CRBSIs), making infection control extremely difficult. It is necessary to strengthen infection control in this medical ICU to reduce the rates of HAIs.

Methods

Before intervention, previous surveillance data of HAIs were carefully reviewed and discussed by the infection control team with the ICU's director and chief nurses. The main problem identified in this large ICU was the lack of a dedicated and experienced professional to look after infection control. To strengthen infection control, a well-trained infection control physician was sent to the ICU and has worked there full time since September 2010. Her duties included performing surveillance on all kinds of HAIs, such as VAP, CRBSIs, and catheter-associated urinary tract infections (CAUTIs); auditing infection control practices; communicating with ICU physicians and nurses on a daily basis; and organizing various training activities. She was supported by a team of infection control practitioners comprising three people who assisted in

---

Sidebar 5-1. Methods for Leaders to Support an IPC Program

- Make IPC a visible priority throughout the organization.
- Allocate staff time and resources to the IPC program, including the appropriate number of IPC professionals who have needed skills; laboratory support; technical support, such as computers and printers; and administrative support, such as data entry and secretarial support. Resource allocation should also include time to implement a system of continuous performance improvement, to educate HCWs, and to work toward enhanced patient safety.
- Facilitate the IPC professional's access to patient records, performance-improvement data, and other systems to support surveillance-data collection and analysis functions, including the reporting of infection-prevention information.
- Support the program by ensuring provision of adequate personal protective equipment (PPE) and supplies, such as alcohol-based hand rubs, gowns, and gloves, that make it easier for HCWs to prevent or avoid infections.
- Attend and actively participate in multidisciplinary IPC meetings.
- Serve as a resource to the IPC department as well as to any multidisciplinary teams addressing IPC issues.
- Publicly acknowledge successes in IPC, such as reduced infection rates, decreased lengths of stay, or cost savings.
- Serve as a role model to HCWs (for example, perform hand hygiene and use appropriate PPE).
- Set expectations for HCWs (for example, follow IPC policies and require attendance at IPC–related classes or training sessions).
- Show support for IPC–related policy changes by supporting HCWs to attend in-services.
- Make timely and appropriate education and training efforts a priority for clinical and nonclinical staff.
- Make compliance with IPC procedures part of performance evaluations and competency reviews.
- Support coordination of IPC efforts within the community and ensure active communication with public health agencies.
- Ensure compliance with regulations and requirements from such authorities as ministries of health.
- Pay specific attention to IPC emergencies when developing the organization's emergency management plan.

Source: Adapted from Olmsted R, Soule BM. The role of leadership in infection prevention and control programs. In Arias KM, Soule BM, editors: *The APIC/JCR Infection Prevention and Control Workbook*, 2nd ed. Oak Brook, IL, and Washington, DC: Joint Commission Resources and Association for Professionals in Infection Control and Epidemiology, 2010, 17–25.

Sidebar 5-2. Clarifying the Economics of IPC Practices

IPC practices can employ simple cost-effective analyses when evaluating or proposing new or changed procedures, purchasing new devices, or allocating additional IPC resources. A cost-effective analysis quantifies the difference between an additional health care expenditure, such as an infection-prevention program, and improved health care outcomes. This method measures how much it costs the organization to achieve an improved clinical or programmatic benefit. For example, some evidence-based practices or procedures, such as using maximal sterile barrier precautions during the insertion of central venous lines, are more costly at the outset but may save money by reducing infections. Extra supplies add costs but have demonstrated reduced instances of catheter-associated bloodstream infections (CABSIs).[1] In another example, using needles and syringes one time for one patient instead of for multiple patients virtually eliminates the risk of transmitting blood-borne infection, and using safety needles, which are often more expensive than regular needles, reduces needlesticks and subsequent cost of infections with hepatitis B and other blood-borne pathogens among HCWs.[2-4]

IPC professionals should have an open dialogue with leaders about the costs of HAIs or outbreaks, the benefits of implementing IPC best practices, and the potential costs for undersourcing an infection-prevention program. Using published studies can serve as a benchmark.[5-10] Providing this valuable information to the leaders and comparing it with the organization's experience can help leaders make decisions about resource allocation that will affect patients and HCWs. The same information can demonstrate the value of investing in and strengthening the IPC program as a highly cost-effective patient-safety strategy. Methods for simple economic analyses can be found in several of the readings and references below.

References

1. Hu KK, et al. Use of maximal sterile barriers during central venous catheter insertion: Clinical and economic outcomes. *Clin Infect Dis.* 2004 Nov 15;39(10):1441–1445.
2. Glenngård AH, Persson U. Costs associated with sharps injuries in the Swedish health care setting and potential cost savings from needle-stick prevention devices with needle and syringe. *Scand J Infect Dis.* 2009;41(4):296–302.
3. Whitby M, McLaws ML, Slater K. Needlestick injuries in a major teaching hospital: The worthwhile effect of hospital-wide replacement of conventional hollow-bore needles. *Am J Infect Control.* 2008 Apr;36(3):180–186.
4. O'Malley EM, et al. Costs of management of occupational exposures to blood and body fluids. *Infect Control Hosp Epidemiol.* 2007 Jul;28(7):774–782.
5. Guanche-Garcell H, et al. Device-associated infection rates in adult intensive care units of Cuban university hospitals: International Nosocomial Infection Control Consortium (INICC) findings. *Int J Infect Dis.* 2011 May;15(5):e357–362.
6. Rosenthal VD, et al. International Nosocomial Infection Control Consortium (INICC) report, data summary for 2003–2008, issued June 2009. *Am J Infect Control.* 2010 Mar;38(2):95–104.
7. Edwards JR, et al. National Healthcare Safety Network (NHSN) report: Data summary for 2006 through 2008, issued December 2009. *Am J Infect Control.* 2009 Dec;37(10):783–805.
8. Pérez CD, et al. The Spanish national health care-associated infection surveillance network (INCLIMECC): Data summary January 1997 through December 2006 adapted to the new National Healthcare Safety Network Procedure-associated module codes. *Am J Infect Control.* 2009 Dec;37(10):806–812.
9. Anderson DJ, et al. Underresourced hospital infection control and prevention programs: Penny wise, pound foolish? *Infect Control Hosp Epidemiol.* 2007 Jul;28(7):767–773.
10. Perencevich EN, et al. Raising standards while watching the bottom line: Making a business case for infection control. *Infect Control Hosp Epidemiol.* 2007 Oct;28(10):1121–1133.

surveillance, provided microbiological data, or randomly monitored cleaning and sterilization, respectively. An assigned infection control link nurse (*see* section on IPC professionals below) also played a significant role in facilitating surveillance, intervention, and education.

In addition, an infectious diseases physician/hospital epidemiologist worked in the ICU for two hours daily as a consultant of infection control and for antimicrobial stewardship. Measures including comprehensive training, strengthened hand hygiene, prevention bundles adapted from the US Centers for Disease Control and Prevention (US CDC) or Society for Healthcare Epidemiology of America (SHEA) guidelines, and regular feedback were implemented, but the ward setting and nurse-bed ratio remained the same. Training covered all HCWs and was carried out every three months; topics covered policies, procedures, and practices of infection control and were further stratified for physicians, nurses, and workers. Alcohol-based hand rubs were placed near each bed and each trolley and in the corridors. Hand-washing posters were made available for each room and displayed in the corridors. Hand-hygiene compliance was monitored by the infection control practitioners. Infections were monitored on a daily basis, and rates of VAP, CRBSIs, and CAUTIs were calculated monthly and then compared to the baseline (rates determined before intervention). Analysis was performed by the infection control team. Feedback on infection rates, compliance with procedures, and any issues associated with infection control for the ward as a whole and for each medical team individually were given once a week via a joint meeting with infection control professionals and ICU core

HCWs (director, chief nurses, attending physicians, chief residents, and senior nurses). Written reports about infection rates were given once a month to the director, chief nurses, and attending physicians of the ICU and were also forwarded to the vice president of the hospital in charge of medical affairs.

Results

Compared to rates before intervention, the overall HAI rates dropped 26% and 38%, calculated based on infected cases and events, respectively. The rates calculated based on cases and events per 1,000 ICU–stay days dropped 53% and 58%, respectively. Significant reductions were also seen in VAP and CAUTI rates (drops of 68% and 70%, respectively). As for CRBSIs, the rate remained virtually unchanged (2.31 per 1,000 catheter-days before intervention and 2.14 after intervention). Usually, one case of CRBSI developed per month, and the unchanged rate was due to the low numerator.

Lessons Learned

This study demonstrated that in a resource-limited setting, the implementation of common measures, such as improving hand hygiene and implementing bundles for prevention, could significantly minimize HAIs, although further reduction might require changes in ward settings and improvement of the nurse-bed ratio.

A dedicated infection control physician working full-time in an ICU is also essential to generate good infection control practices. This "working inside" approach could provide real-time discussion with and feedback to ICU HCWs and therefore contribute to the establishment of a very active partnership between infection control and ICU HCWs.

One limitation of this organization's strategy is the need for a well-trained and inspired infection control practitioner working full-time in the ICU, which may be a luxury for many hospitals in resource-limited countries, as the infection control team is usually inadequately staffed there.

This study has several limitations. First, it was an observational study and was observed for only a relatively short period (eight months). The long-term effect of the intervention is unknown but will be continuously monitored. Second, multiple measures were included, such as the involvement of a full-time infection control practitioner, increased education, improved hand hygiene, and implemented preventive bundles. Therefore, it is difficult to identify which factor or factors really worked and which factor generated the greatest number of benefits.

To keep physicians throughout the organization interested in the IPC program, practitioners can provide them with some of the following information:
- Infection rates for surgical site infections (SSIs), VAP, bloodstream infections (BSIs), and urinary-tract infections (UTIs)
- Antibiograms indicating the organization's rates of multidrug-resistant organisms (MDROs), such as methicillin-resistant *Staphylococcus aureus* (MRSA), vancomycin-resistant *Enterococcus* (VRE), and *Klebsiella pneumoniae* carbapenemase (KPC)
- New or proposed policies that will affect physician practice. It is important to involve leadership in the development of these policies.
- Updated scientific information and new evidence-based guidelines
- Governmental documents and regulations related to IPC
- Surgeon-specific SSI rates to help surgeons reduce SSI rates

IPC Professionals as Leaders

Although strong administrative and physician leadership involvement is crucial to the success of any IPC program (*see* Chapters 3 and 4 for discussion of JCI requirements for IPC leadership), dedicated IPC professionals are needed to manage the day-to-day operations of the program, to identify areas of improvement, and to address new issues that arise. The responsibilities of this individual(s) are numerous[15] and include the following:
- **Risk assessment**—evaluating infection risks continually and proactively by formal and informal means using quantitative or qualitative methods
- **Surveillance and investigation**—developing surveillance system planning and design, data collection, investigation, interpretation, and communication of findings
- **Prevention**—helping develop IPC policies and procedures and implementing IPC strategies for such areas as hand hygiene, equipment and environmental cleaning, disinfection and sterilization, and hazardous waste collection and management
- **Research**—staying abreast of national guidelines, laws, and clinical pathways addressing IPC and researching new and emerging diseases
- **Education and training**—providing all HCWs with training and education on IPC issues. Education efforts might start with the assessment of HCW needs and involve training programs, frequent communication, and evaluation.
- **Response**—responding to infection clusters, outbreak, pandemic, or bioterrorist event. To prepare for such events, this individual should be knowledgeable about cluster- and

outbreak-investigation methods and be involved in emergency-preparedness efforts.

- **Management**—running the day-to-day operations of the IPC program. This could include program implementation and evaluation, regulatory compliance, reporting, and planning for current and future projects.
- **Consulting**—working with HCWs to address IPC questions and to solve problems; collaborating with other departments on policies and procedures (for example, appropriate isolation of patients with communicable diseases and product selection for patient care); providing input on the care of the environment and construction projects to ensure that infection-prevention issues are considered, such as room and floor layout, water-system and air-flow design, access to supplies, hand-washing facilities, and appropriate facilities

Establishing an Effective Infrastructure

How do organizations make sure that IPC programs function effectively and address all the necessary issues? One way is to establish an infrastructure that supports the systems and functions of the program. This can be challenging in settings with limited resources. Several components are essential for a strong infrastructure.[16–18]

Creating a Multidisciplinary Team to Oversee the Program

One of the primary structural elements of an IPC program is a multidisciplinary IPC team, task force, or formal committee that is charged with creating, implementing, and monitoring the IPC program. As discussed in Chapter 3, JCI requires a designated mechanism—the IPC program—that is multidisciplinary and includes at least representatives from nursing, medicine, IPC, and housekeeping. The responsibilities of the oversight group include setting criteria to define HAIs, establishing data-collection (surveillance) methods, implementing risk-reduction strategies, and reporting processes and outcomes. Because infection prevention involves all parts of an organization, coordination activities must involve communicating with the entire organization to ensure that the program is continuous and proactive. In addition to the medical, nursing and housekeeping/environmental services staff who participate in the oversight group, others who may be included, as determined by the organization's size and services, include the following:

- Senior leader from administration
- Central sterile processing representative
- Equipment maintenance personnel (biomedical engineering staff)
- Facilities management, including engineering and maintenance personnel
- Information management staff
- Laboratory personnel, particularly microbiology
- Pharmacists
- Medical staff (for example, department heads or representatives of surgery, pediatrics, medicine, emergency, or other services)
- Nursing leaders and staff from specific clinical specialties
- Patient-safety/performance-improvement specialists

The team should meet regularly, to actively participate in discussion of an agenda of topics, including reports of infections and infection risks, policies and procedures, performance improvement action items with time frames, including responsible parties and other topics. The organization should provide education and training in IPC for the team members as well as clarity about their roles and responsibilities.

The first responsibility of this team is to establish the focus of the organization's IPC program by assessing and analyzing the risks specific to the organization. Following the risk assessment, the team develops a well-defined and specific IPC plan that includes goals and objectives to reduce infection risks.

As part of the infrastructure that nurtures and supports the IPC program, and for optimal function, there should be clear, strong connections and integration of IPC with quality improvement, and patient safety.[19–23] In those organizations with a quality-improvement committee, IPC plans should be reviewed with the committee to obtain feedback and suggestions for improvement and to integrate IPC data with other quality and patient-safety data. This collaboration enhances the use of all the information for the best decision-making process to improve or to maintain patient care and staff safety.

Program Management

In addition to a multidisciplinary team, such as an IPC committee or IPC advisory council, organizations should designate an individual who has experience with IPC to take the lead in creating and managing the program. He or she should be trained in IPC or have the opportunity to be mentored and coached by an experienced person(s). The individual should seek feedback from other areas of the organization during the development of the IPC program, such as the nursing, respiratory therapy, and pharmacy staff. The person who accepts the lead responsibility for coordinating the program will have responsibilities that include working with the IPC committee or others to set criteria for defining HAIs and for establishing the surveillance process and methods for collecting, analyzing, and reporting data. The lead IPC physician is also responsible for communicating with all parts of the organization to make certain that the program is ongoing and proactive. Regardless of who leads the daily IPC activities, it is essential to have representatives from at least medicine and nursing involved in the oversight of the IPC program. The statistician, data-collection staff, central-sterilization manager, microbiology, pharmacy, or operating-theatre supervisor can also provide valuable input. As discussed with the IPC committee, the role of the participants in the oversight group depends on the size and services of the organization.

IPC Professionals

To have the appropriate number and skill mix of IPC professionals, organizations should consider the following factors:

- The scope of the IPC program, including the type of services the organization provides. Organizations providing multiple services (such as hospitals with laboratories) need to design IPC programs that meet the needs of all service areas.
- The scope of responsibilities of the IPC professional and the ratio of IPC professionals to the number of occupied acute care beds for which they are responsible[24]
- The characteristics of patient populations. Different patient populations have varying IPC needs. For example, immunocompromised populations are at higher risk for infection, so organizations that serve predominantly immunocompromised populations need to factor those risks into the allocation of staff resources.
- Economic pressures. Although the ideal number of IPC

staff might not be economically feasible for some organizations, an effort should be made to address the needs of the organizations within the budgets available. Creative ways to do this can include time sharing and resource sharing with other organizations in the community.

- Demographics of the workforce. If a health care organization has a significant number of employees and patients who are not proficient in the region's primary language, efforts should ensure that IPC staff are able to communicate effectively with other HCWs and patients about IPC issues.
- Expansion of IPC staff resources. One method used to expand the IPC resources is the Link Nurse Program, which is common in the UK and other countries.[25–30] A similar approach is the Nurse Liaison Program used in some US hospitals. For both of these methods, staff nurses who are selected or volunteer are provided basic training in IPC and take leadership roles on their units. They become extensions of the IPC practitioner and may perform limited surveillance, help develop policies and procedures, observe practices, and take on other responsibilities.
- Education of IPCs. IPC professionals should have basic knowledge of IPC theories as well as skills and abilities that allow them to implement and to maintain an effective IPC program. There are several ways for IPC professionals to obtain knowledge and skills, including formal training, informal on-the-job mentoring, experience with managing IPC challenges, and working toward and obtaining IPC certification. *See* Table 5-1 for a brief list of training opportunities. For other IPC resources, *see* Appendix 2.

Table 5-1. IPC Professional Training Opportunities

Organization and Website	Selected Formal Training Opportunities
Hospital Infection Society (HIS), the London School of Hygiene and Tropical Medicine (LSHTM), and the Public Health Laboratory Service (PHLS) **http://www.lshtm.ac.uk/**	The Diploma in Hospital Infection Control (DipHIC) was established in 1997 for IPC practitioners, IPC physicians, microbiologists, epidemiologists, and others who complete the requirements of training.
The International Federation of Infection Control (IFIC) **http://www.theific.org**	Basic training course (and a planned distance-learning module for the future)
The Certification Board of Infection Control and Epidemiology, Inc. (CBIC; US–based) **http://www.cbic.org/**	Certification course examination (based on the US practice analysis) in many countries
Valparaiso University, Chile **http://www.uv.cl**	Master's degree in Infection Control and Hospital Epidemiology designed to train professionals in charge of infection control programs or hospital epidemiology from Latin American countries

After the appropriate skill mix and number of IPC professionals are determined for the program, the organization should make sure that all IPC professionals are adequately trained and that their competency is verified routinely. These individuals should know and understand how to apply epidemiological principles to infection prevention. The successful completion of a course in IPC or IPC professional certification might be a benchmark for competence in this area.[30-32]

Policies and Procedures

Policies and procedures are part of the infrastructure for the IPC program. Clear policies that incorporate the basic principles and concepts of IPC provide guidance for patient care, HCW safety, care of the environment, and management of IPC emergencies. Maintaining current policies that are updated on a regular schedule and based on scientific evidence is essential. The policies should be disseminated to all appropriate HCWs, who should receive education to ensure that they understand the policies and can perform the procedures. Periodically, selected policies and procedures are monitored or audited to determine whether they are effective and current and whether HCWs are complying. Both process and outcome monitoring are useful. These methods are discussed in the section "Identifying Risks Through Surveillance, Data Collection, and Analysis," beginning on page 75.

Involving the Entire Organization

The risk of infection occurs throughout a health care organization, and any program designed to prevent and to control infection must involve *all* areas of an organization. Several JCI requirements guide organizations to use an integrated approach to IPC (*see* Chapters 3 and 4, as well as Appendix 1, for more details).

IPC Policies and Procedures That Apply to All Staff

The policies for hand hygiene, maximal sterile-barrier precautions and isolation measures, reprocessing or reusing supplies, immunizations or health screenings for HCWs, and safe needle use apply to all personnel. These policies should be developed by the IPC staff in partnership with the person(s) and the service(s) that will implement or is affected by the policy directives. Service- or disease-specific policies help incorporate appropriate IPC practices in the daily operations of various parts of the organization, such as the operating theatre, interventional radiology, pharmacy, and other key departments. In one study at a children's hospital, investigators looked at how well HCWs adhered to the organization's policy for specific infection-prevention practices. A clear policy along with education resulted in a significant improvement in disposal of sharp objects and hazardous-waste handling, the availability of PPE, and compliance with isolation precautions.[33] In Cape Town, South Africa, transmission of tuberculosis (TB) from patients with a high incidence of comorbidity with human immunodeficiency virus (HIV) and patients with multidrug-resistant TB (MDR-TB) were attributed in part to a lack of a clear TB infection control policy for HCWs to follow.[34] For more information on this initiative, *see* Case Study 5-2.

CASE STUDY 5-2

Reducing Transmission of Tuberculosis to Health Care Workers with an Intensive TB-IPC Education and Awareness Intervention (South Africa)

Shaheen Mehtar, MBBS, MRC Path (UK), FRCPath (UK), FCPath (SA), MD (Lon); W.A. Mentjies, MBChB; DOM; FCPHM(SA) Occ Med; MMed (Occ Med); Idriss Kallon, MTech (Env Health), BSocSc(Hons); Sr. D. Arendse, BSc Nursing (Stell)

Introduction

South Africa has one of the world's highest burdens of tuberculosis (TB).[1] The additional burden of HIV accounts for up to 65% of HIV coinfection among notified TB cases. Between January 2004 and April 2007, more than 11,000 laboratory-confirmed cases of MDR-TB were reported to the National Department of Health, South Africa; 36% of these were from the Western Cape, which has consistently reported 2.6% of all TB cultures as MDR-TB.[2]

Documenting health care–associated transmission for TB in low- to middle-income (LMI) countries is difficult, because the laboratory cost for routine epidemiological-molecular investigation for TB is not funded. However, one of the indicators for transmission of TB in health care facilities is occupationally acquired TB (OATB), which, by law, has to be reported to the occupational health departments for work-related compensation irrespective of whether it was acquired in the workplace.

In South Africa, the prevalence of TB among the general population is approximately 930/100,000 people, which makes skin testing of HCWs ineffective.[2] The aim of the intensified TB infection prevention and control (TB-IPC) program was to improve HCW compliance to the TB-IPC policy and to measure the reduction of transmission to HCWs.

Methods

At Tygerberg Academic Hospital (TBH), Cape Town, South Africa, OATB was used as an indicator for health care–associated transmission. Early notification of HCWs with positive smears or cultures was sent from the microbiology laboratory to the unit for infection prevention and control (UIPC)—a further confirmatory monthly report from Occupational Health Department (OHD), followed with such details as category of HCW, area of work, HIV status if known, and whether the diagnosis was pulmonary or extrapulmonary TB.

An IPC risk assessment of TBH was carried out, which included evaluation of administrative controls (TB-IPC policy implementation), appropriate use of PPE, and engineering controls in the hospital. Isolation rooms in the clinical areas were identified, and their purpose of use, such as clinical or administrative, was documented.

The hospital's TB-IPC policy, which was approved in early 2010, made clear recommendations based on risk assessment of clinical areas. As a result, exhaust fans were installed in some single rooms. The response by the IPC team to any case of TB admitted to TBH was instituted by ensuring the following:

- TB was declared an "alert organism" in June 2010, and all cases of TB, particularly MDR-TB, were to be identified for the UIPC as soon as possible.
- An intense education program on the TB-IPC policy for all HCWs except physicians was undertaken in June 2010. Standard and airborne precautions were reinforced.
- Each patient was visited by the IPC team, and patients were given advice on appropriate transmission-based precautions; the presence of a functioning exhaust ventilation was also noted by the team.
- An IPC "trolley"—a cart on wheels containing PPE and alcohol hand rub—for airborne precautions was provided for each case of MDR-TB, with all the necessary PPE, such as N95 respirators and hand-hygiene supplies. Instructions on implementing airborne precautions and an *aide-mémoire* were provided. The use of the respirators was recorded to evaluate compliance with PPE during the period of the patient's hospitalization.

The burden of disease was established by recording all admissions of TB (new and readmissions), and areas with the highest caseload were identified. The OHD provided information regarding new cases of OATB, and this was matched with the number of patient admissions by specialty and the impact of the intensified TB-IPC program recorded. The data were analyzed for risk ratios using statistical software.

Results

Burden of disease with MDR-TB

The number of patients with MDR-TB–positive isolates (smear and culture) and MDR-TB cases was reported from TBH between 2008 and 2010. Inpatient samples accounted for 48%, 71.7%, and 73% of MDR-TB cases, respectively, reported from the National Health Service Laboratories, reflecting a statistically significant increase in admissions of MDR-TB cases to TBH ($p = 0.46$). MDR-TB cases were identified in all specialties, including surgery and obstetrics and gynecology.

Facilities for the Isolation of TB

Of the 516 single rooms (40.5% of inpatient beds) at TBH, only 20.7% (264/1274 beds) were available for patient use. In total, less than 2% (5/264) of single rooms had negative pressure, and MDR-TB cases were given priority of admission to these. Triage was not always possible, especially in the outpatient department. On the wards, the movements of patients could not be restricted; the space between the beds was more than adequate, and natural ventilation was often possible.

Training

Formal training in TB-IPC was provided by the IPC team annually to between 157 and 180 HCWs (mainly nurses). On-the-spot training and reminders when implementing airborne precautions proved more fruitful. Although many of the HCWs had been dealing with TB patients for most of their working lives, many of them felt inadequately trained to do so.

Personal Protective Equipment

Adequate amounts of PPE were provided, and no clinical area reported being out of stock. According to the TB-IPC policy, surgical masks were indicated when dealing with suspected or known non-MDR-TB cases, while respirators were provided for HCWs managing MDR-TB cases. Only 23.6% of HCWs used surgical masks when dealing with suspected or known TB patients. When entering isolation rooms, surgical masks were worn between 8% and 29% of the time; however, when dealing with known cases of MDR-TB, the use of face covers was 50% and 86%. Nurses were more likely to use PPE (face covers) compared with physicians.

Occupationally Acquired Tuberculosis

The HCWs either worked in dedicated areas (nurses) or in several places (physicians and the allied health professionals). The ancillary staff rotated around the hospital, but some

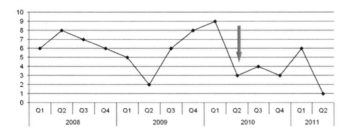

Figure 1. Number of Occupationally Acquired Tuberculosis Cases Reported, 2008 to 2011.

Note: The arrow indicates the point of implementation of an intensified TB-IPC program.

worked in dedicated areas. The number of cases of OATB reported to the OH department is shown in Figure 1. However, in the second quarter of 2011, for the first time in three years, no cases of OATB were reported.

HIV was most common among the ancillary workers compared with the other occupational groups but did not have a significant bearing on OATB. There was no clear correlation between the place of work and acquiring TB. Although the ICUs had the largest number of TB admissions, these were not identified by the HCWs as places where they might have acquired TB. HCWs had a 2.54-times-greater risk of contracting OATB (95% confidence interval [CI]-1.96–3.3) compared with the general population. As for the relative risk of acquiring TB by specialty, internal medicine was 1.6 times higher than the ICU, while for pediatrics, surgery, and obstetrics and gynecology, the relative risk was 2.2, 3.7, and 6.3 times greater, respectively.

Lessons Learned

The burden of TB in hospitals is increasing, particularly those with MDR-TB. Although TB-IPC policies and protocols exist, the implementation is less than satisfactory. Isolation facilities with negative pressure ventilation are inadequate. Despite training in TB-IPC, the use of PPE is inadequate by medical staff dealing with suspected or known cases of TB, which is reflected in the rate of OATB. Consistent implementation of a TB-IPC policy by all staff members can reduce transmission of TB in high-burden countries.

Case Study References

1. World Health Organization. World Health Statistics 2010. Accessed 7 Oct 2011. http://www.who.int/whosis/whostat/EN_WHS10_Full.pdf.
2. Department of Health, Republic of South Africa. Tuberculosis Strategic Plan for South Africa, 2007–2011. Accessed 6 Oct 2011. http://www.info.gov.za/view/DownloadFileAction?id=72544.

Education

Education that reinforces best practices or leads to behavioral changes to improve practice can be a powerful deterrent to spreading HAIs. Each individual affiliated with a health care organization must understand his or her role in IPC efforts. To achieve a clear understanding of the required efforts of each person, organizations must continually educate HCWs about the following topics:

- How infections are transmitted in the health care setting to patients and to staff
- The role of HCWs in preventing and controlling infection transmission, including their role in providing leadership, direct care, or supportive services
- How HCWs can identify potential infection-prevention problems and develop the strategies to address those problems
- How to report infections and related problems, including which information to report and where to report it
- How caregivers can preserve their health to help preserve their patients' safety

An example of one organization's efforts to educate and to communicate with HCWs on an important IPC initiative is found in Case Study 5-3.

CASE STUDY 5-3

Impact of an Infection Control Training Program on the Rates of Ventilator-Associated Pneumonia in a Respiratory Intensive Care Unit (Egypt)

Ossama Rasslan, MD, PhD; Mahmmoud Khalil, MD; Muhammed Abd El Sabour, MD; Maha El Gafarey, MD; Lamia Fouad, MD; Wael Abd El-Fattah, MD

Introduction

HAIs are problematic in the ICU because of their frequency, morbidity, and mortality. The most common ICU infections are pneumonia, BSIs, and UTIs, most of which are device related.[1] Ventilator associated pneumonia (VAP) is an HAI that commonly causes significant morbidity and mortality in mechanically ventilated patients.[2] VAP is preventable, and many practices have been demonstrated to reduce the incidence of VAP and its associated burden of illness.[3]

Leaders at Ain Shams University Specialized Hospital, Abbassia, Egypt, carried out an active baseline surveillance of VAP in its respiratory intensive care unit (RICU). The US CDC's National Nosocomial Infection Surveillance System (NNIS) reported that, in 2004, the median rate of VAP per thousand ventilator-days in NNIS hospitals ranged from

2.2 in pediatric ICUs to 14.7 in trauma ICUs.[4] In other reports, patients receiving continuous mechanical ventilation had 6 to 21 times the risk of developing hospital-associated pneumonia compared with patients who were not receiving mechanical ventilation.[5] This hospital's VAP incidence per 1,000 ventilator-days was 79.8 (64.7–98.1), much higher than rates reported elsewhere.

The hospital's aim was to assess the impact of a training program dedicated to HCWs regarding infection control practices and a bundle approach on the rate of VAP.

Methods

The study was carried out in the following phases from December 2008 through May 2011.

Phase I: December 2008–March 2009

Phase I included active surveillance of the rates of VAP, which was divided into early (≤ 96 hours of admission) and late onset (>96 hours of admission).[5] Designated surveillance forms were used for all patients in the RICU, including patients with and without HAIs. The data were recorded daily on the form of each patient, including administrative data (for example, hospital number, admission date), demographic risk factors (for example, age, gender, severity of underlying illness, primary diagnosis, and immunological status), and interventions (for example, device exposure, surgical procedure, treatments) for infected and for noninfected patients. If a patient acquired VAP, the date of onset, site of infection, microorganisms isolated, and antimicrobial susceptibility were also reported.

A baseline assessment for infection control practices, environmental cleaning and disinfection, and methods for sterilization and disinfection was performed. Hand-hygiene resources and compliance were monitored.

Baseline designated surveillance for VAP was performed, as it has been standardized by the US CDC (NNIS), who provides unambiguous definitions, to detect problems requiring intervention. Assessment of ventilatory circuits and respiratory equipments was performed regarding proper cleaning and sterilization. The VAP bundle application was also assessed.

Phase II: April–July 2009

Education and training for improving hand-hygiene practices were implemented, including the following:
- Data presentations and videos for all staff
- Display of posters calling for use of antiseptic wash and surgical scrubs
- Distribution of handouts describing the initiative to nurses and intensivists

- On-the-job training on hand-hygiene practices for workers, nurses, residents, and intensivists
- Observation of hand-hygiene practices of 15 physicians and 15 nurses throughout the day, with compliance recorded using a checklist
- Restocking of hand-hygiene supplies as follows:
  - Supplies for hand-washing stations were applied in the RICU.
  - Pocket alcohol rub was prepared in the RICU laboratory with the help of a pharmacist and introduced to physicians and nurses to prompt hand-hygiene compliance among HCWs.
  - Each water-supply point was supplied with a liquid dispenser containing liquid soap, a towel dispenser for disposable towels, a pump for liquid surgical-scrub solution, and a basket with a black bag.
  - Posters promoting hand washing were posted at each washing point to remind all staff of the hand-hygiene practices.

In addition, a VAP bundle, supported by educational sessions, was instituted. The bundle included the following elements:
- Stress ulcer prophylaxis via sacrulfate unless contraindicated
- Daily assessment of readiness to extubate
- Continuous open suction from endotracheal tube every two hours via a suction catheter that was changed thrice daily or if visibly soiled; aspiration of secretions via one suction catheter for the mouth and another for the endotracheal suction
- Elevation of head of bed to be between 30 and 45 degrees unless contraindicated
- Deep vein thrombosis prophylaxis (unless contraindicated) via intravenous (IV) heparin
- Exchange of ventilatory circuit (expiratory valve, inspiratory limb, expiratory limb, and water traps) every five days or unless soiled or contaminated with a checklist for accurate follow-up of circuit exchange
- Chest physiotherapy
- Avoidance of unnecessary intubation
- Oral wash via brushing of the mouth every two hours with chlorhexidine

The bundle compliance was assessed weekly via a checklist for its application and patients for VAP reduction.

Phase III: August–December 2009 and January–May 2011

This phase included reevaluation of the intervention phase through surveillance of VAP. Hand-hygiene practices' adherence and compliance with VAP bundle were monitored.

Results

The results of this initiative are displayed in Tables 1 and 2 below.

Table 1. Incidence of VAP Among the Surveyed RICU Patients Admitted, December 2008–December 2009

This table shows that VAP incidence in the surveillance performed during the period of the study is 79.8/1,000 ventilator-days, with higher incidence of infection for late-onset VAP than for early-onset VAP.

Variable	Number of Infections	Patient-Days	Incidence per 1,000 Ventilator-Days (95% CI)
VAP early	25	1,077	23.2 (15.4–34.6)
VAP late	61	1,077	56.6 (43.9–72.6)
VAP total	86	1,077	79.8 (64.7–98.1)

Note: CI = confidence interval

Table 2. Monthly VAP Incidence Rate Among the Surveyed RICU Patients Admitted During All Study Phases

Phase	Months	Number of VAP	Ventilator-Days	Incidence per 1,000 Mechanical Ventilation Days
Pre-intervention Phase I	December 2008	8	92	86.9
	January 2009	6	12	53.6
	February 2009	6	86	69.8
	March 2009	10	105	95.2
Intervention Phase II	April 2009	9	93	96.8
	May 2009	7	86	81.3
	June 2009	3	79	37.9
	July 2009	13	119	109.2
Post-intervention 1, Phase III	August 2009	2	76	26.3
	September 2009	5	89	67.2
	October 2009	6	85	70.5
	November 2009	5	86	58.3
	December 2009	1	45	22.2
Post-intervention 2, Phase III	January 2011	2	91	22
	February 2011	1	31	32.5
	March 2011	1	29	34.5
	April 2011	1	34	29.4
	May 2011	1	50	20

Lessons Learned

Using simple, noncostly methodologies can enhance the knowledge and improve the practices of HCWs, which may have an impact on VAP rates in the RICU.

Case Study References

1. Eggimann P, Pittet D. Infection control in the ICU. *Chest.* 2001 Dec;120(6):2059–2093.
2. Meric M, et al. Intensive care unit-acquired infections: Incidence, risk factor and associated mortality in a Turkish university hospital. *Jpn J Infect Dis.* 2005 Oct;58(5):297–302.
3. Muscedere J, et al. Comprehensive evidence-based clinical practice guidelines for ventilator-associated pneumonia: Prevention. *J Crit Care.* 2008 Mar;23(1):126–137.
4. US Centers for Disease Control and Prevention. National Nosocomial Infections Surveillance (NNIS) Systems Report, Data summary from January 1992 through June 2004, issued October 2004. NNIS. Dec 2004. Accessed 24 Sep 2011. http://www.cdc.gov/nhsn/PDFs/data Stat/NNIS_2004.pdf.
5. Fishman JA. Nosocomial pneumonia. In Fishman AP, Elias AJ, Gippi AM, editors: *Fishman's Pulmonary Diseases and Disorders*, 4th ed. New York: McGraw-Hill, 2008, 2273–2289.

Although most organizations teach infection precautions to HCWs who provide direct care, they sometimes overlook those HCWs who might be exposed to or act as carriers of infection, such as housekeepers who maintain the patient and organizational environment, or those who manage equipment or wastes, such as biomedical technicians, waste and garbage handlers, plumbers, electricians, and delivery personnel.

Direct-care HCWs should know how to identify risk factors for infection in specific patient populations. Older adults—many of whom might suffer from chronic illnesses, lack of mobility, and immunodeficiency—are particularly vulnerable and may show few of the common symptoms, such as fever or elevated white blood count in the presence of infection. Evaluating subtle signs, such as unexpected confusion or lethargy, should be part of the skill set of those who care for this population. Patients with indwelling devices, such as urinary, peripheral, or central venous catheters, and those undergoing invasive therapy, surgery, ventilatory support, and dialysis are considered high-risk populations. HCWs who care for these patients or the equipment or devices used to diagnose disease or to administer therapy should receive education that focuses on the particular risks of the associated care processes. Thus, thorough education for HCWs in an organizationwide IPC program must address the core principles of IPC and the unique infection risks of certain populations, procedures, or pathogens.

Some studies demonstrate the positive effects of training and education. In Thailand, when implementing a new central line–associated bloodstream infection (CLABSI) bundle in a pediatric intensive care unit, compliance was enhanced with education.[35] In another hemodialysis (HD) unit in Khartoum, Sudan, researchers found serious gaps in HD staff knowledge and adherence to infection control recommendations, indicating the need for a more structured training program.[36] It is generally believed that education alone does not always suffice in changing behavior or that the delivery of education may not be effective. This was demonstrated in a hospital in Saudi Arabia, where hand-hygiene compliance reached only 50% after a long educational campaign,[37] and also in China, where nursing compliance with standard precautions was still not optimal after a training program.[38]

Education for HCWs should include an initial orientation, annual IPC updates, and periodic information about new policies or recent developments, such as emerging diseases, resistant organisms, or new methods to prevent infection. It is important for IPC professionals to continually assess the educational needs of HCWs and to use varied teaching and learning methods that include the appropriate verbal and written language and address norms, values, and cultural behaviors.. The education should be followed by an evaluation to determine whether learning has taken place.

Communication

In addition to providing education, organizations must communicate to all physicians, nurses, clinical and support staff, students, and volunteers the IPC goals, objectives, and initiatives and share results of any surveillance data and performance-improvement projects under way. HCWs and leaders must have the most current information so they can apply it to clinical care, protect themselves from acquiring infection, and guide the work of the organization.

It is also important to communicate IPC information to the committees that govern the organization, such as the administrative/leadership committee, patient-safety or quality committee, medical and nursing committees, governing board, and groups that oversee the organization's environment and facilities. Providing these groups and frontline HCWs with information about how a particular initiative has improved safety or reduced infections can go a long way toward ensuring compliance throughout the organization. The communication between HCWs can affect care and patient outcomes. In one study in Michigan that examined the culture of patient safety on three units, nurses from the unit with the least-robust safety culture were also the least satisfied in their communication with physicians.[39] This contextual dissonance can create an environment that may influence infection risk for patients. In addition, as patients move from one part of the hospital to another, to different hospitals within a system, or from a hospital to an outpatient or ambulatory care setting, it is essential to communicate any IPC information to the health care providers at the next level of care. Organizations should develop systems to ensure that this communication occurs. Effective methods for communicating IPC information to HCWs include the following:

- Group in-services
- Formal or informal reports
- One-on-one conversations
- Newsletters
- E-mails, faxes
- Staff meetings
- Intranet sites
- Videos
- Breakroom bulletin boards

Communicating Infection Prevention and Control Data and Information to Families and Visitors

In many settings, the patient's family and other visitors are an integral part of the patient's care team. They participate in hygiene and other daily activities, wound care, moving the patient, and other direct care activities. In some settings, the family members are the primary caregivers, particularly for children. In addition, the family and visitors may bring meals to the patient and even prepare them on site at the hospital. Thus, it is essential that the family be included in the communication program about infection-prevention methods and rules to help them best care for their family member and to protect themselves and others from acquiring or transmitting infection. Brochures, pamphlets (*see* Figure 5-1 for one example), videos, and other means can be used to communicate with families and visitors in addition to one-on-one verbal communication. HCWs should always consider cultural sensitivities, learning capabilities, and skills and language needs as they prepare, disseminate, and provide education to families and visitors in the hospital and to families and patients in the community.[40–42]

Participating in Organizationwide Committees

Committees outside of the IPC program often make decisions that influence IPC practices. In an organizationwide IPC program, IPC personnel should serve on the committees that develop policies and procedures affecting patient care and HCW policies addressing infection risk. IPC personnel can provide data, information, and expert commentary as decisions are made. Such committees might include quality-improvement, patient-safety, and nursing-oversight committees and those groups that address surgery, construction and renovation, product selection, environmental chal-

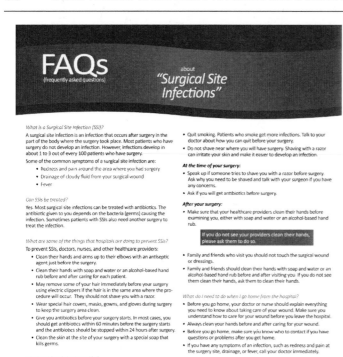

Figure 5-1. Patient and Family Education Brochures

Patient and family educational brochures like the one pictured here are means to communicate important health care issues to patients and their loved ones. This and other patient resources are available at http://www.shea-online.org /ForPatients.aspx.

Source: Society for Healthcare Epidemiology of America (SHEA). Available at http://www.shea-online.org/Assets/files/patient%20guides /NNL_SSI.pdf.

lenges, and accreditation issues. Likewise, the information and decisions from the ICC and other committees and specific groups should be disseminated to appropriate staff as a way to keep them apprised and involved and to continually integrate IPC information throughout the organization.

Building Relationships Within the Organization

Dedicated IPC practitioners along with a physician leader to oversee everyday operations of an IPC program are essential to successful program operation. However, these professionals are only part of the IPC process. A successful IPC program is a product of the participation of many individuals throughout a health care organization working together to prevent the spread of infection. IPC professionals should identify key

people throughout the organization and in the community and communicate frequently with them about IPC activities. These key people might represent the following areas:

- Administrative leaders
- Medical and nursing staff
- Facility management and construction teams
- Housekeeping or environmental services
- Pharmacy, respiratory therapy, laboratory
- Public health officials

Creating Multidisciplinary Performance-Improvement Teams

When vulnerabilities in IPC practice are identified and system issues become apparent, the organization should initiate improvement projects that will result in better care for the patients, safer work environments for staff, and reduced risk for families and visitors. When the issue crosses several departments or more than one type of care setting, the most effective way to address these issues is with a multidisciplinary team. It is important to include those persons who truly understand the work setting or the technical aspects of the care provided and the facility. These individuals are most knowledgeable about the current practices and the barriers in the workplace and can provide valuable input for solutions and improvements.[43–45]

Establishing the Focus of the IPC Program

Performing the Risk Assessment and Creating an IPC Plan

JCI requirements state that the IPC program must address issues that are epidemiologically important to the organization, including important infections, infection sites, and associated devices. This information is used to establish priorities and activities to prevent and to reduce the incidence of HAIs. JCI also requires that the organization identify the procedures and processes associated with the risk of infection and implement strategies to reduce infection risk. It is thus important for an organization to review those processes and, as appropriate, to implement policies, procedures, education, improvement, and other activities to reduce risk of infection. Together, these standards and measurable elements convey a strong message that the organization will be expected to perform some type of risk assessment to determine the priorities of the IPC program.[46–48]

Performing a risk assessment should be one of the first activities of a new IPC program and an ongoing activity of established programs.[47] The risk assessment is the foundation of the IPC program. Optimally, the risk assessment and refocusing of program activities should be performed at least annually and more often if needed due to changes in circumstances, such as the addition of a new service or a change in population or community events.

An IPC risk assessment is a careful, proactive examination of events that could cause infections, harm, or even death to patients, staff, families, or visitors. The plan that evolves from the assessment is based on those risks of the highest priority and identifies methods to minimize, to mitigate, or to manage these risks if they occur.

The risk-assessment process includes an analysis of existing information, such as surveillance data, injuries, or other reports of adverse events; system issues, such as lack of education or communication; population-specific challenges, including patients and staff; and infrastructure or resource limitations. Information is gathered from careful examination of infection experience, such as rates of infections or outbreaks, mortality, information gathered proactively through surveys or focus groups of staff, a review of the scientific literature, and new mandates or requirements. Some risks may be anticipated based on environmental changes, emerging diseases, or events in other health care settings or in the world. For example, in each country, differences in emerging or reemerging infections affect community and hospital populations (*see* Chapter 1). Some conditions, such as the potential for an influenza pandemic, are a risk for which every health care organization in the world should prepare. Natural disasters may be anticipated based on a country's location and climate. There are also different economic realities for health care organizations, depending on the countries in which the organizations are located. Each organization can select its own methodology for performing a risk assessment.

General topics or categories can be considered in a risk assessment. These may include, but are not limited to, the following:

- Geography of organization location and associated risks (for example, floods, earthquakes)
- Community health issues (for example, lack of immunizations, prevalence of disease, inadequate clean water and sanitation)
- Characteristics of the patient populations served by the health care facility
- Results of past studies, surveillance data, audits, or clinical findings
- Type of care, treatment, and services provided
- Facility and environmental issues (for example, cleaning, construction, ventilation)

- Consistent access to needed supplies, equipment, and medications (for example, open versus closed drainage systems, clean versus sterile supplies, reuse of single-use devices, patient-shared equipment, hand-hygiene supplies)
- Locally adopted clinical pathways or practice guidelines
- Risks to HCWs (for example, variable immunization, high prevalence of TB)
- Emergencies affecting the health care settings
- Current local, state, and federal laws
- Education and training for HCWs
- Communication strategies and effectiveness
- Information from the World Health Organization (WHO), ministries of health, US CDC, and other public health agencies

After the general categories have been determined, the organization can identify and analyze specific risk events in each category. For example, one category might be "risks to HCWs," and the individual events may include sharps injuries, exposure to TB or other communicable diseases, or degree of compliance with hand-hygiene or isolation procedures. Another category might be "high-risk infections" and include specific risk events, such as CLABSIs, VAP, postcoronary artery bypass graft surgery, or post–Cesarean section endometritis. Each of these specific potential risk events is assessed as part of the overall risk analysis (*see* Table 5-2).

Here are the two basic questions for assessment of risk:
1. What is the probability (how likely) that a risk event will occur?
2. How severe would the risk event be should it occur?

Additional questions can be posed for deeper analysis. A description of the risk-assessment process is found in Sidebar 5-3. A list of potential risk-assessment queries is found in Sidebar 5-4. The process for completing a risk assessment includes several steps, as indicated in Table 5-3.

The risk-assessment process should be systematic and include at least those persons who are responsible for the IPC program and others who are key leaders or staff who support the program or are affected by it. Adequate time should be allotted to gather data to assess risk events. The IPC team may need information from medical records, risk management, quality and patient safety, finance, special services, or public health agencies in addition to surveillance data.

The method for performing the risk assessment can be quantitative or semiquantitative, using numerical values to rate the risk events, or it can be qualitative, using written descriptions to discuss the risks and their potential harm. Either method will be useful if the persons who are participating and those who will receive the report understand it.

Table 5-2. Examples of Risk Categories and Specific Risk Factors for IPC

Risk Category	Risk Factors
Geographic location	• Natural disasters (tornadoes, floods, hurricanes, tsunami, earthquakes) • Breakdown or absence of municipal services • Broken water main, contaminated water supply, strike or work stoppage by sanitation employees • Accidents in the community (airplane, train, bus; fires involving mass casualties) • Intentional acts (bioterrorism, "dirty bomb," contamination of food and water supplies) • Prevalence of disease linked with vectors, temperature, other environmental factors
Community	• Community outbreaks of transmissible infectious diseases (influenza, meningitis, severe acute respiratory syndrome [SARS]) • Diseases linked to food and water contamination (*Salmonella*, hepatitis A) • Vaccine-preventable illness in unvaccinated population (measles) • Infections associated with immigrant or migrant populations (displaced persons in camps) • Public health infrastructure (vaccine availability) • Socioeconomic levels (income and education)
Organization programs and services	• Cardiac surgery service • Orthopedic service • Neonatology dialysis • Long term care • Ambulatory clinics • Hospice (end of life care) • Home care • Behavioral health care
Special populations served	• Women and children • Frail elderly • Behavioral health care • Long term care • Rehabilitation • Diseases associated with lifestyle • Predisposition for illnesses resulting from cognitive and physical changes • Migratory populations
High-risk patients	• Surgical • Intensive care unit • Neonatal or pediatric intensive care unit • Immunocompromised hosts • Oncology • Dialysis • Transplant • Rehabilitation
HCW risks	• Lack of understanding disease transmission and prevention • Degree of compliance with infection-prevention techniques and policies (hand hygiene) • Use of PPE and isolation • Sharps injuries • Screening for transmissible diseases • Work-restriction guidelines • Practice-accountability issues

Table 5-2. Examples of Risk Categories and Specific Risk Factors for IPC *(continued)*

Risk Category	Risk Factors
Medical procedures	• Invasiveness of procedure • Equipment used for procedure • Knowledge and technical expertise of providers • Adequate preparation of patient • Adherence to recommended infection-prevention techniques • Physical environment where procedure performed
Equipment and devices	• Cleaning, disinfection, transport, and storage for intravenous (IV) pumps, suction equipment, other equipment • Sterilization or disinfection process for flexible and rigid scopes, surgical instruments, prostheses • Complexity of device structure (lumens, channels) • Skill and experience of user • Safety features (user dependent or automatic) • Reuse of single-use devices • Preparation of IV fluids or medications • Open versus closed systems • Injection practices and equipment
Environmental issues	• Construction, renovation, alterations • Utilities performance • Routine environmental cleanliness • Special cleaning procedures • Knowledge of staff • Adequate staff for effective cleaning • Airflow and filtration, humidity • Negative-pressure rooms
Emergency preparedness	• Staff knowledge • Capacity to manage influx of infectious patients • Triaging patients • Space availability • Isolation, barriers, PPE availability • Utilities and supplies • Security issues
Resource limitations	• Staffing limitations for nursing, physicians, clinical support staff, other support staff, environmental services, IPC professionals • Sterile supplies • Congested patient care areas • Negative-pressure rooms • Clean water
Organization's outcome and process surveillance data	• CLABSIs • VAP • CAUTIs • SSIs • Gastrointestinal infections • Sepsis • Compliance with isolation procedures, aseptic technique • Handling of linen and waste • Device-related bundle compliance

Sources: Adapted from Soule B. Risk-based approach to infection prevention: Creating an infection prevention and control plan. In Arias KM, Soule BM, editors: *The APIC/JCR Infection Prevention and Control Workbook*, 2nd ed. Oak Brook, IL, and Washington, DC: Joint Commission Resources and Association for Professionals in Infection Control and Epidemiology, 2010, 37–39; and Joint Commission Resources. *Risk Assessment for Infection Prevention and Control.* Oak Brook, IL: Joint Commission Resources, 2010, 66–68.

In the semiquantitative method, numbers are assigned to each issue to designate the degree of risk (*see* Figure 5-2) The numbers from each category can be added together or multiplied to obtain the score for each individual risk. (If multiplying, do not use any zeros). The risk assessment

---

Sidebar 5-3. The Risk-Assessment Process

- Determine the scope of the assessment and select general-risk categories.
- Identify specific risk factors in each category.
- Determine a methodology and risk-scoring system with clear definitions.
- Collect data for the risk analysis.
- Evaluate and score the risk events.
- Determine and identify the risk priorities for the organization.
- Use prioritized risks as the basis for the IPC plan.
- Disseminate results to staff and leaders.

Source: Adapted from Soule B. Risk-based approach to infection prevention: Creating an infection prevention and control plan. In Arias KM, Soule BM, editors: *The APIC/JCR Infection Prevention and Control Workbook*, 2nd ed. Oak Brook, IL, and Washington, DC: Joint Commission Resources and Association for Professionals in Infection Control and Epidemiology, 2010, 31–32.

Sidebar 5-4. Questions to Analyze Potential Infection-Risk Events

- What are the potential or actual risks that may lead to infections in this organization?
- What is the probability that any given risk event will occur?
- If the risk event occurs, how severe could it be?
- How frequently might the risk event occur?
- What is the organization's ability to identify the risk?
- What is the scope of response that would be required by the organization to reduce or to eliminate the risk?
- How well does leadership support response to the event?
- How prepared is the organization to respond to challenges at this time?
- What effect would the risk have on the environment, fiscal health, or image of the organization?
- How would the risk affect patients and staff?

Source: Adapted from Soule B. Risk-based approach to infection prevention: Creating an infection prevention and control plan. In Arias KM, Soule BM, editors: *The APIC/JCR Infection Prevention and Control Workbook*, 2nd ed. Oak Brook, IL, and Washington, DC: Joint Commission Resources and Association for Professionals in Infection Control and Epidemiology, 2010, 40.

---

team can select which numbers they wish to use and the method of calculation. After the numbers are added or multiplied and the scores are determined, the highest priorities can be indicated on the assessment form by special markings such as color coding or other techniques. A quantitative risk assessment should be performed for the IPC program as a whole and can also be developed for a particular topic such as MDROs.

A sample quantitative risk assessment is provided in Figure 5-2.

For a qualitative assessment, the risk and the rationale are discussed, and the risk is rated using word versus numbers. A risk priority is assigned. A sample of a qualitative risk is shown in Table 5-4.

One qualitative risk assessment used by some groups is the gap analysis, a priority-setting approach in which the organization asks such questions as the following:
- "What is the risk at this time?"
- "Where do we want to be?" or "What is our desired goal?"
- "What is the gap between now and our target?"

Each risk is considered, assessed, and ranked to determine the highest priorities. This leads to an action plan. Table 5-5 is an example of a gap analysis for one significant infection-prevention issue.

When the analysis is completed, the risks considered the highest priority for the organization are selected and presented to the IPC committee or patient-safety and quality committee and administration for approval and support. After the leadership agrees to the selected priorities, they should support the work with the needed resources. Some countries or organizations may not have the infrastructure or monetary resources for all priorities. In those circumstances, leaders can still make the issues highly visible and convey their importance to the organization and staff by ensuring that there are clear policies and procedures, education, and monitoring or auditing to make changes where possible and risks can be addressed sequentially.

Developing the IPC Plan

When the IPC priorities have been designated and approved, the organization uses them to develop the IPC plan. The plan has two main parts: (1) background information about the program, including the scope of services offered by the IPC department; and (2) the action plan for the year.

Background information. For background information, the plan might contain some demographic information about the organization, such as the number of beds, types of services, community served (whether it is teaching or nonteaching or other information that sets the frame-

Table 5-3. Steps in Performing a Risk Assessment

Steps	Details
Form a multidisciplinary group to perform the risk assessment.	Engage IPC practitioners, physicians, nursing, support staff, leaders, others.
Determine the general categories of risks to be addressed.	Consider risks internal to the organization and those that are external, risks that are known, and those that can be anticipated.
Identify the specific risk events in each category.	Develop a list of risk events or risk factors in each category.
Select a method for the analysis (in other words, quantitative or qualitative).	Develop a format and template to support the method selected.
Select a scoring system.	Use numerical ratings for each term, for example, High (5), Medium (3), Low (1); or Life Threatening (9), Severe (7), Moderate (5), or Mild (3).
Collect the information needed to assess each risk event.	Obtain information from the following: • Surveillance data • Medical records • Financial information • Accidents and incidents • Deaths • Admissions or discharges • Other
Score each potential risk event using predetermined criteria or definitions.	See "select a scoring system" above.
Select the highest risks for the organization as the priorities.	Determine which risks pose the greatest threat of harm to patients, staff, and others. Work with a multidisciplinary group to make the determinations.
Obtain approval from leadership.	Present priorities to the IPC committee for formal approval. When high risks selected, seek approval from organizational leaders.
Develop the IPC plan using the risk priorities.	Use the priorities to develop goals, measurable objectives, actions, and an evaluation plan.
Disseminate the results and IPC plan.	Distribute to leadership, clinical units, service or department heads, key staff, and others.

Source: Adapted from Soule B. Risk-based approach to infection prevention: Creating an infection prevention and control plan. In Arias KM, Soule BM, editors: *The APIC/JCR Infection Prevention and Control Workbook*, 2nd ed. Oak Brook, IL, and Washington, DC: Joint Commission Resources and Association for Professionals in Infection Control and Epidemiology, 2010, 31–32.

work for the IPC). The plan can include the mission and the vision or future of the IPC program. For example, the mission might state: "*The infection prevention and control program minimizes risk of infection to promote a high quality of care, safety, and well-being in patients, staff, and visitors.*" A vision might say, "*The IPC program strives to achieve zero infections in all patients.*" The IPC plan can include information about the infrastructure of the IPC program, including the number of staff and their roles; training or certification of the IPC committee; and ways in which medicine, nursing, and other key staff participate in coordinating the program. Often an IPC plan includes a state-ment about the authority of designated individuals (for example, chairman, IPC physician, IPC nurse, or administrator) to make decisions for such actions as placing a patient in isolation, closing a unit, or stopping surgery because of construction risks. The plan may discuss the scope of services that the IPC team offers to the organization, including staff education, surveillance activities and outbreak investigation, development of policies and procedures, oversight of maintenance of the environment and medical equipment, and consultation with staff throughout the hospital for IPC problems. The integration of the IPC program with quality improvement and patient safety and

HAMAD MEDICAL CORPORATION
CORPORATE INFECTION CONTROL RISK ASSESSMENT 2010

RISK EVENT	Probability of Occurrence				Potential Severity of Event				Potential Response Required (Change in Care, Treatment,				Organizational Preparedness			Risk Priority
	High	Med	Low	None	Life Threatening	Permanent Harm	Temporary Harm	None	High	Med	Low	None	Poor	Fair	Good	
Score:	4	3	2	1	4	3	2	1	4	3	2	1	3	2	1	
POTENTIAL INFECTIONS																
VAP		3				3				3				2		54
SSIs		3				3				3				2		54
CLABSIs			2			3				3				2		36
MDROs																
MRSA			2				2			3				2		24
Clostridium difficile			2					1			2			2		8
VRE			2				2			3					1	12
ESBL Gram Negative		3					2			3				2		36
PSA		3					2			3				2		36
ACBA		3					2			3				2		36
EMPLOYEE/PATIENT EXPOSURE RELATED																
Noncompliance for PPE use			2				2				2				1	8
Poor hand-hygiene compliance			2			3					2			2		24
Needle sticks and sharps injuries			2			3				3				2		36
Staff exposure to TB		3					2				2			2		24
Staff exposure to chickenpox		3					2				2			2		24
COMMUNICATION/EDUCATION																
Nonacceptance of IPC guidelines and recommendations		3					2				2			2		24
Lack of patient and family education on IPC			2				2				2			2		16
ENVIRONMENT																
Improper cleaning and disinfection of environment		3				3				3				2		54
Nonavailability of housekeeping		3				3					2			2		36
Improper storage of clean and dirty supplies				1			2				2		3			12
Improper cleaning/disinfection of supplies/equipment/toy			2				2				2			2		16
EMERGENCY PREPAREDNESS																
Nonawareness of staff about emergency prep. plan		3					2			3					1	18
Lack of supplies			2				2		4						1	16
Lack of surge capacity in isolation rooms				1		3				3				2		18
GEOGRAPHICAL LOCATION AND COMMUNITY ENVIRONMENT																
Tuberculosis		3					2				2			2		24
Meningitis			2				2				2				1	8
Salmonella			2				2				2				1	8
Chickenpox			2				2				2				1	8
Dust storm			2				2				2				1	8
Labor camp			2				2				2				1	8

Figure 5-2. Infection Prevention and Control Risk Assessment

In this risk assessment tool, risk levels are assessed by probability, severity, required response, and preparedness and those scores are multiplied to produce an overall risk priority. The highest priorities for performance improvement (VAP and SSIs) are highlighted for emphasis.

Source: Hamad Medical Corporation, Doha, Qatar. Used with permission.

the educational offerings are also appropriate topics for the IPC plan. The plan may address the availability and appropriate use of gloves, masks, soap, and disinfectants; which surveillance cultures are collected; and the training of staff who clean the environment. The plan may also explain how the IPC program uses current scientific knowledge, accepted practice guidelines, and applicable regulations to guide activities and policy development.

Annual action plan. The second part of the IPC plan is the section that describes the priorities, goals, objectives, and evaluation process for a given time period. This is also where the organization identifies strategies to reduce infection risk that evolve from the risk priorities, goals, and objectives. The key to having a useful and dynamic plan is to keep it simple and to state clearly how goals will be accomplished and measured. The grid in Table 5-6 provides one example for capturing the key elements of the IPC plan in a way that is easy to monitor, to update, and to describe. Using a grid like this can also provide a tool for teaching, describing, and marketing the program to the organization and external agencies as well as for developing reports. Other formats may also be useful.

Implementing Strategies to Reduce Infection Risk

The IPC team develops risk-reduction strategies on an ongoing basis. Some strategies are short term, developed based on surveillance data or in response to consultations with the staff, observations of the environment during rounds, or observations of care practices. Some interventions evolve from known areas of risk based on published research and the experience of other IPC programs. Adverse outcomes may also stimulate new strategies or indicate the need for change in other areas.

Table 5-4. Sample Qualitative Infection Prevention and Control Risk Assessment

Population at Risk	Risk Event	Rationale	Risk of Event	Potential Severity	Potential for Prevention	Overall Priority
Intensive Care Unit (ICU) Patients	High rate of VAP in ICU patients, particularly those who are long term, or immunologically immature, or have extremely severe illness Rates currently at 75th percentile of National Healthcare Safety Network (NHSN) in some ICUs	Ventilators present risk of associated pneumonia because they bypass normal body defense mechanisms for the respiratory system. **Measure:** Reduce to 25th percentile or less of NHSN comparative data and target zero VAP rates in at least 2 ICUs for 6 consecutive months during 2012.	Medical ICU Cardiac Care ICU Trauma ICU Neonatal ICU Burn ICU	**Serious** **Serious** **Serious** *Life Threatening* *Life Threatening*	Moderate Moderate Moderate Low Low Preventability depends on strict compliance with infection guidelines by all staff all the time.	Medium Medium Medium *Urgent* **High**
Operating Theatre Employees	Sharps injuries with needles and lancets in surgery Risk of blood-borne pathogen infections such as hepatitis or HIV Sharps injury rates have been increasing during past year— 12% increase.	Many sharps are used during a surgical procedure; sometimes not handled carefully. Hollow needles particularly risky for transmitting blood-borne pathogens if patient infected. **Measure:** Decrease from 20 to 2 or fewer sharps injuries per quarter by June 2012.	Staff performing or assisting in surgery	**Serious**	High preventability if proper precautions are used per policy Staff must be well trained; appropriate technique used at all times	Moderate

Key:
Severity   Mild, Moderate, **Serious**, *Life Threatening*
Prevention   Low, Moderate, **High**, *Highly Likely*
Priority   Low, Medium, **High**, *Urgent*

Source: Barbara M. Soule. Used with permission.

At least annually, as the organization establishes the focus of the IPC program, the IPC team develops more long-term intervention strategies based on the risk assessment and the goals and objectives that have been selected for that year.

Several strategies can help IPC professionals choose the most beneficial interventions. First, it is essential to be aware of and to use relevant evidence-based practice guidelines. Many guidelines exist and are discussed throughout this book. WHO, the US CDC, the Institute for Healthcare Improvement (IHI), SHEA, the Infectious Disease

Table 5-5. Sample Gap Analysis for Infection Prevention and Control Risk Assessment

Area/Issue/Topic/Standard	Current Status	Desired Status	Gap (Describe)	Priority: High, Medium, Low
Incomplete implementation of WHO Hand Hygiene Guidelines (IPSG.5)	• Guideline approved by ICC • Required elements not implemented throughout the organization	Full implementation of required elements throughout the organization by January 2012 (for example, Categories 1A, 1B, 1C)	• Only 40% of units and services are following WHO HH Guidelines and organizational policy. • Lack of ownership of hand-hygiene implementation by staff and staff leaders	High

Source: Adapted from Soule B. Risk-based approach to infection prevention: Creating an infection prevention and control plan. In Arias KM, Soule BM, editors: *The APIC/JCR Infection Prevention and Control Workbook*, 2nd ed. Oak Brook, IL, and Washington, DC: Joint Commission Resources and Association for Professionals in Infection Control and Epidemiology, 2010, 33.

Association of America (IDSA), APIC, the International Federation of Infection Control, and others have analyzed and synthesized research to make thoughtful recommendations, most of which can be found online. For example, IHI has identified care bundles that include a selected number of evidence-based care processes that, when performed together, can result in dramatically reduced infection rates. Examples of care bundles and their components include the following:

Central-Line Bundle[49]
- Hand hygiene
- Maximal sterile-barrier precautions for insertion
- Chlorhexidine skin antisepsis
- Optimal catheter-site selection, with subclavian vein as the preferred site for nontunneled catheters
- Daily review of line necessity, with prompt removal of unnecessary lines

Ventilator Bundle[50]
- Elevation of the head of the bed
- Daily "sedation vacations" and assessment of readiness to extubate
- Peptic ulcer disease prophylaxis
- Deep venous thrombosis prophylaxis

The Compendium of Strategies to Prevent Infections in Acute Care Hospitals synthesizes the guidelines from the Healthcare Infection Control Practices Advisory Committee (HICPAC) for CAUTIs,[51] SSIs,[52] CLABSIs,[53] VAP,[54] MRSA,[55] and *Clostridium difficile*.[56]

A second strategy is to use surveillance data to guide action. For these data to be helpful, they must be valid and reliable. Data are *valid* when they measure what they were intended to measure, and they are *reliable* when they consistently measure the event they were designed to measure over time.[57] Reliability and validity can be determined by having two different persons using the same criteria review the same patient information. In an ICU, the comparison might be made by an IPC professional and a dedicated ICU specialist. When the decision about whether the patient has an HAI is consistent between the two persons, this agreement validates the surveillance process. If there is a large disparity between findings, then the surveillance criteria or assessment methodology should be examined.

It is essential to use the surveillance data to make changes. If data are collected and analyzed but not used to guide IPC activities, they are useless, and the surveillance process involves wasted resources. One of the key roles of the IPC practitioner is to translate data and information into practice-improvement strategies and to function as an interventionist to initiate and to guide improvement activities.[58] Principles of surveillance are discussed in the following section.

A third strategy is to integrate factors that contribute to successful and sustained change into planning and execution. For example, evaluating peoples' opinions about a change before implementation can assist in stimulating acceptance rather than resistance. When planning for change, including experienced, competent staff in the change process who are respected will encourage acceptance by others. Considering the organizational culture and attitudes toward patient safety and working toward a culture that supports innovation and advocates for improvement should help increase success. When an organization makes the appropriate supplies available and provides time for implementation of new changes, these efforts will also support the goal.

Table 5-6. Sample Annual Hospital IPC Action Plan

Risk Priority	Organizational Goal	IPC Measurable Objective	Method(s)	Evaluation	Participants
High VAP rates in surgical intensive care unit—above 75th percentile of National Health-care Safety Net-work (NHSN) benchmark	Provide safe, excellent quality of care for all patients.	Rates at or below 25th percentile NHSN by Mar 2012 Strive for zero infections for a minimum of 3 months.	Use evidence-based practices to reduce VAP. Initiate VAP Bundle and performance-improvement (PI) team.	Monitor monthly. Report quarterly to staff and Infection Control Committee (ICC)	ICU nurse ICU physician Respiratory therapy Infection prevention and control Quality improvement
12% increase in sharps injuries (scalpel) among the operating theatre (OT) staff from previous year	Provide safe work environment for employees.	Reduce scalpel injuries to OT staff from 20 per quarter to fewer than 2 per quarter by June 2012. Strive for zero sharps injuries for a minimum of 3 months.	PI Team—develop process-improve-ment tools; review equipment; review existing policy; update as necessary.	Monitor monthly, Report monthly to OT staff and quar-terly to ICC and Employee Health.	OT staff Employee health nurse/physician Surgeons Environmental Services Infection preven-tion and control
Expected influx of patients with com-municable disease to emergency department during epidemic	Prepare organiza-tion for emergency situations.	Triage and care for up to 100 patients per day for 3 days with respiratory illness related to epidemic or pandemic.	Develop triage and surge plan for ED and hospital by June 2012. Educate staff on roles by Sept 2012. Obtain supplies by Sept 2012. Test plan and revise based on findings by Oct 2012.	Test three times by June 2013 with increasingly suc-cessful results in managing influx based on triage times, available supplies, and staff performance. Report results to ICC and employee safety committee.	Emergency room nurses and physicians Administration Admitting Safety Infection control Pharmacy

Source: Barbara M. Soule. Used with permission.

Intervention strategies may include such efforts as reducing a high rate of CLABSI[53] or infections after sur-gery[52]; decreasing the incidence of VAP[54] or CAUTIs[51]; reducing infections from other invasive devices; minimizing sharps injuries in HCWs; addressing epidemiologically important organisms, such as *Clostridium difficile*,[56] MRSA,[55] or highly resistant gram-negative organisms; or preventing TB transmission in the acute or ambulatory care setting. Educating staff, making changes in policies and procedures, or reinforcing existing ones and providing feed-back on current activities help improve performance. Often it is necessary to use all these methods simultaneously. *See* Cases Studies 5-4, 5-5, and 5-6 for strategies used by sev-eral organizations to reduce infection from invasive patient-care devices.

CASE STUDY 5-4

Reducing External Ventricular Drain–Related Infection Through the Implementation of a Routine of Care at a Neurology Intensive Care Unit (Brazil)

Eduardo F. Camacho RN, MSc; Ícaro Boszczowski MD, MSc *(SHEA International Ambassador);* Silvia Figueiredo Costa MD, PhD

Introduction

In 2007 the neurology ICU's incidence of external ventricular drain–related infection (EVDRI) at Hospital das Clínicas, University of São Paulo, Brazil, was above the 90th percentile

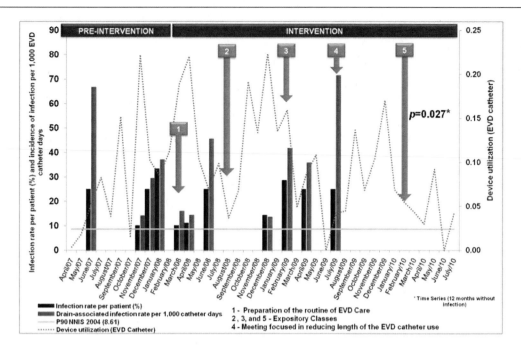

Figure 1. Infection Rate per Patient and Incidence of Infection per 1,000 EVD Catheter-Days and EVD Catheter Utilization Data

- Checking for cerebrospinal fluid (CSF) leakage at the end of procedure
- Daily dressing care using MBP. Specifics of incision care included cleansing with a saline solution, application of alcohol and chlorhexidine, covering with sterile gauze, and wrapping the head.
- Obtaining CSF only if infection is suspected
- Replacing the system whenever it was violated
- Removal of the catheter as soon as possible

based on the former National Nosocomial Infection Surveillance System (NNISS) 2004 benchmarks. In response, the infection control department, in partnership with the neurosurgery department, implemented a strict protocol of external ventricular drain (EVD) care.

Method

The department compared EVDRI rates during preintervention (April 2007 to July 2008) and intervention (August 2008 to July 2010).

Intervention

Routine of Care

The following items were described in a written protocol:

- Hand hygiene before and after handling the EVD catheter
- Catheter insertions performed in operating rooms with use of maximal barrier precaution (MBP; cap, mask, and sterile gown/gloves; large sterile drapes covering the patient's head and trunk)
- Hair removal with clippers (electric razor) immediately before the surgical procedure
- Preparation of the scalp with chlorhexidine followed by an alcohol-based agent
- Perioperative antimicrobial prophylaxis with cefuroxime
- Tunneling a 5 cm EVD catheter skin-insertion site and the trepanation site

Education

The department's approach to prevention included targeted educational sessions. Specific issues included the following:

- Reducing the length of ventricular catheterization
- Training sessions on hand hygiene for all staff
- Focus on aseptic technique and preserving integrity of the system whenever handling the EVD
- Education on aseptic technique for dressing changes for all medical residents who are assigned this task

Results

During the study, 178 patients were submitted to 194 procedures, corresponding to 1,217 catheter-days and 12 infections related to EVD. The patients' average age was 48, and 62% of patients were females. Crude mortality was 35% (42% in the preintervention phase and 30% in the intervention phase, $p = 0.09$). Perioperative antimicrobial prophylaxis was given in 80% of the procedures during all study periods (85% in the preintervention phase and 77% in the intervention phase, $p = 0.2$). Five observations of EVD care were made, one observation of hand hygiene, one meeting for writing down the routine of care, three training sessions with expository classes, and one intervention (meeting with neurosurgical staff) to reinforce reducing the permanence of the EVD catheter, with a total of five interventions, as shown in Figure 1.

One hundred twenty-one HCWs (92%) were trained at the first intervention, 94 HCWs (72%) at the second intervention, and 86 HCWs (66%) at the third intervention. During the observations of care in the preintervention period, it was noted that in 98% of the opportunities, dressings were not performed correctly, and 66% did not follow practices for scalp hygiene. After the routine of care implementation and education sessions, the organization achieved 100% adherence to dressings and scalp hygiene.

Infection rates of EVDRI during the study were reduced from 9.5% to 4.8%, and the incidence of EVDRI went from 14 to 7 infections per 1,000 catheter-days ($p = 0.027$). The rates of clinical meningitis/ventriculitis (that is, without an identified agent) were 11% ($n = 8$) and 11% ($n = 11$; $p = 0.90$) during the preintervention and intervention periods, respectively. During the whole year following the fourth intervention, no microbiologically documented infections were present.

Lessons Learned

Educational intervention proved to be a simple and low-cost tool, with a significant impact on the reduction of infection indicators related to EVD in the process of adding quality to good practices in the implementation and maintenance of EVD. The embedding of a routine of care along with multi-professional continued-education programs proved effective in preventing these infections.

CASE STUDY 5-5

Effectiveness of a Prospective Multifaceted Infection Control Program to Reduce Central Line–Associated Bloodstream Infections in Neonatal Intensive Care Units of 10 Developing Countries: Findings of the International Nosocomial Infection Control Consortium (INICC) (Argentina, Colombia, India, Mexico, Morocco, Peru, Philippines, El Salvador, Tunisia, and Turkey)

Victor D. Rosenthal, MD, CIC, MSc; Regina Berba, MD; Lourdes Dueñas, MD; Canan Aygun, MD; Martha Sobreyra-Oropeza, MD; Amina Barkat, MD; Mandakini Pawar, MD; Khaldi Ammar, MD; María Eugenia Rodríguez-Calderón, MD; Teodora Atencio-Espinoza, RN; Cheong Yuet-Meng, MD; Gulden Ersoz, MD; Tanu Singhal, MD; Josephine Anne Navoa-Ng, MD; Davut Ozdemir, MD; Marena Rodríguez-Ferrer, MD

This multinational, multicentric prospective surveillance study is the first to demonstrate the positive impact of the multidimensional infection control approach in the neonatal intensive care units (NICUs) of developing countries.

Introduction

CLABSIs are associated with increased morbidity and mortality, extra length of stay and costs, and bacterial resistance.[1,2] In developing countries, CLABSI rates are reported to be three to five times higher than in US ICUs.[3-5] Intrinsic factors contribute to higher rates in developing countries, primarily related to their lower socioeconomic levels and lack of resources.[6]

Successful device-associated health care–associated infection (DA-HAI) preventive strategies have been described in the literature.[7,8] However, approaches for CLABSI reduction have not been assessed in the NICUs from developing countries.

Method

This study analyzed the impact of a multidimensional infection control approach developed by the INICC to reduce the CLABSI rate in patients hospitalized in NICUs from 15 cities in 10 developing countries—Argentina, Colombia, India, Mexico, Morocco, Peru, Philippines, El Salvador, Tunisia, and Turkey.

A before-and-after prospective CLABSI surveillance study was performed on a cohort of 6,942 patients hospitalized in 15 NICUs during 91,391 bed-days. The study was divided into two phases. In Phase 1 (baseline), active surveillance was performed. In Phase 2 (intervention), the INICC multidimensional approach was implemented. CLABSI rates obtained in Phase 1 were compared with rates in Phase 2.

The INICC strategy for CLABSI prevention was based on the recommendations published by SHEA and the IDSA in 2008.[9] It included the following components:
1. Central-line care bundle of infection control interventions
2. Education
3. Outcome surveillance
4. Process surveillance
5. Feedback of CLABSI rates
6. Performance feedback of infection control practices

The central-line care bundle included the following elements[9]:
- Performance of active surveillance for CLABSI
- Education of HCWs involved in the insertion, care, and maintenance of central lines on CLABSI prevention
- Use of a catheter checklist to ensure adherence to infection-prevention practices at the time of central-line insertion
- Hand hygiene before catheter insertion or manipulation[10]
- Use of an all-inclusive catheter cart or kit
- Use of MBP precautions during central-line insertion
- Disinfection of catheter hubs, needleless connectors, and infection ports before accessing the catheter

Table 1. Hand-Hygiene and Catheter-Care Process Improvements, Phases 1 (Baseline Period) and 2 (Intervention Period)

	Phase 1 (Months 1–3)	Phase 2	Relative Risk (95% Confidence Interval)	P Value
Number of hand-hygiene observations	1,451	5,175	NA	NA
Hand-hygiene compliance % (*n*)	63% (911)	79% (4,106)	1.26 (1.18–1.36)	0.0001
Number of inserted catheters	3,631	25,705	NA	NA
% of catheters with sterile dressing	45% (1,628)	72% (18,572)	1.61 (1.53–1.70)	0.0001
% of catheters with sterile dressing in good conditions	57% (2,064)	81% (20,848)	1.43 (1.36–1.49)	0.0001

Table 2. Infection Rates of Patients Hospitalized in the Neonatal Intensive Care Units in Phase 1 (Baseline Period) and in Phase 2 (Intervention Period)

	Phase 1 (Months 1–3)	Phase 2	Relative Risk (95% Confidence Interval)	P Value
Number of CLABSIs	60	272		
Number of central-line days	3,314	22,460		
Central-line use, mean	0.20	0.30	1.53 (1.48–1.59)	0.001
CLABSI rate per 1,000 central-line days	18.1	12.1	0.67 (0.51–0.88)	0.0045

- Removal of nonessential catheters
- Performance of direct observation of hand-hygiene compliance; placement and condition of sterile gauze or sterile polyurethane dressing on the insertion site; recording of the date of central-line insertion and last administration set change; gauze-dressing replacement every 48 hours; replacement of transparent semipermeable membrane dressings at least every 7 days, with the date and time of the dressing replacement recorded; use of structured observation tools at regularly scheduled intervals[8]

Processing of surveillance-assessed compliance with key infection control practices, such as compliance rates for hand-hygiene practices and specific measures for prevention of CLABSI.[7]

Performance feedback was provided to HCWs by communicating the rates resulting from the assessment of practices routinely performed in the NICU. The infection control team reviewed these rates at monthly meetings. In addition, statistical graphs and visuals were posted inside the ICU to provide an overview of DA-HAI rates and rates of compliance with infection control practices.[7]

Results

The analysis of our surveillance data during baseline showed a high incidence density of CLABSI in the NICUs, which was reduced by 34% after the implementation of the multidimensional infection control strategy. The organization enrolled 6,942 patients hospitalized in 15 NICUs for 91,391 days, for a total of 25,730 central-line days.

All hospitals were from countries with low and middle-low socioeconomic levels. The type of hospital was not found to be an independent factor to explain the high CLABSI incidence, as most of the patients were from academic and private hospitals, and only 11% were from public hospitals, whose DA-HAI rates were reported to be typically influenced by major resource limitations.[6] In both phases, patients' characteristics, such as gender, were similar; but age was slightly lower and gestational age slightly longer in Phase 2.

During Phase 2, a significant improvement was noted in the performance of infection control practices. Hand-hygiene compliance rose from 63% to 79%. Catheters with sterile gauze or transparent dressing rose from 49% to 78% (relative risk [RR]-1.61, 95% confidence interval [CI]-1.53–1.70, *p* = 0.0001), and sterile gauze or transparent dressings in good condition rose from 57% to 81% (RR-1.43, 95% CI-1.36–1.49, *p* = 0.0001). *See* Table 1.

Regarding CLABSI rates, during Phase 1, 3,291 central-line days were recorded, for a central line–use mean of 0.20. There were 60 CLABSIs, for an overall CLABSI baseline rate of 18.2 CLABSIs per 1,000 central-line days.

In Phase 2, we recorded 22,439 central-line days, for a central line–use mean of 0.30. After implementing the multi-dimensional approach, there were 272 CLABSIs, for an incidence density of 12.1 per 1,000 central-line days. These results showed a CLABSI rate reduction from baseline of 34% (18.2 to 12.1 CLABSIs per 1,000 central-line days; RR-0.66, 95% CI-0.50–0.88, p = 0.0039). *See* Table 2.

The IPC multidimensional approach fostered by the INICC will likely be increasingly adopted in the developing world to achieve successful reductions in DA-HAIs.[8]

Lessons Learned

This analysis showed that the CLABSI rate reduction in the NICUs was related to the effectiveness of the multidimensional strategy. A significant improvement was noted in hand-hygiene compliance and in the central-line care bundle. Likewise, in a study conducted by the INICC in 15 developing countries, the implementation of a program focused on surveillance, education, and performance feedback resulted in higher compliance with hand hygiene and adherence to infection control measures, which also coincided with significant reductions in the CLABSI rate.[8] These measures can be effectively adopted as a comprehensive bundle strategy, feasible for limited-resource NICUs. The rates, however, revealed opportunities for improvement, as they are still higher than those from developed countries.[3]

The multidimensional approach is a fundamental tool to fight against the burden of CLABSIs in the NICUs of limited-resource settings.

Case Study References

1. Rosenthal VD, et al. The attributable cost, length of hospital stay, and mortality of central line-associated bloodstream infection in intensive care departments in Argentina: A prospective, matched analysis. *Am J Infect Control.* 2003 Dec;31(8):475–480.
2. Higuera F, et al. Attributable cost and length of stay for patients with central venous catheter-associated bloodstream infection in Mexico City intensive care units: A prospective, matched analysis. *Infect Control Hosp Epidemiol.* 2007 Jan;28(1):31–35.
3. Edwards JR, et al. National Healthcare Safety Network (NHSN) report: Data summary for 2006 through 2008, issued December 2009. *Am J Infect Control.* 2009 Dec;37(10):783–805.
4. Rosenthal VD, et al. International Nosocomial Infection Control Consortium (INICC) report, data summary of 36 countries, for 2004–2009. *Am J Infect Control.* Epub 2011 Sep 10.
5. Rosenthal VD, et al. Device-associated nosocomial infections in 55 intensive care units of 8 developing countries. *Ann Intern Med.* 2006 Oct 17;145(8):582–591.
6. Rosenthal VD, et al. Socioeconomic impact on device-associated infections in limited-resource neonatal intensive care units: Findings of the INICC. *Infection.* 2011 Oct;39(5):439–450.
7. Rosenthal VD, et al. Effectiveness of a multidimensional approach to reduce ventilator-associated pneumonia in pediatric intensive care units of five developing countries: International Nosocomial Infection Control Consortium findings. *Am J Infect Control.* Epub 2011 Nov 2.
8. Rosenthal VD, et al. Impact of International Nosocomial Infection Control Consortium (INICC) strategy on central line-associated bloodstream infection rates in the intensive care units of 15 developing countries. *Infect Control Hosp Epidemiol.* 2010 Dec;31(12):1264–1272.
9. Marschall J, et al. Strategies to prevent central line-associated bloodstream infections in acute care hospitals. *Infect Control Hosp Epidemiol.* 2008 Oct;29 Suppl 1:S22–30.
10. Rosenthal VD, Guzman S, Safdar N. Reduction in nosocomial infection with improved hand hygiene in intensive care units of a tertiary care hospital in Argentina. *Am J Infect Control.* 2005 Sep;33(7):392–397.

Study Participants (listed by country of origin):

Argentina: Victor D. Rosenthal, MD, CIC, MSc; Sandra Guzman, RN; Ariel Boglione, RN; Oscar Migone, RN

Colombia: María Eugenia Rodríguez-Calderón, MD; Marena Rodríguez-Ferrer, MD; Nayide Barahona-Guzmán, RN; Alfredo Lagares-Guzmán, MD; Guillermo Sarmiento-Villa, MD

El Salvador: Lourdes Dueñas, MD; Ana Concepción Bran-de-Casares, RN; Lilian de Jesús-Machuca, RN

India: Mandakini Pawar, MD; Amit Gupta, MD; Narinder Saini, MD; Tanu Singhal, MD; Sweta Shah, MD; Vatsal Kothari, MD

Mexico: Martha Sobreyra-Oropeza, MD

Morocco: Amina Barkat, MD; Naima Lamdouar Bouazzaoui, MD; Kabiri Meryem, RN

Peru: Teodora Atencio-Espinoza, RN; Favio Sarmiento-López, MD

Philippines: Regina Berba, MD; Glenn Angelo S. Genuino, MD; Rafael J. Consunji, MD; Jacinto Blas V. Mantaring III, MD; Josephine Anne Navoa-Ng, MD; Victoria D. Villanueva, RN; María Corazon V. Tolentino, RN

Tunisia: Khaldi Ammar, MD; Nejla Ben-Jaballah, MD; Asma Hamdi, MD

Turkey: Canan Aygun, MD; Sukru Küçüködük, MD; Gulden Ersoz, MD; Ali Kaya, MD; Necdet Kuyucu, MD; Davut Ozdemir, MD; Mehmet Faruk-Geyik, MD; Mustafa Yildirim, MD; Selvi Erdogan, RN; Hakan Uzun, MD

CASE STUDY 5-6

Catheter-Associated Urinary Tract Infection Bundle at Bangkok Hospital Medical Center (Thailand)

Arisara Suwanarit, RN, BSN, MS

Introduction

Bangkok Hospital Medical Center (BMC) consists of three hospitals—BMC, Bangkok Heart Hospital, and Wattanosoth Cancer Hospital—with 550 beds and a daily census of 3,000 outpatients and 9,500 patient-days per month.

The Infection Control Committee (ICC) of BMC was founded in 1986. Recently, the ICC has focused increased attention on prevention of HAIs, particularly CAUTIs.

Data gathered in 2008 revealed six individual months during which the CAUTI rate was greater than the National Healthcare Safety Network (NHSN) benchmark of 3.3 incidents per 1,000 catheter-days (pooled mean).

Methods

BMC's infection control nurses (ICNs)—who have been certified in infection control from Mahidol University (Faculty of Medicine, Ramathibodi Hospital, Mahidol University,

Bangkok)—reviewed medical records and visited the ICUs, the cardiac care units, and the intermediate care units to collect additional facts, specifics, and case studies to present to the ICC. The ICC was a multidisciplinary committee consisting of all stakeholders in the infection-prevention process, including subcontract participants and the following:

- Hospital CEO
- Infectious-disease physician
- ICNs
- Nurse management
- Total Quality Control Director
- Pharmacist
- Representative from Safety, Occupational Health, and Environment
- Subcontractors, including the following:
  - Housekeeping
  - Laboratory
  - Pathology
  - Food Service
  - Central Sterile Supply Department

Over the course of several meetings, the ICC developed a fishbone diagram of the BMC CAUTI process. As a result, the following changes were made to the process:

- Using new urinary catheter bags to ensure a closed system (a closed system uses a collapsible bag and a port for injection, including a one-way valve, to prevent backup into the bladder)
- Initiating a CAUTI bundle, with the following components:
  - WHO's Five Moments for Hand Hygiene[i]
  - Aseptic technique
  - Fixed urinary catheter
  - Closed-system urine bag suspended below bladder
  - Discontinuation of catheter at the earliest opportunity
- Instituting and promoting a new BMC hand-hygiene campaign
- Designating ICNs to closely monitor results

Results

CAUTI rates improved through 2009, but August and September of 2009 were in excess of the NHSN benchmark, prompting a review of data and patient case studies. Focused, targeted discussion by the ICC identified external sources that would have an effect on CAUTIs:

- Inadequate perineum care
- Urinary catheter not attached in a secure position
- Neglecting to clean device with anti-septic
- Collection and measurement of urine to empty catheter bag not at a scheduled time
- Failure to observe catheter tubing for unobstructed urine flow

Subsequent reviews of patient medical records demonstrated a high portion of medically complex patients with the following complicating factors:

- Diabetes
- Benign prostatic hyperplasia (BPH)
- Receipt of steroid therapy
- Renal failure
- Long duration of indwelling catheter > 10 days
- Prolonged hospital stay > 30 days
- Extended antibiotic use

Table 1. CAUTI Incident Rate by Month and Year, 2009–2010	
Month and Year	**Incident Rate per 1,000 Catheter-Days**
December 2009	1.23
January 2010	1.96
February 2010	1.24
March 2010	0
April 2010	1.03
May 2010	2.24
June 2010	0
July 2010	2.44
August 2010	0
September 2010	1.15
October 2010	0
November 2010	1.04

When the November 2009 data again exceeded the benchmark (6.87 incidents per 1,000 catheter-days), an action plan was immediately developed and implemented in December 2009 to concentrate on complex cases with comorbid conditions and emphasizing the following steps:

- Inserting a catheter only when indicated
- Following guidelines for perineum care
- Ensuring proper hand-washing and aseptic technique with sterile equipment
- Developing an adhesive clamp that holds the catheter in place to maintain unobstructed urine flow
- Developing a written multidisciplinary care plan promoting discontinuation of the catheter as soon as medically indicated
- Emphasizing that nurses are responsible for 24-hour management of the urinary catheters and that ICNs must reeducate nurses on proper catheter practice and techniques. ICNs continued to monitor the results.
- Submitting monthly reports to the ICC on the following:
  - CAUTI infection rate
  - Risk factor for each variance case
  - Results of compliance with CAUTI bundle

Since that time, with one exception (November 2010; 6.87 incidents per 1,000 catheter-days), the incident rates declined below the benchmark rate, as shown in Table 1 above.

Moreover, compliance with all aspects of the bundle has remained at or near 100%.

Continuing goals of the BMC CAUTI program include the following:

- To decrease the number of CAUTIs per 1,000 patient-days (via internal benchmarking)
- To maintain the number of CAUTIs per 1,000 patient-days below the NHSN benchmark from the pooled mean to a percentile of 25%
- To decrease unnecessary catheter use, such as for convenience
- To develop an algorithm to evaluate continuing indications for catheter use

Lessons Learned

- **Teamwork**—A major contributing factor to implementation was the involvement of the multidisciplinary team, including contract employees. The scope of the HCWs involved must be all-inclusive. Teamwork and full participation are key factors for performance and the realization of the action plan.
- **Compliance**—Without full compliance with the CAUTI bundle, optimal outcomes will not be achieved. Specialized Infection Control Ward Nurses focus daily on unit compliance issues.
- **Medical Advances**—The organization must keep abreast of the newest developments and advances in medical theory, medical equipment, and new medications to apply a proactive response to the ongoing issue of CAUTIs.
- **Sustainability**—All gains will be lost if this program is not sustainable and consistent throughout the hospital. The CAUTI bundle is the foundation upon which to build. Training during orientation, annual competency, audits, and monitoring must be scheduled and in position to maintain the improvements into the future.

Case Study Reference

1. World Health Organization. Five Moments for Hand Hygiene. Accessed 22 Sep 2011. http://www.who.int/gpsc/tools/Five _moments/en/.

Identifying Risks Through Surveillance, Data Collection, and Analysis

Surveillance is a fundamental aspect of an effective IPC program and an essential activity to determine high-risk areas that call for intervention strategies.[59–63]

Surveillance involves collecting data about infections and care practices for a variety of purposes, including to:

- assess an organization's risks for infection for patients, staff, and the environment;
- identify areas that need further investigation, such as areas where patients seem to be at higher risk;
- search for cases of a specific disease;
- identify cluster or outbreaks of infections and then to intervene;
- determine whether processes used to prevent and to control infections are effective and whether revisions or improvements to systems are necessary;
- determine education and policy needs;
- check the success of any changes made to a system or process; and
- identify any problems, such as the emergence of new infections or outbreaks.

Because infection risks change over time, data collection and analysis must be a dynamic process. Although constant monitoring is resource intensive, it can be clinically and financially effective because it allows a program to be proactive in identifying and preventing or mitigating multiple infection risks (many preventable), and in turn to prevent morbidity and mortality or use of valuable resources. The quantitative information an organization gets from surveillance-data collection and measurement of activities can help determine whether an IPC program is actually reducing infections and adding value to the organization.

The German national HAI surveillance system, Krankenhaus-Infektions-Surveillance-System (KISS), was instrumental in identifying and analyzing infections from a new ventricular device in Case Study 5-7.

CASE STUDY 5-7

Reducing Ventriculostomy-Associated Infections After the Introduction of a New Ventricular Device (Germany)

Petra Gastmeier, MD; Christine Geffers, MD

Introduction

Ventricular devices are used frequently in neurosurgery for cerebrospinal fluid drainage in patients with raised intracranial pressure. The major complication of this procedure is a ventriculostomy-associated infection (that is, meningitis or ventriculitis).[1] (Here, *meningitis or ventriculitis* is defined as any meningitis or ventriculitis according to US CDC defi-

Table 1. Device-Associated Infection Rates (per 1,000 Device-Days) in Neurosurgical Intensive Care Unit A (ICU A) Versus Reference Data

Type of Infection	Infection Rate in ICU A	Reference Data (Infections per 1,000 Device-Days)		
		Pooled mean	75th percentile	Median
UTIs*	2.4	5.1	4.3	9.4
Primary BSIs#	2.1	1.7	1.1	3.0
Pneumonia*	7.6	7.5	5.3	10.0
Meningitis/Ventriculitis#	7.2	4.7	3.8	7.2

Note: *Reference data of the ICU component of KISS for neurosurgical ICUs (20 neurosurgical ICUs participating)*
* Period January 2006 to December 2010
# Period January 2008 to December 2010

nitions associated with ventricular device use in the previous 48 hours.) Surveillance of ventriculostomy-associated infections was established at a neurosurgical ICU A of Charité Universitätsmedizin Berlin in January 2008 according to the methods recommended by the German national HAI surveillance system, KISS. The ventriculostomy-associated infection rate was on the level of the 75th percentile of the national data in 2010. For other device-associated infections, the rates were below the 75th percentile (*see* Table 1).

In April 2011 a significant increase of ventriculostomy-associated infections was observed. Ten cases occurred during a period of the first six months of 2011 (*see* Figure 1), resulting in an increase of the ventriculostomy-associated infection rate to 22.7 in the first half of 2011.

Methods

The data were discussed with senior physicians and nurses of the neurosurgical unit to identify possible explanations. The neurosurgical department introduced a new ventricular device at the beginning of 2011, because the head of the department was convinced that this new device had some mechanical advantages. The nurses mentioned that handling and using the new device was more difficult than using the former device, which may explain the increase of ventriculostomy-associated infections.

The development of infection rates on ICU A, together with the national reference data, convinced the neurosurgeons that an intervention was necessary. The team discussed returning to the old device or improving methods of using and handling the new device to exploit its possible advantages. Changes in antibiotic prophylaxis and the use of impregnated devices were also considered, as was the need for a rigid sterile protocol for device placement.

Results

Physicians of the infection control department along with physicians and nurses of the neurosurgical department created a working group to reduce infection rates. The teams decided to train staff for proper handling of these new devices with a focus on the following infection control aspects:

- The standard operating procedures were evaluated, and an additional training was initiated.
- A special focus was placed on hand hygiene. Alcohol-based hand-rub consumption data of ICU A was compared with national reference data, and it was determined that hand-rub consumption on ICU A (140 mL per patient-day) was above the 75th percentile of the national reference data (129 mL per patient-day).
- More frequent and strategic use of gloves was also discussed.
- WHO's Five Moments for Hand Hygiene[2] (*also see* Figure 6-1) was taught using case situations.
- Infection control nurses performed hand hygiene–compliance observations in conjunction with infection control practitioners, who were also designated to monitor subsequent infection rates.

Discussion

Data on ventriculostomy-associated meningitis and ventriculitis are scarce, and discussions on the subject are controversial. Comparison with reference data is important to identify the institution's position and to stimulate further infection control measures. The introduction of new medical devices is often associated with handling problems and should be accompanied by surveillance activities.

Lessons Learned

Surveillance of HAIs is an important means to identify the impact of new medical devices. Surveillance of HAIs in neu-

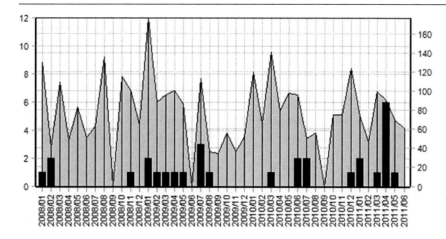

Figure 1. Occurrence of Ventriculostomy-Associated Meningitis/Ventriculits in ICU A, January 2008–June 2011

Black bars = number of infections per month (axis on the left side)
Grey bars = ventricular-days per month (axis on the right side)

rosurgical ICUs should focus not only on VAP, central venous CABSIs, and CAUTIs but also on ventriculostomy-associated infections.

Case Study References

1. Tängdén T, et al. Neurosurgical gram-negative bacillary ventriculitis and meningitis: A retrospective study evaluating the efficacy of intraventricular gentamicin therapy in 31 consecutive cases. *Clin Infect Dis.* 2011 Jun;52(11):1310–1316.
2. World Health Organization. Five Moments for Hand Hygiene. Accessed 27 Jul 2011. http://www.who.int/gpsc/tools/Five_moments/en/.

What to Collect

The surveillance data an organization collects and analyzes can establish infection trends. Surveillance should be simple and practical. IPC professionals have many duties and responsibilities, and their resources should be focused on the surveillance that will be most useful in improving patient safety and care outcomes. Although total surveillance may be ideal, particularly for a new program to obtain baseline data, it is not usually feasible to survey everything in most organizations. Focusing data-collection efforts on infections that place patients at highest risk provides the most benefit from surveillance activities. For example, instead of tracking all UTIs, organizations might consider monitoring those UTIs involving indwelling catheters in specific high-risk patient populations. Alternatively, organizations should consider tracking all central lines regardless of whether the patient is in an intensive care unit or on a general medical or surgical service.

There many approaches to surveillance. The two most common general types of surveillance are described below.[57]

The first type is process monitoring. Process monitors examine IPC processes or procedures *before and as* they are implemented (for example, practices that are established in the organization to reduce infection risk). A process monitor measures the frequency and consistency with which staff perform procedures, such as hand hygiene; how often physicians or nurses use appropriate barriers when inserting peripheral or central intravenous lines or indwelling urinary catheters; the use of the appropriate PPE for isolation; or the timing of the administration of preoperative antibiotics prior to the surgical incision. The purpose of a process monitor is to determine whether policies and best practices are being followed by staff. The results of process monitors can guide education where gaps are identified and can reinforce best practices where they exist.

The second type of surveillance reviews outcomes. Outcome measures examine the results of IPC processes, patient-care practices, or other procedures *after* they are implemented and performed. Outcome measures include the rates of UTIs, SSIs, VAP, and BSIs, particularly those related to peripheral, central venous, or arterial lines. These rates indicate the effectiveness of infection-prevention and patient-safety efforts.

Process and outcome measures are helpful in evaluating HCW performance and environmental conditions. For example, the number of HCWs who convert from negative to positive TB skin tests is an outcome measure and may be correlated with process measures to prevent the transmission of TB, such as appropriate isolation procedures, ventilation patterns and negative-pressure rooms, and administration of proper TB medications for patients with active pulmonary TB to whom the staff are exposed. If HCWs are converting their skin test statuses and there is lack of compliance with TB–prevention protocols, this may be contributing to the increase in conversions. Needlestick and sharps injuries are an outcome of the processes in place to prevent these accidents, such as safe disposal of sharps and safety needles. The number or percentage of staff who develop hepatitis B or C or HIV from sharps injuries represents one outcome of infection-prevention procedures.

Many variations of surveillance can measure processes or outcomes. Some of these measures are described below.

Focused incidence surveillance. Incidence surveillance looks at all new infections in a given time period (for example during one month, one quarter, or one year). Infections can be compared from one period to another when rates are calculated using denominators of persons at risk for the infection, days of device use, or number of procedures and a numerator of those who actually get the infection. Incidence surveillance can be performed in a number of ways, including the following:

- **Targeted surveillance**—concentrates on specific patient populations or procedures. For example, in a chronic care organization, targeted surveillance might involve monitoring patients who receive enteral or parenteral feedings and who suffer a higher-than-expected incidence of diarrhea; or in an acute care setting, surveillance may be targeted to infections of patients in ICUs, patients with selected surgical procedures, or those at risk for BSIs. Data from these targeted surveillance efforts can identify areas that need improvement.

- **Problem-oriented surveillance**—focuses on identified infections and measures the occurrence of these specific infections. When a group of patients has the same illness, surveillance efforts should involve an in-depth assessment to determine whether an ongoing problem exists and what control measures can be applied to address the problem. For example, when a cluster of patients who have had primary joint replacement develop joint infections, more detailed surveillance should further examine all the circumstances involved in the surgical procedure.

Prevalence surveillance. Prevalence surveillance monitors all infections (existing and new) during a given time period, such as one day, one week, or one month. For example, the IPC practitioner may want to look at the prevalence of VAP in a single ICU during a three-month period or the number of patients who come to an ambulatory or primary health center with new or continuing malaria in one week. A prevalence survey is like a photograph that captures one point or period in time. A single prevalence survey can be used to develop IPC interventions but IPC professionals must understand that a single survey may not be a reliable indicator of ongoing infection risk. However, repeated prevalence surveys of the same infection performed over time add validity to the data, increasing confidence. Prevalence surveillance is very intensive during the period being monitored, but, because the time period can be limited, this method provides opportunity for other IPC activities and is a cost-effective use of IPC practitioner resources.[64,65] Many countries or large groups of hospitals use this form of surveillance to assess the state of infections in the country.[66,67,68] In one prevalence study, conducted in 36 Vietnamese hospitals using a standardized questionnaire on a designated day during February–December 2008, results highlighted the need for a national HAI data-

base and reporting system using standardized surveillance definitions to monitor HAI trends and patient outcomes.[68]

Although the types of data an organization collects during its surveillance efforts will depend on the organization's patient populations and services provided, the following list suggests some common organisms, areas, and groups to monitor or to audit during surveillance efforts:

- MDROs, such as MRSA, VRE (particularly in critical care areas), *Clostridium difficile*; multidrug-resistant gram-negative organisms, such as *Acinetobacter baumanii*, KPCs, or extended spectrum beta lacatamases (ESBL); *pseudomonas*; or others specific to the country or the organization. Procedures that are often monitored include the following:
  - SSIs (all or selected procedures)
  - Infections related to implanted devices
  - Infections related to indwelling devices, such as urinary catheters and central intravenous lines
  - Sharps or needlestick injuries in staff
- Emerging pathogens, such as H1N1 influenza or Chikunguyea
- Hepatitis B or C infections in hemodialysis units
- Infections among immunocompromised patients
- Infections among patients with extremes of age (premature infants to frail older adults)

In choosing what data to collect, an organization should consider not only its patient population and services provided but also what data are available, accessible, and meaningful. Organizations can use their own staff as resources to identify areas of concern and to look internally and externally for suggestions of common areas to monitor. Many of these areas will be identified in the risk assessment (*see* pages 60–64). The organization might choose to perform surveillance on process measures, such as the use of isolation procedures, the cleaning of patient environments, appropriate barrier precautions during construction or renovation, or the use of appropriate procedures to prevent VAP. As described above, monitoring the rate of infections will provide the organization with outcome data. Employees can also provide valuable information on which activities put them and their patients at risk for infections (for example, whether a large number of staff members sustain needle sticks or acquire HAIs during the course of their work). One process monitor might assess whether nurses and nurse aides are using proper isolation precautions in a long term care facility.

The US CDC's HICPAC guidelines for infection prevention as well as the Compendium of Strategies for the Prevention of Infections in Acute Care Hospitals have included suggestions for process and outcome measures for use by IPC programs. Table 5-7 presents some of these measures.

Table 5-7. IPC–Related Process and Outcome Measures

Measure	Process Measures	Outcome Measures
From CDC Guidelines for Prevention of Catheter-Associated Urinary Tract Infections		
Device-related care	Compliance with documentation of indication for indwelling urinary catheter placement: Conduct random audits of selected units and calculate compliance rate • Numerator: Number of patients on unit with catheters with proper documentation of indication • Denominator: Number of patients on the unit with catheter in place • Standardization factor: 100 (for example, multiply by 100 so the measure is expressed as a percentage)	Rate of CAUTIs • Numerator: Number of persons with CAUTIs • Denominator: Number of days of indwelling urinary catheters • Standardization factor: Multiply by 1,000 catheter-days
From CDC Guidelines for Disinfection and Sterilization in Health Care Facilities		
Disinfection and sterilization	Adherence to high-level disinfection or sterilization policy for endoscopes • Numerator: Number of persons who comply with all policy requirements for the management of endoscopes • Denominator: Number of persons observed performing cleaning and HLD or sterilization of endoscopes • Standardization: Multiply by 100 observations	Rate of infections attributed to inadequate cleaning or disinfection of endoscopes (specify type of endoscopes) • Numerator: Number of endoscope-related infections • Denominator: Number of endoscopic procedures (specify type of procedure) • Standardization: Multiply by 100
From CDC Guidelines for the Prevention of Intravascular Catheter-Related Infections		
Central line–associated bloodstream infections (CLABSIs)	Compliance with documentation of daily assessment regarding the need for continuing central venous catheter (CVC) access Measure the percentage of patients with a CVC where there is documentation of daily assessment • **Numerator:** Number of patients with CVCs who have documentation of daily assessment • **Denominator:** Number of patients with CVCs • Multiply by 100 so the measure is expressed as a percentage	CLABSI rate • **Numerator:** Number of CLABSIs in each unit assessed (using standardized definitions) • **Denominator:** Total number of catheter-days in each unit assessed (using standardized definitions) • Multiply by 1,000 = number of CLABSIs per 1,000 catheter-days • **Risk adjustment:** Stratify CLABSI rates by type of patient-care unit

Sources: Adapted from Gould CV, et al., Healthcare Infection Control Practices Advisory Committee. *Guideline for Prevention of Catheter-Associated Urinary Tract Infections 2009.* Atlanta: Centers for Disease Control and Prevention, 2009; Rutala WA, Weber DJ, Healthcare Infection Control Practices Advisory Committee. *Guideline for Disinfection and Sterilization in Healthcare Facilities, 2008.* Atlanta: Centers for Disease Control and Prevention, 2008; O'Grady NP, Healthcare Infection Control Practices Advisory Committee. *Guidelines for the Prevention of Intravascular Catheter-Related Infections, 2011.* Atlanta: Centers for Disease Control and Prevention, 2011.

Risk stratification of data. An important concept in the surveillance of infection data is stratification. Stratifying data arranges it in groups and subgroups to allow for more precise analysis and problem identification. For example, infections in neonates are often risk-stratified by birth weight. Babies who weigh less are generally at higher risk of infection, because their bodies and immune systems may not be fully developed. Examining infections by birth weight allows the IPC staff to pinpoint the babies who are getting infections and to implement the appropriate prevention strategies. The NHSN looks at infections in babies by weight in grams (g). They stratify by those babies who are less than or equal to 750 g, 751 g–1,000 g, 1,001 g–1,500 g, 1,501 g–2,500 g, and greater than 2,500 g.[69]

It is also valuable to stratify risk variables to account for the dynamic process that leads to SSIs. For many years, the NHSN[69] has promoted risk stratification using the following three dichotomous variables to score each surgical procedure:
1. Microbial exposure levels (for example, clean, clean contaminated, contaminated or dirty)
2. Duration of the surgical procedure (greater than the 75th percentile of time designated for the specific surgery)
3. Host characteristics (American Society of Anesthesiologists [ASA] score)

The NHSN has recently published a set of new risk models that improve the predictive performance for SSIs, compared with the traditional NHSN risk index stratification.[70]

An IPC program can also stratify process or outcome measures by population, age, gender, site of care, days of stay, type of ICU, type of device,[70] and other factors.[69,71]

How to Collect the Data

As there are several sources for IPC data, there are also several methods to collect it. The following are some practical suggestions on how to collect data for IPC efforts.

Reporting systems. These systems allow staff to phone, to e-mail, or to write reports about patients with infections. Individual infections are reviewed on an ongoing basis to look for serious individual infections and patterns, clusters, or outbreaks. If a cluster of infections is identified, IPC professionals must act promptly to address the infection(s) and to control the spread to other patients. Reporting systems are a passive approach to surveillance that rely on health care or laboratory personnel to report issues, so when using this method, underreporting is a frequent limitation. For organizations to overcome underreporting, they must make it easy for staff to report potential infections, avoid punishing staff members who report infection (avoid blaming them for the issues), and respond to reports. Staff members must believe that by reporting, they are helping

improve the safety of patients and helping decrease infections across the organization. Providing feedback to staff members who report potential infections will help establish value and strengthen their commitment to this process. The more proactive approach to identifying infections is for IPC practitioners to actively seek out infections, using laboratory reports, clinical reviews, and observation as described below.

Record review. There are a variety of sources from which organizations can collect data regarding infections, including the following:
- Admission logs
- Employee health records
- Incident reports
- Laboratory reports
- Patient records
- Billing or cost data
- Pharmacy records
- Reports on numbers/types of diagnostic workups and care-recipient disposition
- Treatment plans
- Mortality reports

Practitioners can review records for surveillance data using manual or other means. The choice of method will depend on the size and scope of the organization's activities and the resources available. Computers and software can ease the data-collection process. Even when data are collected manually, electronic programs can sort and analyze data and generate rates, graphs, charts, and reports.

Walking rounds. This data-collection method allows IPC practitioners to collect infection data on weekly or daily rounds, depending on the organization's size. On walking rounds, the practitioners consult with other staff and make clinical observations. The practitioners can also review charts, laboratory or radiology reports, treatment plans, and antibiotic or culture reports.

Forms. Many organizations create simple tools to collect surveillance data. For example, an organization can create a form on which staff members note their use of antibiotics. Information from this form can be converted into a chart or graph that, when taken in aggregate, will quickly reveal antibiotic-use trends over time. Pharmacists can generate similar data and are invaluable partners in these efforts. One such form is presented in Figure 5-3.

Data mining. This is a newer method that employs information technology systems that has become important for infection surveillance. Data mining uses a variety of data sources, such as patient records, pharmacy and medication records, laboratory information, and incident reports, and applies rules of association to link patients, their specimens, organisms, antibiotic susceptibilities and other information. This process allows the identification of important patterns and potential infections.[72] The use of a specialized computer program reveals trends sometimes not shown by traditional record-review methods. Data mining can be quite helpful to the infection control practitioner or hospital epidemiologist but does not eliminate the need for some record review to ensure that potential infections identified are true infections.

ANTIBIOTIC AUDIT REPORT

Patient Information

Name_____	Admit Date_____
Record No._____	Unit_____
DOB/Age_____	Service_____
Gender_____	Admit Source_____
Age_____	Allergies_____
Weight (kg)_____	_____

Clinical Information

Admitting Diagnosis _____

Prior Medical History _____

_____

_____

Recent Antibiotics   Y / N   _____

Immunocompromised   Y / N   _____   Septic   Y / N

Suspected Site of Infection: Lungs   Abdomen   Urine/Bladder   Bloodstream

Other:_____

Tmax_____   WBC_____   CrCl_____

Culture Results	Date	Site	Pathogen
	_____	_____	_____
	_____	_____	_____
	_____	_____	_____
	_____	_____	_____

Antibiotic Information

Date	Agent	Dose	Route	Prescriber
_____	_____	_____	_____	_____
_____	_____	_____	_____	_____
_____	_____	_____	_____	_____

Audit Summary

Abstractor _____   Abstraction Date_____

Evaluation of Antibiotic Use: Appropriate   Not Appropriate

Rationale_____

_____

_____

Feedback/Action_____

_____

_____

Remarks/Notes_____

_____

_____

Figure 5-3. Antibiotic Audit Report

Source: The Joint Commission. *What Every Health Care Executive Should Know: The Cost of Antibiotic Resistance.* Oak Brook, IL: Joint Commission Resources, 2009.

Box 5-1. Steps in an Outbreak Investigation

- Verify the diagnosis.
- Confirm the outbreak.
- Create a case definition.
- Use descriptive epidemiology.
- Develop a hypothesis.
- Test the hypothesis.
- Implement control measures.
- Refine the hypothesis and execute additional studies.
- Write and distribute a report.

Literature reviews. Although internal data are important in the discovery of infections, IPC professionals should also review the IPC literature and information from IPC organizations and governmental agencies for important HAIs that are occurring and emerging in other organizations or countries. Reliable sources for this type of information are included in Appendix 2.

From this type of research, IPC professionals can determine whether their organization should be collecting internal data on these new infections and what, if any, control measures need to be in place.

Outbreak Investigation

Periodically, most organizations will experience clusters or outbreaks of infections. These represent an incidence of infections above the normal, expected, endemic rate. When monitoring SSIs, for example, the IPC practitioner may see several infections in primary total hip replacements, which signals a potential problem. Or the hospital epidemiologist reviewing medical ICU data may identify several incidents of VAP that occur around the same time and have the same pathogenic organism, such as a cluster of *Acinetobacter baumanii* VAP infections in ICU patients. In these circumstances, the IPC staff must undertake an investigation to determine whether the infections are related and the cause(s). Infection clusters or outbreaks should be investigated using a systematic approach that includes verifying whether there is an outbreak, creating a case definition, gathering data, reviewing the cases to determine similarities or differences, and analyzing the findings. Box 5-1 outlines the typical steps in an outbreak investigation. The investigation usually requires a multidisciplinary team of professionals who are familiar with the type of infection, the processes of care, and with data analysis and statistics. Case Studies 5-8 and 5-9 describe examples of how organizations reacted to outbreaks in their facilities.

CASE STUDY 5-8

Risk Factors in an Outbreak of Clostridium difficile *Infection* (Chile)

Pola Brenner, RN, MSC; Patricio Nercelles, MD

Introduction

Leadership, including supervisors and IPC practitioners at Hospital Carlos Van Buren in Chile, noted a large number of *Clostridium difficile* infections (CDI) among internal medicine patients during June and July 2010. Leadership sought to understand the epidemiology and risk factors associated with CDI and to describe the strategies implemented for control.

Findings

The CDI outbreak affected 15 patients in the internal medicine ward during June and July 2010, with an overall attack rate of 29.4%.

Among case patients, the average age was 73.9 years; 66% were male. Prior to admission, 67% were in the community, 20% were on another ward in the same hospital, and 13% came from another hospital. Underlying medical issues included cerebrovascular disease (33%) and pneumonia (27%). On average, onset of diarrhea occurred 21.3 days after hospitalization (with a range of 4 to 40 days). All the cases had antimicrobial therapy for an average of 10.7 days prior to developing diarrhea. The most common antibiotics used were clindamycin and cefotaxime. When compared to controls without CDI, previous use of clindamycin was independently associated with CDI ($p = 0.0006$). Length of stay was three times higher among case patients compared with noninfected controls.

Interventions

The strategies adopted to control the outbreak included the following:
- Cohorting patients
- Isolating with contact precautions, including the following:
  - Enhancing hand-hygiene compliance
  - Wearing PPE (such as aprons and gloves)
  - Disinfecting surfaces, including use of chlorine 1,000 ppm, four times a day
  - Restricting visitors
  - Limiting educating students in the affected wards, such as during teaching rounds
- Restricting clindamycin use

The compliance with each strategy differed. In the case of cohorting and restriction of teaching, there was no compliance at first, probably due to lack of awareness of appropriate procedures among physicians and staff. Regarding PPE, staff adhered to the use of gloves but not to apron use, perhaps due to lack of resources. In general, there was good compliance with hand hygiene, clindamycin restriction was generally observed, and very good compliance was noted for visitor restriction. Disinfection of surfaces was evaluated by ATP (bioluminiscence), and shortcomings were demonstrated in the cleaning of the bed rails.

As the outbreak continued after the initial implementation of the control strategies, leadership decided to implement a bundle approach, which included five measures:
1. Cohort isolation
2. Contact precautions
3. Dedicated equipment used exclusively for one patient
4. Continuing the current procedure for surface disinfection
5. Permitting only one person (personnel or visitor) in the patient's room at a time.

Leadership also ensured the availability of resources to comply with these strategies.

Results

CDI cases did not decrease with the initial control strategies. However, after implementation of a bundle approach, the outbreak was controlled, and no new CDI cases had occurred after one week of the bundle's implementation in August 2011.

Lessons Learned

- Ensuring appropriate use of antimicrobials is an ongoing task; compliance with policies should be audited routinely.
- Implementing an alert system when patients with CDI are identified is essential to initiating early strategies to prevent larger outbreaks.
- Including emergency physicians in the educational programs is crucial.
- Establishing the bundle approach at the beginning of similar outbreaks is recommended.
- Institutions must ensure quantity and quality of resources to comply the strategies.
- Leadership and collaboration among clinical services is essential to ensure compliance with strategies, including restriction of use of clindamycin.

CASE STUDY 5-9

Control of an Outbreak of Carbapenem-Resistant Klebsiella pneumoniae in a Tertiary Care Medical Center (Colombia)

Ana Lucia Correa, MD (SHEA International Ambassador);
Andrea Restrepo, MD (SHEA International Ambassador);
Luz María Mazo, RN; Mónica Valderrama, RN; John Jairo Zuleta, MD

Introduction

During the final week of January 2008, Hospital Pablo Tobon Uribe's microbiology laboratory coordinator reported the presence of three clinical cultures that grew carbapenem-resistant *Klebsiella pneumoniae* (CRKP). Leaders identified the index case that corresponded to a patient from Israel who came to the hospital for liver transplantation one week earlier. Further molecular analysis showed that the *K. pneumoniae* clone predominating in this outbreak was the same as the KPC-3 clone identified previously in Israel.[1]

The organization's approach to control this outbreak during a three-year period is described below.

Methods

The following measures were implemented in a progressive manner.

Control Measures

All three infected patients were located in the adult intensive care unit (AICU). Initially they were placed in contact isolation and a single room. Soon after, contact isolation was extended to all AICU patients regardless of colonization or infection status. Later, as the outbreak was spreading, the same procedure was implemented in other critical units. Single-use gowns were mandatory for HCWs in these areas. Also, surfaces were cultured to identify any common source.

Patients were cohorted progressively. First, the patients were allocated to a dedicated zone of the AICU, with no physical barrier to separate one zone from the other; subsequently, a door separated the two areas. Initially, when patients were discharged from the ICU, they were placed in a single room in a ward with other patients infected by other multidrug-resistant bacteria. Finally, at the end of the first year, a special ward was assigned exclusively to patients colonized or infected with CRKP. The cohorting also included a dedicated operating room assigned to these patients in which anesthetic recovery took place.

Entrance to the units with widespread contact precautions was restricted to visitors, HCWs in training, and students. Sharing of medical equipment between patients was not allowed.

Surveillance cultures from rectal swabs and tracheal aspirates were obtained from all patients in AICU, initially 48 hours after admission and, subsequently, at admission and every 7 days. No further surveillance cultures were obtained from patients identified as colonized or infected. When noncolonized or infected patients were discharged from the AICU, they were placed in a single room, and contact precautions were withdrawn when two surveillance cultures were negative.

Hand-hygiene practices were encouraged and reinforced. Surveillance cultures were performed on HCWs with dermatitis, and HCWs with severe cases were excluded from patient care.

Cleaning and disinfection processes were standardized, and infection-prevention nurses supervised cleaning staff. Daily clorhexidine baths for colonized patients were introduced at the end of 2008.

Administrative Measures

Periodic meetings were held with the administrative HCWs during the outbreak. All interventions were discussed in these meetings, and hospital management supported all decisions. Other interventions included the following:

- Elective surgeries and transplants that required ICU care were postponed.
- Patient electronic medical records were labeled "colonized or infected by CRKP" to guarantee immediate institution of contact precautions in case of readmission.
- The local health authority was informed of the outbreak. Advice from national and international experts was requested. Importation of colistin was initiated, because the antibiotic was not available in Colombia at that time.

Educational Measures

All HCWs from the above units were retrained in contact-precaution procedures and hand hygiene. In periodic meetings, the HCWs were informed about the outbreak, mechanism of transmission, and risk factors for developing infection. HCWs received continuous counseling to lower their stress levels. In addition, cleaning staff were trained in the new standardized procedures.

Results

From January 2008 through June 2011, 244 patients were affected by CRKP. From the whole group, 76 patients, including 17 (22.4%) children, were confirmed to have clinical infections. Their mean age was 42.5 years (standard deviation 28.1); 37 (48.7%) were women. More than half the infected patients (42; 55.3%) were hospitalized in ICUs. Before developing infections, 33 of the 76 (43.4%) infected individuals were identified by surveillance cultures as being colonized.

Figure 1 shows the number of colonized and infected patients per 1,000 patient-days distributed by quartiles. During the study, there were 40,504 hospital-discharged patients, with a mean hospital stay of 7.8, 8.2, and 8.8 days, respectively, for each year analyzed.

The hospital achieved a reduction of the rate of new CRKP–infected and –colonized patients per 1,000 patient-days, from 1.27 in the second trimester of 2008 to 0.08 in the second trimester of 2011 ($p < 0.001$).

Discussion

Basic control measures were not enough to contain the outbreak. Very early, the organization started doing surveillance cultures, and still the outbreak was uncontrolled. Only when complete patient and staff cohorting was assured could leaders and HCWs control transmission in a significant way, thereby decreasing the number of colonized and infected patients.

The highest rate of affected patients per 1,000 patient-days was 1.27, which was observed in the second trimester of 2008. The outbreak was considered controlled when the rate dropped to 0.08. These rates are exceedingly lower than the rates reported by other groups in the world. Kochar et al. described a CRKP outbreak in a New York hospital during 2006.[2] During this outbreak, the maximum rate was 14 affected patients per 1,000 patient-days, and the organization considered it controlled when the rate dropped to between 4 and 6.[2]

Lessons Learned

To control any outbreak, it is important to acknowledge existing guidelines and previous experiences reported by other groups, but it is more important for the infection-prevention group to be creative in order to guarantee the acceptance and implementation of these measures in each institution. Administrative support, problem comprehension, and voluntary adherence from the staff are essential.

Case Study References

1. Lopez JA, et al. Intercontinental spread from Israel to Colombia of a KPC-3-producing *Klebsiella pneumoniae* strain. *Clin Microbiol Infect.* 2011 Jan;17(1):52–56.
2. Kochar S, et al. Success of an infection control program to reduce the spread of carbapenem-resistant *Klebsiella pneumoniae*. *Infect Control Hosp Epidemiol.* 2009 May;30(5):447–452.

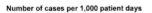

Benchmarking

Although it is important to collect data, it is even more important to do something with the data after they are collected. Data without analysis are not useful and a waste of resources. One effective way to analyze surveillance data is through benchmarking. The benchmarking process compares the organization's data with a reliable, scientifically based set of data that the organization believes represents best practice. Benchmarking, with data feedback to clinicians and quality-management professionals, accounts for the most significant and enduring changes for improvement in managing infections.[73,74]

Organizations can benchmark against themselves and also with external sources, such as WHO's *Weekly Epidemiological Record*[75] or the US CDC's NHSN[69] (formerly the Nosocomial Infections Surveillance [NNIS]) reports. Internal sources help illustrate success in improving performance over time, whereas external benchmarking can help reveal higher-than-average rates of complications that can highlight larger issues.

Internal benchmarking. The first step in effectively benchmarking data is to establish performance rates. This begins with generating baseline information to which subsequent data can be compared. To compare data over time, the organization must calculate rates, which control for differences in the number of population at risk during different time periods. By comparing data to the initial baseline and over time periods, an organization can see whether the infection rate is increasing or decreasing. Rates are

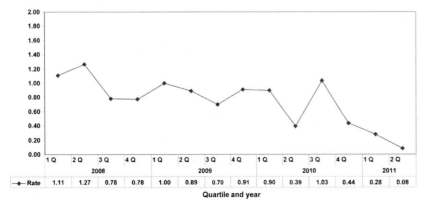

Figure 1. Cases of Carbapenem-Resistant *Klebsiella pneumoniae* (Infected and Colonized) per 1,000 Patient-Days, 2008–2011

critical in tracking performance, trending variance, measuring statistical significance, and calculating an acceptable target rate. Internal benchmarking can be used to compare rates for the organization as a whole or to look at rates over time within services.

External benchmarking. External benchmarking is the comparison of the organization's data with external data sources. Comparison with the following may be useful:

- Comparable health care settings or populations
- Medical practices literature or other professional, recognized standards of practice
- Established databases, including the following:
  - WHO's *Weekly Epidemiological Record*
  - Specific country databases (for example, KISS)[71,76]
  - NHSN database at the US CDC[77]

To successfully benchmark with internal or external data, an organization must use standardized and uniform definitions and methods for infection identification, data collection methods, and risk adjustment. This allows the organization to compare "apples to apples" for an accurate picture of how well its IPC program is doing. It is also important to benchmark against the highest standards so the organization continues to strive to meet and to exceed the best benchmarks.

In some cases, such as within certain behavioral health care organizations, comparisons with the rates of other similar organizations might not be effective because of case-mix variation. In this situation, comparing rates internally over time within the organization has more impact on evaluating what is really happening.

Whenever an organization revises a process or creates a new one, it should determine how its effectiveness can be measured. It is important to use process surveillance indicators directly applicable to the new or revised practice. Examples of this type of thinking appear in the IPC guidelines available from WHO and the US CDC. In its newer infection-prevention guidelines, HICPAC includes performance measures to help organizations evaluate the usefulness of those recommendations.[78,79]

Note: Although benchmarking is a useful method for organizations to evaluate their statuses in relation to best performers, all organizations should continually strive to minimize infections and to work toward achieving zero infections whenever possible (*see* Chapter 7).

Reporting Data to External Agencies

In addition to collecting data for internal improvement processes, it is important to gather information to aid in the early identification of high-risk infections, infection clusters, outbreaks, bioterrorist threats, or new diseases.

Public health or national agencies in some countries perform their own monitoring activities to help with early identification For example, the Ministry of Health in Saudi Arabia requires all hospitals to report within 24 hours all cases of meningococcal meningitis. These reports are received by the 24-hour on-call Ministry of Health staff, who promptly initiate contact tracing and preventive vaccination to all possible contacts. Public health agencies also rely on organizations to rapidly report unusual trends and patterns, such as several cases of measles if the endemic rates are very low. If an organization does not have an effective system in place for reporting to public health organizations, the likelihood of rapid disease and outbreak identification is diminished. To make sure that trends and patterns are reported to the appropriate authorities, organizations should have policies and procedures that comply with local reporting laws.

International Library of Measures. JCI's Quality Improvement and Patient Safety (QPS) standards*—which require organizations to participate in performance-measurement activities, such as benchmarking, including defining measures, collecting data, analyzing data, and using this information to improve performance—also require organizations to select five clinical measures from the International Library of Measures and incorporate them into their performance-measurement efforts. In addition, Clinical Care Program Certification standards require programs to choose at least two of their four measures from the International Library of Measures.

These standardized measures help organizations collect and benchmark data on several critical clinical issues related to the following infection-prevention topics:

- Pneumonia (I-PN)
- Surgical Care Improvement Project (I-SCIP)

The goal of the library is to create consistency in international data collection by standardizing the measures that are collected and the processes by which they are collected. Organizations can use this information to benchmark their performance internally—for example, between health care provider specialty groups or between specific patient care units—over time in order to identify opportunities for improvement. Organizations will also be able to benchmark their performance against other like or similar organizations, as well as compare their performance to other professional and accrediting bodies. The measures most applicable to this publication are listed in Table 5-8.

Standards are effective as of this book's publication date of January 2012. Consult your current JCI accreditation manual for updated standards.

Table 5-8. JCI Measures Related to Infection Prevention and Control

ID	Name
Pneumonia (I-PN)	
I-PN-2	Pneumococcal Vaccination
I-PN-7	Influenza Vaccination
Surgical Care Improvement Project (I-SCIP)	
I-SCIP-Inf-1d	Prophylactic Antibiotic Received Within 1 Hour Prior to Surgical Incision (hip arthroplasty)
I-SCIP-Inf-1e	Prophylactic Antibiotic Received Within 1 Hour Prior to Surgical Incision (knee arthroplasty)
I-SCIP-Inf-2d	Prophylactic Antibiotic Selection for Surgical Patients (hip arthroplasty)
I-SCIP-Inf-2e	Prophylactic Antibiotic Selection for Surgical Patients (knee arthroplasty)
I-SCIP-Inf-3d	Prophylactic Antibiotics Discontinued Within 24 Hours After Surgery End Time (hip arthroplasty)
I-SCIP-Inf-3e	Prophylactic Antibiotics Discontinued Within 24 Hours After Surgery End Time (knee arthroplasty)

Source: Joint Commission International. International Library of Measures. Accessed 1 May 2011. http://www.jointcommissioninternational.org/News/2010/8/20/International-Library-of-Measures.

Evaluating the Infection Prevention and Control Program: Goals, Objectives, and Strategies

Periodically (at least annually), the goals, objectives, strategies, and results of the IPC program should be evaluated by the IPC team and the IPC committee to ensure that prevention methods are working and that infections and infection risks are being kept to the minimum. The evaluation process identifies which activities have been successful and which should be changed to achieve better results.

The evaluation should be performed as a multidisciplinary effort in a systematic and purposeful manner. First, the IPC committee should determine the evaluation time line and method to be used and how the results will be disseminated and integrated into the next risk and planning cycle prior to beginning the evaluation process. Next, to perform the evaluation, the team will have to collate the results and data related to each of the objectives and strategies. In addition to the formal objectives, the evaluation should include an analysis of any clusters or outbreaks, significant policy changes, unusual deaths, and other pertinent events. Using this collective information, the team can perform the evaluation, record the findings, prepare a report, and disseminate the information to the staff and leadership of the organization. As with the risk assessment, numbers, discussion, or both can be used to evaluate the program (*see* Figure 5-4).

Conclusion

By employing a planned approach to address and to minimize or eliminate infection risk, an organization can develop an effective IPC program. Using evidence-based prevention and control strategies and evaluating how these approaches affect infection outcomes are crucial to success. When the program is in place, the organization must exercise continual vigilance for new and ongoing issues that must be assessed and dealt with to prevent HAIs. Maintaining focus on IPC is a continuing challenge that requires multiple approaches to accomplish goals. Chapter 6, "Maintaining and Sustaining an Effective Infection Prevention and Control Program," provides strategies to help IPC professionals succeed in achieving program goals.

References

1. Saint S, et al. The importance of leadership in preventing healthcare-associated infection: Results of a multisite qualitative study. *Infect Control Hosp Epidemiol.* 2010 Sep;31(9):901–907.
2. Goeschel CA. Nursing leadership at the crossroads: Evidence-based practice 'Matching Michigan-minimizing catheter related blood stream infections.' *Nurs Crit Care.* 2011 Jan–Feb;16(1):36-43.
3. Damschroder LJ, et al. The role of the champion in infection prevention: Results from a multisite qualitative study. *Qual Saf Health Care.* 2009 Dec;18(6):434–440.
4. Arthur D, et al. Hospital-acquired infections: Leadership challenges. Panel discussion. *Hosp Health Netw.* 2008 Oct;82(10):56–65.
5. Shewchuk M. Leaders' role in infection prevention and control: Fighting the invisible and invincible . . . if only. . . . *Can Oper Room Nurs J.* 2004 Jun;22(2):18, 21–22, 36.
6. Sriratanaban J, Wanavanichkul Y. Hospitalwide quality improvement in Thailand. *Jt Comm J Qual Saf.* 2004 May;30(5):246–256.

7. Association for Professionals in Infection Control and Epidemiology. APIC-Premier Survey on HAI Prevention Strategies. Accessed 8 Jul 2011. http://www.premierinc.com/about/news/08-sep /SurveySummary_09122008.pdf.

8. Perencevich EN, et al. Raising standards while watching the bottom line: Making a business case for infection control. *Infect Control Hosp Epidemiol.* 2007 Oct;28(10):1121–1133.

9. Stone PW, et al. The economic impact of infection control: Making the business case for increased infection control resources. *Am J Infect Control.* 2005 Nov;33(9):542–547.

10. Dunagan WC, et al. Making the business case for infection control: Pitfalls and opportunities. *Am J Infect Control.* 2002 Apr;30(2):86–92.

11. Zejda JE. [Professional profiles of physicians certi- fied in epidemiology in the view of hospital man- agers in the Silesian Voivodeship of Poland]. *Przegl Epidemiol.* 2003;57(1):1–8.

12. Dembry LM, Hierholzer WJ Jr. Educational needs and opportunities for the hospital epidemiologist. *Infect Control Hosp Epidemiol.* 1996 Mar;17(3): 188–192.

13. Norrby SR, Carbon C. Report of working group 3: Specialist training and continuing medical educa- tion/professional development in the infection dis- ciplines. *Clin Microbiol Infect.* 2005 Apr;11 Suppl 1:46–49.

14. Voss A, et al. The training curriculum in hospital infection control. *Clin Microbiol Infect.* 2005 Apr;11 Suppl 1:33–35.

15. Manning ML. Expanding infection preventionists' influence in the 21st century: Looking back to move forward. *Am J Infect Control.* 2010 Dec;38(10):778–783.

16. Borg MA, et al. Survey of infection control infrastructure in selected southern and eastern Mediterranean hospitals. *Clin Microbiol Infect.* 2007 Mar;13(3):344–346.

17. Struelens MJ, et al. Status of infection control policies and organisation in European hospitals, 2001: The ARPAC study. *Clin Microbiol Infect.* 2006 Aug;12(8):729–737.

18. Cunney R, et al. Survey of acute hospital infection control resources and services in the Republic of Ireland. *J Hosp Infect.* 2006 Sep;64(1): 63–68.

19. Pittet D, et al.: Infection control as a major World Health Organization priority for developing countries. *J Hosp Infect.* 2008 Apr;68(4):285– 292.

20. Yokoe DS, Classen D. Improving patient safety through infection con- trol: A new healthcare imperative. *Infect Control Hosp Epidemiol.* 2008 Oct;29 Suppl 1:S3–S11.

21. Burke JP. Infection control—A problem for patient safety. *N Engl J Med.* 2003 Feb 13;348(7):651–656.

22. Gerberding JL. Hospital-onset infections: A patient safety issue. *Ann Intern Med.* 2002 Oct 15;137(8):665–670.

23. Soule B. Patient safety. In Friedman C, Newsom B, editors: *IFIC Basic Concepts of Infection Control,* 2nd ed. (Revised 2011). Portadown UK: International Federation of Infection Control, 2011, 1–15. Accessed 29 Nov 2011. http://theific.org/basic_concepts/Chapter1.pdf.

24. O'Boyle C, Jackson M, Henly SJ. Staffing requirements for infection control programs in US health care facilities: Delphi project. *Am J Infect Control.* 2002 Oct;30(6):321–333.

25. Cooper T. Educational theory into practice: Development of an infec- tion control link nurse programme. *Nurse Educ Pract.* 2001 Mar;1(1):35–41.

26. Ching TY, Seto WH. Evaluating the efficacy of the infection control liaison nurse in the hospital. *J Adv Nurs.* 1990 Oct;15(10):1128–1131.

27. Roberts C, Casey D. An infection control link nurse network in the care home setting. *Br J Nurs.* 2004 Feb 12–25;13(3):166–170.

28. Dawson SJ. The role of the infection control link nurse. *J Hosp Infect.* 2003 Aug;54(4):251–257.

29. Teare EL, Peacock A. The development of an infection control link- nurse programme in a district general hospital. *J Hosp Infect.* 1996 Dec;34(4):267–278.

30. Goldrick BA. The Certification Board of Infection Control and Epi- demiology white paper: The value of certification for infection control professionals. *Am J Infect Control.* 2007 Apr;35(3):150–156.

31. Memish ZA, Soule BM, Cunningham G. Infection control certification: A global priority. *Am J Infect Control.* 2007 Apr;35(3):141–143.

32. Soule B, Memish Z. Infection control practice: Global preparedness for future challenges. *J Chemother.* 2001 Apr;13 Suppl 1:45–49.

33. Chatterjee A, et al. Impact of surveillance rounds on adherence to infec- tion control policies and procedures at a children's hospital. *Infect Con- trol Hosp Epidemiol.* 2004 Sep;25(9):786–788.

34. Sissolak D, Marais F, Mehtar S. TB infection prevention and control experiences of South African nurses—A phenomenological study. *BMC Public Health.* 2011 Apr 25;11:262.

35. Chuengchitraks S, et al. Impact of new practice guideline to prevent catheter-related blood stream infection (CRBSI): Experience at the Pediatric Intensive Care Unit of Phramongkutklao Hospital. *J Med Assoc Thai.* 2010 Nov;93 Suppl 6:S79–83.

36. Elamin S, et al. Staff knowledge, adherence to infection control recom- mendations and seroconversion rates in hemodialysis centers in Khar- toum. *Arab J Nephrol Transplant.* 2011 Jan;4(1):13–19.

37. Bukhari SZ, et al. Hand hygiene compliance rate among healthcare pro- fessionals. *Saudi Med J.* 2011 May;32(5):515–519.

38. Luo Y, et al. Factors impacting compliance with standard precautions in nursing, China. *Int J Infect Dis.* 2010 Dec;14(12):e1106–1114.

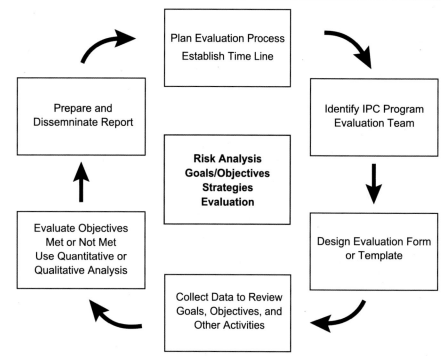

Figure 5-4. Annual Evaluation Process

Source: Barbara M. Soule. Used with permission. This figure first appeared in Arias K, Soule B, editors: *The APIC/JCAHO Infection Control Workbook.* Oakbrook Terrace, IL, and Washington, DC: Association for Professionals in Infection Control and Epidemiology, and Joint Commission Resources, 2006, 86.

39. Manojlovich M, et al. Developing and testing a tool to measure nurse/physician communication in the intensive care unit. *J Patient Saf.* 2011 Jun;7(2):80–84.

40. Bloomfield S, et al. Prevention of the spread of infection—The need for a family-centered approach to hygiene promotion. *Euro Surveill.* 2008 May 29;13(22):pii: 18889.

41. Petrovic K, Maimbolwa M, Johansson E. Primiparous mothers' knowledge about mother-to-child transmission of HIV in Lusaka, Zambia. *Midwifery.* 2009 Dec;25(6):e1–10.

42. Hutchinson AF, et al. Communicating information regarding human H1N1-09 virus to high-risk consumers: Knowledge and understanding of COPD patients in Melbourne, Australia. *Collegian.* 2010;17(4):199–205.

43. Geubbels EL, et al. Reduced risk of surgical site infections through surveillance in a network. *Int J Qual Health Care.* 2006 Apr;18(2):127–133.

44. Weinberg M, et al. Reducing infections among women undergoing cesarean section in Colombia by means of continuous quality improvement methods. *Arch Intern Med.* 2001 Oct 22;161(19):2357–2365.

45. Son C, et al. Practically speaking: Rethinking hand hygiene improvement programs in health care settings. *Am J Infect Control.* Epub 12 Jun 2011.

46. Joint Commission International: *Joint Commission International Accreditation Standards for Hospitals*, 4th ed. Oak Brook, IL: Joint Commission Resources, 2010.

47. The Joint Commission: *Risk Assessment for Infection Prevention and Control.* Oak Brook, IL: Joint Commission Resources, 2010.

48. Larson E, Aiello AE. Systematic risk assessment methods for the infection control professional. *Am J Infect Control.* 2006 Jun;34(5):323–326.

49. Institute for Healthcare Improvement. Implement the IHI Central Line Bundle. Accessed 8 Jul 2011. http://www.ihi.org/IHI/Topics/Critical Care/IntensiveCare/Changes/ImplementtheCentralLineBundle.htm.

50. Institute for Healthcare Improvement. Implement the IHI Ventilator Bundle. Accessed 8 Jul 2011. http://www.ihi.org/IHI/Topics/Critical Care/IntensiveCare/Changes/ImplementtheVentilatorBundle.htm.

51. Lo E, et al. Strategies to prevent catheter-associated urinary tract infections in acute care hospitals. *Infect Control Hosp Epidemiol.* 2008 Oct;29 Suppl 1:S41–S50.

52. Anderson DJ, et al. Strategies to prevent surgical site infections in acute care hospitals. *Infect Control Hosp Epidemiol.* 2008 Oct;29 Suppl 1:S51–S61.

53. Marschall J, et al. Strategies to prevent central line-associated bloodstream infections in acute care hospitals. *Infect Control Hosp Epidemiol.* 2008 Oct;29 Suppl 1:S22–30.

54. Coffin SE, et al. Strategies to prevent ventilator-associated pneumonia in acute care hospitals. *Infect Control Hosp Epidemiol.* 2008 Oct;29 Suppl 1:S31–40.

55. Calfee DP, et al. Strategies to prevent transmission of methicillin-resistant *Staphylococcus aureus* in acute care hospitals. *Infect Control Hosp Epidemiol.* 2008 Oct;29 Suppl 1:S62–80.

56. Dubberke ER, et al. Strategies to prevent *Clostridium difficile* infections in acute care hospitals. *Infect Control Hosp Epidemiol.* 2008 Oct;29 Suppl 1:S81–92.

57. Nadzam DM, Soule BM. Performance measures. In Carrico R, editor: *APIC Text of Infection Control and Epidemiology*, 3rd ed. Washington, DC: Association for Professionals in Infection Control and Epidemiology, 2009, 9-1–9-9.

58 Murphy DM. From expert data collectors to interventionists: Changing the focus for infection control professionals. *Am J Infect Control.* 2002 Apr;30(2):120–132.

59. Arias K. Surveillance. In Carrico R, editor: *APIC Text of Infection Control and Epidemiology*, 3rd ed. Washington, DC: Association for Professionals in Infection Control and Epidemiology, 2009, 3-1–3-17.

60. Lee TB, et al. Association for Professionals in Infection Control and Epidemiology. Recommended practices for surveillance: Association for Professionals in Infection Control and Epidemiology (APIC), Inc. *Am J Infect Control.* 2007 Sep;35(7):427-40.

61. Pottinger JM, Herwaldt LA, Peri TM. Basics of surveillance—An overview. *Infect Control Hosp Epidemiol.* 1997 Jul;18(7):513–527.

62. Haley RW. The scientific basis for using surveillance and risk factor data to reduce nosocomial infection rates. *J Hosp Infect.* 1995 Jun;30 Suppl:3–14.

63. McLaws ML. Surveillance. In Friedman C, Newsom B, editors: *IFIC Basic Concepts of Infection Control*, 2nd ed (revised 2011). Portadown, UK: International Federation of Infection Control, 2011, 41–55.

64. Balkhy HH, et al. Hospital- and community-acquired infections: A point prevalence and risk factors survey in a tertiary care center in Saudi Arabia. *Int J Infect Dis.* 2006 Jul;10(4):326–333.

65. Sodano L, et al. [The prevalence survey of nosocomial infections: A very informative tool in a big hospital setting]. *Ann Ig.* 2004 Sep–Oct; 16(5):647–663.

66. Klavs I, et al. Prevalence of and risk factors for hospital-acquired infections in Slovenia—Results of the first national survey, 2001. *J Hosp Infect.* 2003 Jun;54(2):149–157.

67. Gikas A, et al. Prevalence study of hospital-acquired infections in 14 Greek hospitals: Planning from the local to the national surveillance level. *J Hosp Infect.* 2002 Apr;50(4):269–275.

68. Thu TA, et al. A point-prevalence study on healthcare-associated infections in Vietnam: Public health implications. *Infect Control Hosp Epidemiol.* 2011 Oct;32(10):1039–1041.

69. Centers for Disease Control and Prevention. NHSN Patient Safety Component Manual. Accessed 7 Sep 2011. http://www.cdc.gov /nhsn/TOC_PSCManual.html.

70. Mu Y, et al. Improving risk-adjusted measures of surgical site infection for the National Healthcare Safety Network. *Infect Control Hosp Epidemiol* 2011 Oct;32(10):970–986.

71. Dudeck MA, et al. National Healthcare Safety Network (NHSN) Report, data summary for 2009, device-associated module. *Am J Infect Control.* 2001 Jun;39(5):349–367.

72. Gastmeier P, et al. Benchmarking of urinary tract infection rates: Experiences from the intensive care unit component of the German national nosocomial infections surveillance system. *J Hosp Infect.* 2011 May;78(1):41–44.

73. Brossette SE, Hymel PA Jr. Data mining and infection control. *Clin Lab Med.* 2008 Mar;28(1):119–126, vii.

74. Richards C, et al. Promoting quality through measurement of performance and response: Prevention success stories. *Emerg Infect Dis.* 2001 Mar–Apr;7(2):299–301.

75. Gaynes R, et al. Feeding back surveillance data to prevent hospital-acquired infections. *Emerg Infect Dis.* 2001 Mar–Apr;7(2):295–298.

76. World Health Organization. The Weekly Epidemiological Record (WER). Accessed 7 Sep 2011. http://www.who.int/wer/en/.

77. Geffers C, Gastmeier P. Nosocomial infections and multidrug-resistant organisms in Germany: Epidemiological data from KISS (the Hospital Infection Surveillance System). *Dtsch Arztebl Int.* 2011 Feb;108(6):87–93.

78. Centers for Disease Control and Prevention. National Safety Healthcare Network Data & Statistics. Accessed 31 Aug 2011. http://www.cdc.gov/nhsn/datastat.html.

79. Gould CV, et al. Healthcare Infection Control Practices Advisory Committee. *Guideline for Prevention of Catheter-Associated Urinary Tract Infections 2009.* Atlanta: Centers for Disease Control and Prevention, 2009.

80. Sehulster L, Chinn RYW. *Guidelines for Environmental Infection Control in Health-Care Facilities.* Washington, DC: National Center for Infectious Diseases, 2003.

Maintaining and Sustaining an Effective Infection Prevention and Control Program

By
Barbara M. Soule, RN, MPA, CIC, FSHEA
Prof. Ziad A. Memish, MD, FRCPC, FRCPE, FACP, FIDSA
Preeti N. Malani, MD, MSJ

Chapter Six

Once an infection prevention and control (IPC) program has been established and the essential components are in place, organizations must continue to proactively assess infection risks, to implement prevention practices, and to evaluate processes and outcomes. This chapter describes some of the common elements of a successful IPC program that are applicable in all care settings and discusses methods to address deficiencies in care and to improve performance.

Please note: The terms *IPC practitioner* and *IPC professional* are used interchangeably throughout this chapter to identify IPC specialists. In some areas of the world, the preferred term for this same role is *infection preventionist*.

Specific Interventions to Reduce the Spread of Infection

Depending on the organization and its unique characteristics, a variety of interventions will be necessary to address infection prevention issues. The following section discusses some typical IPC interventions and strategies for implementation.

Hand Hygiene

Hand hygiene is widely considered one of the most effective ways to prevent the spread of infection.[1,2] The Institute for Health Care Improvement (IHI) estimates that hospitals could save thousands of lives each year if they imposed a zero-tolerance policy for workers failing to perform hand hygiene when indicated.[3] In a culture that establishes patient safety as a priority, it is essential that each health care organization create an effective hand-hygiene program to achieve and to sustain compliance with recommended practices. Excellent evidence-based guidelines exist,[1,2] but achieving high rates of hand-hygiene compliance has eluded many organizations. This may be due in part to a lack of leadership commitment for reducing health care–associated infections (HAIs), the absence of an organized approach to change behavior, or lack of resources for establishing an institutionwide hand-hygiene program that is successful and sustainable over the long term. Cookson and colleagues have reviewed the published literature to identify the best methods to improve compliance with hand hygiene.[4] The investigators found a lack of strong, methodically sound research to inform caregivers about which interventions are most effective. They did observe that single, brief educational sessions were not likely to be successful, a finding consistent with work from Pittet, Allegranzi, and others demonstrating success with a multifaceted approach to hand hygiene.[5,6]

In 2004 the World Health Organization (WHO) launched its Global Patient Safety Challenge to address adverse events that affect patient care. The first project selected for the challenge was *Clean Care Is Safer Care*, with the cornerstone of hand hygiene and the objective to "achieve an improvement in hand-hygiene practices worldwide to promote strong patient safety culture."[7,8] More than 120 Member States have pledged support of the program, have addressed barriers, and have capitalized on strengths.[9] As of September 2011, more than 13,000 hospital and other health care organizations are participating in this initiative.[10] For further discussion about WHO's approach, *see* Chapter 2.

Since 2008 The Joint Commission's Center for Transforming Healthcare has led a systematic and intense approach to improving hand hygiene.[11] Working with eight hospitals to collect baseline hand-hygiene data using a standardized approach, most of the participants found that their rates of compliance were lower than they had thought. The project then helped organizations design a systematic approach to improvement using teams and data-collection processes, analyzing potential barriers for performing hand hygiene, and developing solutions to improve compliance. The Targeted Solutions Tool™ (TST) provides a systematic methodology and the tools for this project. More details on this initiative can be seen on the Center for Transforming Healthcare's website at http://www.centerfortransforminghealthcare.org/projects/detail.aspx?Project=3 or in Chapter 3 of this book.

In addition to providing safe care, strong economic arguments also support improved hand hygiene. One study found that an increase of only 1% in hand-hygiene compliance saved the institution nearly $40,000 in reduced infection costs.[12] Another study found that there were economic benefits in following hand-hygiene guidelines.[13] Other examples are cited by WHO in the *WHO Guidelines on Hand Hygiene in Health Care* published in 2009.[2] Among those discussed by WHO are the following[2]:

- The excess use of hospital resources associated with only four or five HAIs of average severity may equal the entire annual budget for hand-hygiene products used in inpatient care areas.
- A single severe infection of a surgical site, lower respiratory tract, or bloodstream may cost the hospital more than its entire annual budget for antiseptic agents used for hand hygiene. An illustrative example is a cost analysis from a neonatal intensive care unit (NICU) in the Russian Federation, where the excess cost of one health care–associated bloodstream infection (BSI; US$1,100) would cover 3,265 patient-days of hand-antiseptic use (US$0.34 per patient-day). The alcohol-based hand rub applied for hand hygiene

in this unit would be cost-effective if its use prevented only 8.5 pneumonias or 3.5 BSIs each year.

The hands of health care workers (HCWs) are a major source of infectious agents.[1,2] Microorganisms can be transmitted from such obviously contaminated sources as purulent sputum or drainage from an infected wound and can also be spread through contact with less obvious sources, such as normal intact human skin; items in the patient environment, such as urinals and bedpans; over-bed tables and personal items; and devices used in the care setting, including computer keyboards and phones.[14–20] These latter sources may not be visibly soiled and, therefore, not viewed as reservoirs of organisms, but in some cases they may be implicated in disease transmission. Some "clean" activities, such as taking a pulse or blood-pressure reading or lifting a patient, may also result in acquiring significant transient organisms on hands that can be transmitted to others.

Hand hygiene is a major factor in breaking the chain of infection. Hand hygiene is a simple act, but achieving acceptable HCW compliance rates can be difficult. Some studies have measured mean baseline rates of 5% to 81% and an overall average of 40%.[5] Although HCWs do not generally or intentionally avoid washing their hands, they may perceive they are "too busy," may be distracted, experience skin irritation, or may not value the importance of rigorous hand hygiene enough to engage in the activity as they should.[21,22] Hand hygiene is a requirement of Joint Commission International's (JCI's) International Patient Safety Goal 5. Organizations should implement WHO or US Centers for Disease Control and Prevention (US CDC) guidelines—or another evidence-based set of guidelines that is published and generally accepted—to ensure proper hand hygiene within the organization (*see* Chapters 2 and 3 for more information on this topic).

Monitoring hand-hygiene compliance and providing HCWs with feedback regarding their performance are considered integral to a successful hand-hygiene promotion program. Direct observation of care providers by trained personnel has been considered the gold standard. Advantages of this method are the ability to determine whether hand hygiene is being performed at the correct times and with the correct technique and to establish compliance rates by HCW type, location, and shift. However, observation is extremely time-consuming and only permits observation of a small fraction of all hand-hygiene opportunities. Comparison of compliance rates obtained through observation surveys is problematic due to lack of standardization of criteria for compliance, and observation techniques' interrater reliability may be weak. Self-reporting of compliance is not suf-

ficiently reliable to be useful.[22] Monitoring the use of hand-hygiene products requires much less time, can be performed continually, and is less complicated. However, it does not provide information about the appropriateness and quality of hand-hygiene practices or compliance rates by HCW type. Furthermore, it is not clear how product usage correlates with compliance established by observational surveys. In one study, a comparison of nearly 2,500 hand-hygiene observations did not significantly correlate with the amount of product used per patient-day.[23] Electronic and other newer methods for monitoring hand-hygiene compliance are of great interest throughout the world. They seem promising but require further evaluation before they can be routinely recommended.[24,25]

Given all the methodological and behavioral challenges, how can organizations improve the hand-hygiene practices of their HCWs and move toward high levels of compliance with proper hand hygiene organizationwide? Several strategies are listed below.

Educate HCWs. In some cases, HCWs are not aware of the activities that cause hand contamination. Dressing an open wound is a procedure for which HCWs would likely wash their hands (in addition to wearing gloves). Less obvious procedures, such as touching the patient's immediate care environment, might not be viewed as requiring hand hygiene. Because there is a delay between improper hand hygiene and the emergence of an infection, many HCWs do not see the cause-and-effect relationship between thoroughly cleaning their hands and preventing infection. For HCWs to realize the importance of proper hand hygiene and to engage in it at appropriate times, organizations should provide information on when hand hygiene is appropriate, data and research that illustrate the importance of hand hygiene and feedback about their performance. This information can be incorporated into HCWs' in-services, on posters displayed in patient rooms and in clinical and public areas, in HCW break areas, or through organization newsletters and bulletins. Multiple educational approaches should be used simultaneously to maximize behavior change, and approaches should be reinforced with other activities in a multimodal approach to behavior change.[5,25–27]

WHO's Five Moments of Hand Hygiene (*see* Figure 6-1) is an example of bringing a systematic approach to the HCWs for hand-hygiene opportunities. IPC practitioners should consider and incorporate the different learning preferences of health care personnel into their teaching methods. For example, some HCWs will learn better by hearing the information (verbal or linguistic method); others learn from visual input, such as in images, pictures, graphics, photos, and videos; some prefer an abstract learning style of self-discovery[27]; still others need to perform the action by practicing or participating in return demonstrations to learn (kinesthetic methods).[28]

Even if HCWs see value in hand hygiene, they may experience some confusion as to when it is appropriate to use hand rubs versus hand washing. Organizations should educate HCWs about the appropriate times to wash their hands versus using an alcohol-based hand rub. For example, when hands are visibly dirty, contaminated with proteinaceous material, or visibly soiled with blood or other body fluids or

after using the toilet, HCWs should wash their hands with soap and water. If hands are not visibly soiled, HCWs can use soap and water or an alcohol-based hand rub for routinely decontaminating hands.[1,2]

In some situations, the choice of agent is not clear. For certain organisms that exist in spore forms (for example, *Clostridium difficile*), hand washing has generally been recommended to mechanically remove the spores.[29,30] However, some organizations have continued to allow alcohol-based hand rubs for *Clostridium difficile* in spite of their lack of activity against the spore, citing the benefit of high rates of hand-hygiene compliance as an offset of the potential inactivity against the spores. Studies have shown that the routine use of alcohol-based hand rubs does not significantly increase rates of *Clostridium difficile*.[31] The Society for Healthcare Epidemiology of America (SHEA)/Infectious Disease Society of America (IDSA) Compendium of Strategies to Prevent Healthcare Associated Infections notes that the use of alcohol-based hand rubs in this situation remains an area of controversy.[30]

Create a culture that promotes hygiene. For HCWs to regularly comply with hand-hygiene procedures, an organization should foster a culture of safety—individual and group values, attitudes, perceptions, competencies, and patterns of behavior create commitment to preventing errors and are characterized by communications, mutual trust, and shared perceptions of the importance of safety.[32] Some use the term *zero tolerance* to promote an organizational culture to prevent infections. This type of culture already exists in certain areas of health care. For example, in the operating theatre, surgeons do not perform surgery and nurses or technicians do not assist without first having performed carefully designed preoperative scrubs. This same strict culture of safety is often absent in other settings, and HCWs may be quite reluctant to challenge those with more authority to comply with hand-hygiene protocols. To achieve full compliance, a culture of expectation and support must be reinforced by leadership. Studies have shown that when administrative and key

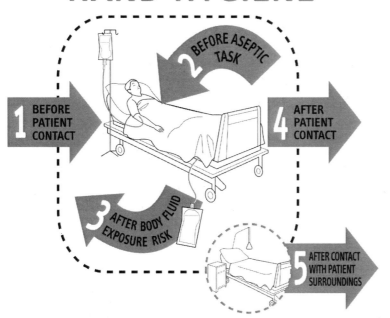

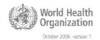

Figure 6-1. WHO's Five Moments of Hand Hygiene

clinical leaders make overt and strong statements that hand hygiene is important, behavior is more likely to change.[33,34]

Organizations cannot expect overnight transformation, as behavioral changes are difficult to initiate and take time to become part of the workplace culture. To track changes in culture and to identify areas for continued work, it is important to periodically monitor hand-hygiene adherence with observational studies and to provide feedback to personnel about their performance. In addition to the culture of the organization, those who are planning a hand-hygiene promotion program for their facility must consider the values, norms, and religious beliefs of the persons who will be affected by a hand-hygiene policy, which will influence compliance and should be integrated into the policies and educational programs.[35]

Make hand hygiene convenient. Where high workload is given as a major factor in noncompliance, an organization should carefully consider what products it provides for hand hygiene. Alcohol-based hand rubs have been shown to require less time than washing with soap and water and thus can save nursing time, which may contribute to increased overall hand-hygiene compliance.[1,2] Organizations can make an alcohol-based hand rub available at the bedside, inside the entrance to the patient's room. or in other convenient locations as well as in individual pocket-sized containers to be carried by caregivers. Containers of alcohol-based hand rub can be attached to trolleys or carts that move from patient to patient to deliver supplies or treatments. Similar containers should be placed in all HCW areas.

Do not rely on gloves. Gloves play an important role in preventing the spread of infection but are not a substitute for hand hygiene. Many gloves have tiny perforations that allow pathogens to reach the skin. Bacteria can be spread from one part of the body to another if soiled gloves are not replaced between tasks. Washing gloves as if they were skin is not satisfactory. Used gloves should also be removed before HCWs touch such surfaces as door handles or telephones. HCWs should be educated about appropriate glove use, and hand washing or hand antisepsis should be carried out before and after contact with every patient, regardless of whether gloves are used.[36]

Enlist clinical and administrative leader support. Clinical and administrative leaders, formal and informal, set the tone for caregivers. When these leaders are observed performing hand hygiene on a regular basis, this behavior encourages other HCWs to follow their example and also to feel more comfortable speaking up when they notice noncompliance. Studies have shown that when respected HCWs wash their hands before touching the patients, the other HCWs making rounds also wash their hands. This role modeling from the clinical setting can be extended to many infection-prevention processes in which persons of influence set the tone for expected behavior.[25,37]

Encourage patient involvement. Organizations should provide education to patients about hand hygiene and support patients and families in performing hand hygiene. Patients can also be encouraged to remind their HCWs to wash their hands. Although this simple reminder can be an important infection-prevention strategy, many patients may be fearful of challenging HCWs on this topic. Other means, such as signs in patient rooms or peer accountability and even video scans, can be used to encourage hand hygiene and also to get patients involved.[38]

Case Study 6-1 below (*also see* Case Study 3-2 in Chapter 3) gives examples of how hand-hygiene compliance—including using the Five Moments of Hand Hygiene—can be a part of overall strategies to improve patient outcomes and performance-improvement initiatives.

CASE STUDY 6-1

An Effective Hand-Hygiene Intervention in the Prevention of Health Care–Associated Infections in Three Provincial Hospitals* (Vietnam)

Nguyen Viet Hung MD, PhD; Truong Anh Thu, MDL; Thi Thanh Thuy, MD; Tran Quy, MD; Hiroshi Ohara, PhD; Lennox K. Archibald, MD, PhD

Introduction

HAIs are associated with significant morbidity and mortality in tertiary care and provincial hospitals across Vietnam. In their efforts to address the issue head on, the Vietnamese Ministry of Health has deemed the control and prevention of HAIs a public health priority. Although appropriate hand hygiene (HH) with soap and water or an alcohol-based hand rub is the single most important measure for the prevention and control of HAIs, various observational studies carried out by infection control personnel in Hanoi demonstrate HCW compliance with HH at only 13% in facilities across the region. Infection control and hospital-epidemiology personnel have found that the factors that contribute to such low HH compliance among HCWs include (a) lack of basic knowledge among HCWs about the modes of transmission of health care–associated pathogens and the infection control

*Note: The three hospitals in this case study have not been named; therefore, no organizational information, as supplied in the other case studies, is provided here.

Table 1. The Compliance with HH Before and During HH Campaign

	Before campaign	During campaign			
		08/2005	09/2005	10/2005	11/2005
Compliance (%)	10/159 (6.3%)	120/316 (38.0)	435/662 (65.7)	473/706 (67.0)	391/595 (65.7)
AOR		9.1	28.5	24.2	28.5
p-value		< 0.001	< 0.001	< 0.001	< 0.001

Table 2. Crude HAI Rates Before and During HH Campaign

	Before campaign	During campaign			
		08/2005	09/2005	10/2005	11/2005
HAI rate (%)	42/246 (17.1)	20/286 (7.0)	24/290 (8.3)	17/264 (6.4)	13/271 (4.8)
AOR		0.4	0.4	0.3	0.2
p-value		< 0.001	< 0.01	< 0.001	< 0.001

Table 3. The Correlation Between HCW HH Compliance and HAI Rate

Variable	Precampaign	Postcampaign	*p* value
HH compliance	10/159 (6.3%)	391/595 (65.7%)	< 0.001
Crude HAI rate	42/246 (17.1%)	13/271 (4.8%)	< 0.001

practices and procedures necessary for prevention and (b) the frequent unavailability of HH facilities in patient rooms. Thus, this study was conducted (a) to determine the prevalence of HAIs in patients in high-risk areas of provincial hospitals and the rate of HH adherence among designated HCWs and (b) to ascertain whether an educational program might help reduce HAI rates in these facilities.

Methods and Findings

During the study period, May–November 2005, an educational/training program to promote HH practices was initiated in the surgical and obstetrics departments and the intensive care unit (ICU) at three provincial general hospitals in Vietnam. This HH program was the only infection control intervention implemented at these facilities during the study period and comprised the following components:
(a) Writing and justification of HH policies for the facilities
(b) Hand-hygiene training for designated HCWs
(c) Introduction of a locally produced alcohol-based hand rub
   The indications and justification for HH activities followed guidelines instituted by the US CDC. Compliance was

ascertained through observational studies conducted on a daily basis by a trained infection control team at each hospital and hospital epidemiologists from Bach Mai Hospital, the main teaching hospital in Vietnam. HAI rates were determined through monthly point prevalence surveys using US CDC case definitions for HAI and a prevalence survey tool that was also designed at the US CDC. Results of HH compliance observational studies were reported back to HCWs in the respective units on a weekly basis.

   Data were analyzed using statistical software packages. Logistic regression analysis was used to control factors known to be associated with noncompliance, and HAI occurrence and adjusted odds ratios (AOR) were computed.

   At the start of the study, the overall mean HCW compliance with HH practices was 6.3%. By November 2005—4 months after initiating the campaign—HH adherence had increased to 65.7%; this increase in compliance was statistically significant (*see* Table 1). In parallel, HAI rates decreased from 17.1% before the campaign to 4.8% by the fourth month of the campaign (*p* < 0.001; *see* Table 2). The correlation between improved HH compliance and fall in crude HAI rate was statistically significant (*p* < 0.001; *see* Table 3).

Interventions

Through the auspices of the Vietnam Ministry of Health, the head of the infection control committee and hospital epidemiologist at Bach Mai Hospital has spearheaded similar interventions in hospitals across Vietnam and raised awareness of the clinical and public health implications of HAI. In addition, there has been an overhaul of infection control policies in hospitals at all levels, including tertiary care and provincial hospitals.

Results

There has been increased awareness of the role played by HH within the chain of transmission of health care–associated pathogens. This has been reflected in continued reductions in

HAI rates in health care facilities in Hanoi and surrounding regions as well as improvement among health care personnel in the recognition and ascertainment of HAIs using updated infection control policies.

Lessons Learned

An intervention consisting of education and enhancement of HH hand hygiene among HCWs using a locally produced alcohol-based hand-sanitizer formulation contributed significantly to a reduction of HAIs in three provincial hospitals in Vietnam. To maintain continued reduction in HAI rates, other health care facilities across Vietnam should consider implementation of a similar multimodal and multidisciplinary approach, using readily available, affordable alcohol-based HH products together with routine observation of HH adherence and feedback of the data to the relevant HCWs. Further studies of the effectiveness of HH in the prevention of HAIs need to be conducted in the other medical and surgical services in tertiary care, regional, and provincial health care facilities.

Ensuring the Appropriate Use of Antimicrobial Agents

Antimicrobials are used prophylactically to prevent infections and therapeutically to treat infections. Patients having surgery often receive antimicrobials preoperatively and during long procedures to reduce the risk of postsurgical infections. Certain patient populations (such as those in the ICU) who are compromised with multiple or chronic illnesses, are using invasive devices, and are susceptible to infection may receive significant quantities and several types of antimicrobials.

Antimicrobial use is complex. During the past decades, the incidence of multidrug-resistant organisms (MDROs) has increased, and HAIs with these organisms are seen in critically ill patients and those who are significantly less ill. If antimicrobials are used inappropriately, organisms can develop resistance to them, and the therapeutic usefulness of specific agents will decline. For a few diseases and infections, very few agents can treat the problem successfully, including selected gram-negative organisms (for example, carbepenam-resistant *Klebsiella pneumoniae* [CRKP], *Acinetobacter*, and extended spectrum beta lactamase [ESBL] that have developed significant resistance with very few options for treatment). Patients with ventilator-associated pneumonia (VAP), burns, or other infections caused by MDROs such as *Acinetobacter baumanii* may experience significant morbidity with severe consequences.[39,40] Newer emerging resistance patterns in some organisms, such as the New Delhi metallo-beta-lactamase (NDM-1) gene, have further decreased the usefulness of antimicrobial agents and added to the burden

of resistant HAIs.[41] Such situations as these are very serious for patients and highlight how imperative it is to minimize resistance through appropriate antimicrobial use. Outbreaks with highly resistant organisms such as CRKP, have become more common in recent years. Case Study 6-2 describes one such outbreak. (*See* Case Study 5-9 on pages 83–84 for another organization's story about a similar outbreak.)

CASE STUDY 6-2

Outbreak of Carbapenem-Resistant Klebsiella pneumoniae (Israel)

Matan J. Cohen, MD, MPH (*SHEA International Ambassador*); Carmella Schwartz, RN, MPH; Shmuel Benenson, MD

Introduction

At the close of 2005, an outbreak of CRKP was identified at Hadassah-Hebrew University Medical Center in Jerusalem, Israel. During 2006, recognizing the failure of standard infection control protocols (isolation precautions) to contain the outbreak, leadership persistently lobbied for a cohorting intervention, including appropriate allocation of space, HCWs, and equipment.

Methods

As of March 2007, cohorting was performed separately for the medical wards and for the surgical wards, rotating between the departments. After this intervention led to a halt in outbreak progression, hot spots were identified for proactive screening and promoted screening interventions, focusing on areas where there was increased pathogen transmission (ICUs and the surroundings of newly discovered colonized/infected patients) or introduction of new carriers to our medical facility (newly admitted patients from the emergency room).

The key players who developed the institutional action were the members of the infection control team. They were supported by the heads of the clinical-microbiology laboratory and the infectious-disease department. Buy-in was important, and the administration agreed to allocate appropriate HCWs, space, and equipment to the initiative. This was followed by an institutionwide intervention in which CRKP patients were identified and immediately relocated to designated cohorting wards, where HCWs were dedicated to care only for the CRKP patients. All HCWs caring for patients were required to comply with the institutional intervention requiring CRKP patients to be in contact isolation and to perform screening of patients' stool according to department-specific criteria.

Results

One month after beginning the cohorting intervention—and after close to 14 months of steady increases in the incidence of CRKP carriers and infected patients—a reversal in the incidence-rate trend was observed (Figure 1A, *p* value < 0.001). Additional interventions of proactive screening led to additional reduction in the institutional incidence and prevalence of CRKP. As seen in Figure 1B, after cohorting began, incidence soon halted. In addition, the burden of the increased workload resulting from the cohorting affected only one department at a time, allowing others to maintain regular work flow.

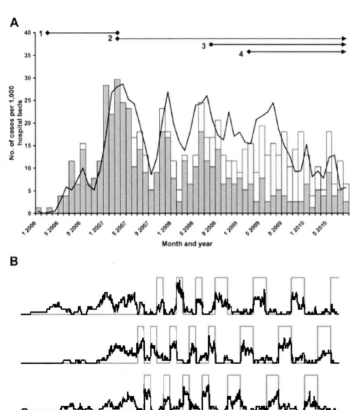

Figure 1. Monthly Institutional and Ward-Specific Carbapenem-Resistant *K. pneumoniae* (CRKP) Rates

Panel A presents clinical samples (gray columns), incident cases detected using surveillance stool samples (white column), and monthly mean institutional prevalence (solid line). **Panel B** shows prevalence rates in the three internal medicine departments for CRKP among hospitalized patients. Each chart represents a department, and the gray boxes mark periods when each department hosted the cohorting. It is clear that each department, while hosting its patients, had a marked increase in prevalence, allowing the other departments to be free of patients requiring cohorting. There are also cases patients with CRKP were not detected in time or were not transferred to the cohorting department.

Source: Cohen MJ, et al. Institutional control measures to curtail the epidemic spread of carbapenem-resistant *Klebsiella pneumoniae*: A 4-year perspective. *Infect Control Hosp Epidemiol.* 2011 Jul;32(7):673–678. Used with permission.

Lessons Learned

Cohorting of patients and nursing staff, along with focused active surveillance strategies, allowed containment of this outbreak. Cohorting decreased infection within the hospital, and active surveillance helped detect asymptomatic carriers.

Infection-prevention programs should have proactive, organized plans in place to minimize MDROs. Two approaches are effective in achieving this goal: antimicrobial stewardship programs to ensure the appropriate use of antimicrobial agents and IPC programs that reduce the risk of infections and prevent transmission.

Although some patients are admitted to a hospital colonized or infected with MDROs, many patients acquire MDROs in the health care setting as a result of cross-transmission from contact with people or the health care environment[42,43] A portion of the patients who become colonized with MDROs will develop infections, some of which result in death.[42,44-46] Interrupting three primary routes of transmission can yield dramatic reductions in the incidence of MDROs in health care settings. *See* Figure 6-2 for more details.

Interruption of the spread of MDROs via these routes includes the following strategies:

- **Achieving high rates of compliance with hand hygiene and barrier precautions.** Consistent and timely application of hand hygiene and isolation barriers and precautions prevents colonized or infected patients from serving as primary sources of organisms and reduces the likelihood of transmission. This includes systems to rapidly identify patients who may be colonized or infected with MDROs and to expeditiously implement appropriate isolation.[47-48] Some organizations have undertaken proactive surveillance cultures of all or selected patients to rapidly identify patients who are colonized with MDROs but may not exhibit signs or symptoms of infection. This process has been effective in some countries,[49,50] but in other countries, active surveillance is still considered controversial,[51] with mixed results in the effectiveness of the screening process. Overall studies suggest that this screening process can be helpful in reducing rates of methicillin-resistant *Staphyloccus aureus* (MRSA) or vancomycin-resistant *Enterrococcus* in certain hospitals and populations depending on the local epidemiology. When the screening indicates patients should be isolated, compliance with isolation policies should be monitored to evaluate whether HCWs are following all the requirements of contact precautions or other types of isolation.[52]

- **Enforcing effective environmental hygiene, including cleaning and disinfection of inanimate surfaces (fomites).** Microorganims can reside on these surfaces, whether moist or dry, for long periods of time. The hands of HCWs come in contact with the surfaces frequently during care of one patient and can be transmitted to other patients. One strategy to reduce this route of transmission is to educate HCWs about touching the patient's immediate environment: It is similar to touching the patient's skin, because both can be colonized with an MDRO. Another approach is to ensure that all "high-touch" surfaces in the patient care areas are thoroughly cleaned, including such items as over-bed tables, bed rails, door knobs, and the toilet areas.

For an example of how one organization monitored the effectiveness of cleaning its high-touch objects, *see* Case Study 6-3.

CASE STUDY 6-3

Lessons from Six-Month, Districtwide Use of Fluorescent Target Monitoring of High-Touch Objects (Australia)

Cathryn Murphy RN, PhD, CIC; Deborough Macbeth RN, PhD, CICP

Introduction

Recent Australian reports of highly resistant epidemiologically important potential pathogens and increasing consumer and government involvement in infection control issues highlight the need for Australia to improve its HAI prevention efforts generally. The absence of clear, unambiguous, jurisdictional guidance regarding hospital cleaning, a growing appreciation of the role of the inanimate environment in HAI risk and acquisition, and the need to prepare well for relocation to a new, larger campus in 2013 compelled the Queensland Health Service District to consider local applicability and usefulness of novel international approaches to monitoring and to achieving sustained improvement in cleaning. The specific purpose of this study was to evaluate covert use of a fluorescent targeting tool, education, and feedback for assessing and improving high-touch-object (HTO) cleaning in a typical Australian inpatient hospital setting.

Methods

Starting in January 2011 and lasting for 17 weeks, a three-phase prospective quasi-experimental, before-after, covert study of seven standardized HTOs was undertaken in the hospital wards of Queensland Health Service District hospitals with the highest proportion of inpatients known to be positive for at least one MDRO. The HTOs included the bedroom light switch, inside bedroom door knob, bedroom soap dispenser, toilet grab rail, and toilet flush button. The HTOs were selected after reviewing the international literature and inspecting the surface of HTOs routinely and permanently fixed in an inpatient room at both hospitals. The center of each specific HTO was identified as the site for marking. Only investigators trained in the use of the fluorescent marker marked the HTOs.

Forty-eight hours after application, investigators used a black (ultraviolet) light to determine the presence or removal of each placed mark. In Phase 1 only, immediately following initial assessment, each HTO was cleaned, remarked, and reassessed after 48 hours. After all marked targets in the room were evaluated, investigators removed all residual marks using an alcohol-free multisurface general cleaning wipe and black light to ensure all surfaces were clean and mark-free.

Between Phases 1 and 2, investigators provided results and standard education to environmental services staff at both hospitals. Education was not provided between Phases 2 and 3. At the time of marking and assessing each room, a work card was completed, noting the ward, bed number, date, time, medical-record number of the occupant, and which specific objects were marked, read, and cleaned.

The study was approved by the District's Infection Control Committee, and, as no human subjects were involved, the study was considered exempt from ethics or similar committee approval. Investigators agreed that only aggregate, nonhospital, and non-ward-specific data would be reported to avoid inadvertent identification of any specific cleaning staff and their associated levels of cleaning.

Results

A total of 986 marks was evaluated. In Phases 1 through 3, cleaning scores ranged from 9.4% to 77.8%, 10.8% to 93%, and 13.5% to 67.7%, respectively. In Phase 3, three HTOs scored lower than their Phase 1 levels. The mean overall cleaning scores for Phases 1 through 3 were 34%, 53%, and 41%, respectively.

Consistent with international experience, fluorescent-target monitoring of HTOs provided an easy and time-efficient tool to assess HTO cleaning in Australian inpatient rooms. It facilitated relevant feedback and education to environmental-services staff.

Lessons Learned

Fluorescent targeting proved to be an easy and time-efficient method to assess and to improve the level of cleaning in a series of 48-hour periods in wards with high MDRO occupancy and frequent patient turnover. However, without ongoing education, preliminary improvements were unsustained. The study enabled investigators to build relationships with environmental services and to begin dialogue with them. Those relationships and conversations have enabled organizations to better understand the opportunities to improve cleaning policy, practice, and education. This information is critical to develop, to implement, and to sustain improvements in hospital cleaning. As staff prepare for relocation to a larger, more complex, new facility in 2013, they are keen to maximize the quality of cleaning, particularly given its role as an adjunct to other standard infection-prevention measures, such as hand hygiene, early identification, and isolation of infectious patients.

This study is the first Australian attempt to assess the use of fluorescent targeting to evaluate cleaning. It has the potential to raise clinician, environmental-services, and other staff awareness and appreciation of cleaning as a strategy for reducing HAI risk in Australian hospitals and also to encourage other countries to explore the suitability of this approach for their own local and national cleaning-improvement initiatives.

Antimicrobial Stewardship

To help reduce infections and MDROs, organizations should have specific policies and monitoring systems in place for antimicrobial use. Antimicrobial stewardship programs (ASPs) can be effective methods to promote best practices, to encourage or to require the use of the most cost-effective drugs, and to guide prudent use to minimize the evolution of antimicrobial-resistant organisms. Organizations that have effective ASPs have reduced the use of antibiotics. In one study from a tertiary care pediatric medical center, an approach using the World Wide Web (WWW) resulted in an 11% decrease in doses prescribed.[53] Overall, in the United States, organizations have achieved between 22% and 36% reductions.[54] Prudent use of antimicrobials through stewardship programs has been shown to reduce infections.[54,55] If possible, a multidisciplinary team or committee should design and monitor the policies.

The team should include an infectious disease physician, medical staff from all services, a clinical pharmacist(s)—potentially one who specializes in infectious diseases—a microbiologist, and the infection control physician or practitioner. There should be active communication from the ASP, which often reports to the pharmacy and therapeutics committee of the medical staff or to the infection control committee. The use of decision algorithms and international, national, or organizational guidelines to develop antimicrobial-use policies can be helpful.

Suggestions for designing an effective ASP include the following[54,55]:

- Assess the current status of antimicrobial prescribing in the organization.
- Provide education and resources, such as articles and training sessions, on new and existing antimicrobial options to prescribing HCWs.
- Provide mandatory in-services about proper use of antimicrobials in surgical and nonsurgical situations. Clinical education can be effective when it is intensive, repeated, and combined with other modalities.
- Engage a clinical pharmacist if one is available to make rounds with physicians. In many cases, a pharmacist can identify prescribing errors and suggest alternatives. If no clinical pharmacist is available, a pharmacist with an interest in the field may substitute.
- Create a formulary that requires approval of restricted drugs. This option can be highly effective in reducing the prescription of targeted drugs but may be unpopular among some physicians and, in some cases, may result in the increased use of nonrestricted drugs. Restricted formularies should be reassessed often.
- Provide a prophylactic antibiotic "forcing function" to ensure proper administration. A forcing function is a feature of a designed intervention that must be performed before another specific action can occur.[56] In the case of prophylactic antimicrobial agents before surgery, a forcing function might be a dedicated nursing professional who screens all surgical patients for prophylactic antimicrobials prior to surgery to determine a patient's candidacy for antimicrobials and to ensure that the proper drugs and doses are given in the correct time frame.
- Develop checklists to make sure that appropriate consideration is made before prescribing an antimicrobial and that the drugs are administered in a timely manner (for example, before surgical incision or within a specified time limit after admission).
- Use a computer-assisted decision system. Although potentially valuable, this type of system can be quite expensive. Organizations should conduct a cost-benefit analysis on this type of system before purchasing one.[57]
- Compare rates with acceptable databases. Track antimicrobial prescribing patterns and administration patterns to monitor rates and to benchmark them against rates in external organizations. Data should be provided periodically to the clinical and leadership staff.

- Create a comprehensive program with multiple strategies designed for the unique characteristics and culture of the organization

For more information on antimicrobial stewardship programs, see The Cost of Antibiotic Resistance, a free toolkit available for download at the Joint Commission Resources site at http://www.jcrinc.com/MDRO-Toolkit/. SHEA also offers several MDRO related resources, including the following:

- SHEA Featured Resources on Antimicrobial Stewardship, http://www.shea-online.org/GuidelinesResources/Featured TopicsinHAIPrevention/AntimicrobialStewardship.aspx

- SHEA/IDSA Joint Guidelines on Antimicrobial Stewardship (2003 and 2007), http://www.shea-online.org /GuidelinesResources/FeaturedTopicsinHAIPrevention /AntimicrobialStewardship/Guidelines.aspx

- Antimicrobial Stewardship in Practice: An Online Educational Series for Healthcare Professionals, https:// www.extendmed.com/antimicrobial/home.html?

For an example of how one organization employed antibiotic stewardship to reduce unnecessary antimicrobial prescription without changing mortality rates and improving quality of patient care, *see* Case Study 6-4.

Animate Transmission

Patient A → Health Care Worker → Patient B

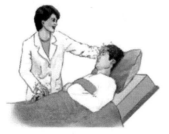

Inanimate Transmission

Patient A → Health Care Worker's Stethoscope → Patient B

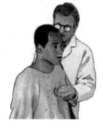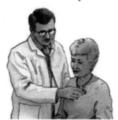

Interaction Between Animate and Inanimate Transmission

Patient A → Infusion Pump → Health Care Worker → Patient B

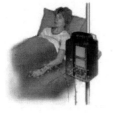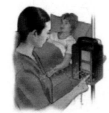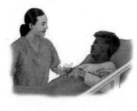

Figure 6-2: Animate Transmission, Inanimate Transmission, and Interaction Between Animate and Inanimate Transmission

Source: Weber S, Soule BM, editors: *What Every Health Care Executive Should Know: The Cost of Antibiotic Resistance.* Oak Brook, IL: Joint Commission Resources, 2009; adapted from Pittet D, et al. Evidence-based model for hand transmission during patient care and the role of improved practices. *Lancet Infect Dis.* 2006 Oct;6(10):641–652.

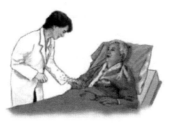

CASE STUDY 6-4

Antimicrobial Stewardship and Impact on Antimicrobial Prescription, Antimicrobial Resistance, and Mortality (Thailand)

Romanee Chaiwarith, MD, MHS *(SHEA International Ambassador)*; **Peninnah Oberdorfer, MD, PhD; Parichat Salee, MD; Chaicharn Pothirat, MD; Nontakan Nuntachit, MD; Lalita Norasethada, MD; Kaweesak Chittawatanarat, MD; Yaowapha Shaijarernwana, BSc, MSc; Manasanant Bunchoo, MSc; Aree Goonna, MNS; Atcharaporn Angsuratanawech, MSc; Wattana Nawachareon, MD**

Introduction

Antimicrobial resistance is now a major issue confronting health care providers and patients. We performed a surveillance study of antimicrobial resistance among bacterial pathogens isolated from hospitalized patients at Chiang Mai University Hospital, Muang, Chiang Mai, Thailand, from 2006 to 2009. Gram-negative bacilli were the majority pathogens isolated from clinical specimens (75%). The three most common pathogens were *Escherichia coli*, *Pseudomonas aeruginosa*, and *Acinetobacter baumannii*.

Ceftazidime-resistant *P. aeruginosa* was found in 41.8% (in 2006), 36.0% (in 2007), 33.3% (in 2008), and 34.9% (in 2009). Carbapenem resistant *A. baumannii* was found in 67.1% (in 2006), 74.2% (in 2007), 68.9% (in 2008), and 74.3% (in 2009). Among carbapenem-resistant *A. baumannii*, the isolates were susceptible to cefoperazone/sulbactam in 66.0% (in 2006) and 93.4% (in 2007), and then declined to 37.4% (in 2008) and 20.5% (in 2009). Extended-spectrum-lactamase (ESBL)–producing

Enterobacteriaceae was more prevalent in *E. coli* (53.3%–62.4%) than in *Klebsiella pneumonia* (52.2%–56.5%). MRSA was found in 34.8% (in 2006), 34.8% (in 2007), 39.5% (in 2008), and 44.3% (in 2009). Clinical isolates from the ICUs and intermediate care units had higher rates of resistance to various antimicrobial agents than clinical isolates from general units.

Increasing antimicrobial resistance, high costs of new antimicrobial agents, and toxicity of old antimicrobial agent (colistin), limit the option for treating patients infected with multidrug-resistant bacteria, which resulted in unfavorable outcomes. Antimicrobial stewardship is one of the promising interventions to reduce antimicrobial resistance. We, therefore, implemented an antimicrobial stewardship program to determine the effect on antimicrobial prescription, antimicrobial resistance, and mortality rate in our hospital.

An antimicrobial stewardship committee was first established at the end of 2009. The core of the committee was comprised of the heads the Divisions of Infectious Diseases of the Department of Medicine and Pediatrics. The rest of the committee was comprised of representatives from the Department of Medicine (the divisions of infectious diseases, pulmonology, critical care, immunology, and hematology), the Department of Pediatrics (the division of infectious diseases), the Department of Surgery, the Department of Orthopedic Surgery, pharmacists, clinical microbiologists, infection preventionists, and information technologists.

Methods

A quasi-experimental study was conducted from January 2008 to December 2009. The study consisted of a 12-month baseline observation period (1 January 2008–31 December 2008; period 1), followed by a 12-month intervention period (1 January 2009–31 December 2009; period 2). The intervention was implemented as a hospitalwide measure. The intervention included 2 strategies: (1) educating health care personnel on antimicrobial prescribing, including antimicrobial selection, dose optimization, de-escalation of therapy, and parenteral to oral conversion; and (2) antimicrobial approval for six antimicrobial agents, including the carbapenems (meropenem, imipenem), piperacillin/tazobactam, cefoperazone/sulbactam, colisitn, and vancomycin, using antimicrobial order forms and health care information technology. All cases that needed these six antimicrobial agents were reviewed by infectious disease specialists, critical care physicians, and pulmonologists. Discussion and feedback about the appropriate use of

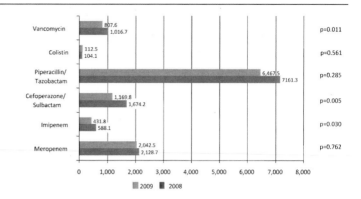

Figure 1. The Monthly Prescription (grams) of Restricted Antimicrobial Agents

restricted antimicrobial agents was carried out with the prescribers as necessary. The antimicrobial susceptibility patterns of isolates and mortality of patients infected or colonized with these six pathogens were monitored; namely, *P. aeruginosa*, *A. baumannii*, ESBL–producing *K. pneumoniae* and *E. coli*, MRSA, and enterococci.

Outcomes included (1) prescription of antimicrobial agents, (2) the antimicrobial susceptibility patterns of the six pathogens, and (3) mortality of patients infected or colonized with those six pathogens.

Statistical analysis

All data were presented in numbers (%); mean and standard deviation (SD) as appropriate. Comparisons of data were performed using Student's *t*-test. A two-sided test at a *p* value of < 0.05 was used to indicate statistical significance. All statistical analyses were performed using statistical data software.

Results

Antimicrobial Prescription

The monthly hospital antimicrobial dosages in period 2 were reduced as compared to period 1 by 30% (*p* = 0.005) for cefoperazone/sulbactam, 26.6% for imipenem (*p* = 0.03), and 20.6% for vancomycin (*p* = 0.011). The dosage reduction was not statistically significant for piperacillin/tazobactam, meropenem, and colisitn (*see* Figure 1).

The reduction in antimicrobial prescription translated into a savings of more than US$30,000 per month, or a total of approximately US$400,000 per year. We also monitored nonrestricted antimicrobial prescription, including ceftazidime, ciprofloxacin, ertapenem, and fosfomycin. There was no statistically significant change in these antimicrobial prescribed between period 2 and period 1, all *p* values being > 0.05.

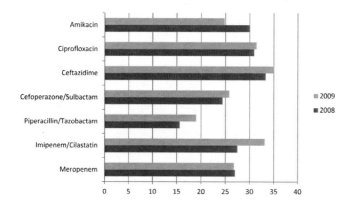

Figure 2. Percentage of Various Antimicrobial Resistances for *P. aeruginosa*

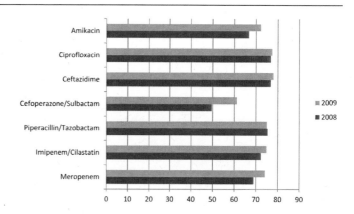

Figure 3: Percentages of Various Antimicrobial Resistances for *A. baumannii*

Antimicrobial Susceptibility Patterns of 6 Pathogens

There were no differences in antimicrobial susceptibility patterns between period 1 and period 2 for *P. aeruginosa* (Figure 2) and *A. baumannii* (Figure 3). The percentages of ESBL–producing *K. pneumoniae* were not different between the 2 periods. ESBL–producing *E. coli* decreased from 61.6% in 2008 to 53.3% in 2009. The percentages of MRSA increased from 39.5% in 2008 to 44.3% in 2009, but the change did not reach statistical significance.

Mortality rate

The mortality rates in period 1 and period 2 were not different for all sentinel pathogens (all *p* values > 0.05)

Discussion

Our study demonstrated the effectiveness of an antimicrobial stewardship program in a 1,500-bed, tertiary care hospital in Thailand. It reduced antibiotic prescriptions by 20%–30%, which translated into a large amount of cost savings. This finding corresponded to previously published reports. However, the antimicrobial resistance patterns were not affected by the program. A longer period of follow-up is needed to determine the ecology changes of these pathogens. The crude mortality rate of patients infected with these particular pathogens was not increased after the implementation.

Limitations

This study has several limitations. First, due to scarcity of the personnel who can evaluate the appropriateness of antimicrobial uses in each case, we did not measure the appropriateness of antimicrobial prescription after the implementation of the program, which is one of the interesting outcomes from antimicrobial stewardship. Second, we did not adjust for other confounding factors regarding mortality rate. We plan

to continue this program, and will explore more data regarding those missing issues.

Conclusions

This finding suggested that antimicrobial stewardship resulted in reduction in unnecessary antimicrobial prescription, without change in mortality rates. Antimicrobial stewardship is one of the programs that improve quality of patient care. This program should be implemented in the hospitals, particularly the tertiary care hospitals, where patients are seriously ill and many broad-spectrum antibiotics are available.

Lessons Learned

An effective antimicrobial stewardship program needs the support and collaboration of hospital administration, and it requires a multidisciplinary team of staff members.

Ensuring HCW Health

A critical aspect of any health care organization's IPC program is having effective policies to protect the health of its HCWs. For example, every year, outbreaks of influenza cause millions of people to get sick. HCWs are not exempt from disease and can develop influenza and other infections that, untreated, can cause significant risk to them and harm to their patients.[58,59]

One way to address this problem is to have strict policies in place that outline when an employee can and, more importantly, *cannot* report for work. For example, if an employee has an elevated temperature or infected wound, policies should dictate that he or she stay away from work until the temperature is normal for a designated period of time or until the wound heals and there is no drainage. If an employee is exposed to varicella, the organization should have policies that can be used by managers, employee health services, and the IPC team to evaluate the exposure risk, to determine diagnostic tests, and to implement restriction guidelines to protect the HCWs and to prevent exposure to others. WHO[60] and the US CDC[61] have published guidelines designed to provide methods for reducing the transmission of infections from patients to HCWs and from HCWs to patients. These guidelines include recommended periods of absence from work, restrictions in the workplace, and time frames for returning to work based on the pathogen or disease.

Employee health programs include several key elements, such as the following:

- Management of job-related illnesses and exposures, including postexposure follow-up
- Work restrictions for HCWs who acquire communicable diseases that can be transmitted to other HCWs, patients, or visitors[61]
- Designated authority for restricting HCWs from the organization when necessary and monitoring return-to-work policies
- Counseling for HCWs about personal infection risks, preventing the acquisition of work-related infections, and postexposure counseling[62]
- Records and documentation of HCW conditions
- Vaccinations for preventable communicable diseases, such as influenza, measles, varicella, hepatitis A and B, and other infections relevant to infection risks in specific countries or locales. The US CDC has issued several guidelines on immunizations for HCWs in the United States, most recently in 2011.[63]

The collaboration of employee health and infection prevention is critical to protecting HCWs from infections. Working together to ensure an effective tuberculosis prevention program or to evaluate an exposure situation, such as from a norovirus outbreak or meningococcal exposure, helps.

Cleaning, Decontaminating, Disinfecting, and Sterilizing Equipment and Supplies

In addition to the hands of HCWs, such equipment as surgical instruments and endoscopes can transmit pathogens to patients[64–67], and supplies such as bed linens and mattresses can have high counts of microorganisms and serve as reservoirs for potential transmission of organisms.[68–69] Individuals responsible for maintenance and repair of the equipment, cleaning, disinfection, or sterilization procedures are at risk of exposure to infectious organisms. To ensure that best practices are implemented at all times in all areas where equipment and supplies are processed, these functions should be centralized whenever possible. One organization's work in this area is examined in Case Study 6-5.

CASE STUDY 6-5

Centralization of Instrument and Equipment Reprocessing (Canada)

Sandra Callery, RN, MHSc, CIC

Introduction

It is a Sunnybrook Health Sciences Centre (SHSC; Toronto, Ontario, Canada) policy to verify that all equipment being reprocessed at SHSC is reprocessed in accordance with hospital policies and Canadian standards, per the Canadian Standards Association.

Each medical program and department manager is responsible for verifying that all equipment reprocessed in his or her area is being reprocessed appropriately for that equipment and in accordance with SHSC policies. Canadian guidelines recommend that, wherever possible, reprocessing should be performed in a centralized area that complies with the physical and human-resource requirements for reprocessing.

The annual review of practices and processes identified multiple hospital areas and outpatient clinics that were reprocessing their own equipment. However, the annual review also revealed that many were unable to maintain adequate cleaning and disinfection requirements. There were limitations with the work space and ventilation. HCW turnover made ongoing education and training a challenge and inhibited full compliance with protocols.

Based on these reports from the Reprocessing Steering Committee, the IPC Committee recommended that wherever possible, all instrument reprocessing be centralized.

Methods

A checklist was distributed to all managers to determine what type of cleaning, disinfection, and sterilization of instruments and equipment was in place in their department.

Staff and departments involved included representation from senior leadership and the following teams and departments: IPC, operating room, ambulatory care, central reprocessing, and materials management. The steering committee had a reporting structure to the IPC Committee and the hospital's Medical Advisory Committee.

Scheduled walkabouts were conducted by the managers of the Centralized Sterilization and Disinfection Service (CSD) and IPC. Walkabouts observed physical space allocated to the cleaning and disinfection process. Areas for storing the clean and sterile instruments were also inspected. Documentation of disinfection or sterilization processes was verified. Based on the observations and compliance with best practices, areas were prioritized for centralization.

Meetings were conducted with the manager or team leader of the area involved as well as the medical and operations directors to explain the centralization process and delivery. Turnaround time for equipment and instruments and additional inventory to be purchased was also discussed. The CSD educator and senior technician were also part of the discussions to ensure familiarity with the instruments involved and to validate the manufacturers' recommendations for sterilization methods.

Once the centralization was complete, daily feedback and follow-up with the end users was delivered, and any significant breakdown in any part of the reprocessing process that potentially compromised patient care was documented through an electronic incident record.

Results

Centralization has occurred over the course of three years. With the exception of three clinics, all areas of the hospital are now centralized for cleaning and sterilizing reusable instruments and equipment. Due to high equipment turnover, three outpatient clinics continue to reprocess their scopes at point of care. The utility spaces were reviewed, and these spaces were retrofitted as required to meet best-practice guidelines and occupational health regulations when using chemicals for high-level disinfection. For the very busy endoscopy suite, the CSD department is now responsible for the reprocessing staff in endoscopy, providing ongoing training and biannual recertification. Upgrades in washers and disinfectors in the CSD have also occurred during this time, creating safe efficiencies. Overall feedback from the staff has been favorable, with seamless delivery of sterile supplies and instruments.

Lessons Learned

Centralization of sterilization processes must be done with open discussion and collaboration with the end users. It is important to provide education and awareness about reprocessing requirements to the patient care areas. Reassurances of good quality-control measures and accountability help encourage compliance with the new process. Mechanisms for communication and incident documentation are critical.

To ensure that equipment and supplies are cleaned properly, organizations should have policies and procedures in place that address the following issues:

- Which equipment and supplies can be cleaned and reused, as opposed to those that are disposable?

- When and how often must equipment and supplies be cleaned?
- What are the most effective cleaning, disinfection, and sterilization processes and agents?
- How will disposable equipment—that is, single-use devices (SUDs)—that must be reused be cleaned, disinfected, or sterilized?
- What SUDs can never be reused?
- Who will keep the records of reused SUD processing?

Guidelines exist for cleaning, disinfecting, and sterilizing health care equipment, including recommended evidence-based practices, options for agents, monitoring processes, storage and transport practices,[70] and protocols to follow when there is a failure to follow disinfection and sterilization principles.[71]

All HCWs who clean, disinfect, sterilize, repair, and maintain equipment should be involved in developing the policies that define practices for their areas of responsibility. Organizations without on-site services that contract with external vendors should nevertheless develop procedures and policies that ensure that these persons are protected from contamination and disease transmission.

Cleaning and disinfecting equipment. Equipment should be cleaned and disinfected before and after each patient use as well as when it passes from one department to another. For example, all equipment should undergo appropriate decontamination before reaching an equipment-maintenance department and then again before returning to the direct-care environment.

Four types of processing can help remove dirt, body fluids, and pathogens from equipment. Depending on the type of equipment and its intended use, one of the following methods should be used to process equipment[71]:

- Cleaning—removes all visible dust, soil, and any other visible material that microorganisms might find favorable for continued life and growth. This is usually done by scrubbing with hot water and detergent.
- Decontamination—removes disease-producing organisms, rendering equipment safe to handle
- Disinfection—destroys most disease-producing organisms but not all microbial forms. There are three levels of disinfection:
  1. High level—kills all organisms except high levels of bacterial spores
  2. Intermediate level—kills mycobacteria, most viruses, and bacteria
  3. Low level—kills some viruses and bacteria
- Sterilization—destroys all forms of microbial life, including bacteria, viruses, spores, and fungi

Sidebar 6-1. Processing Endoscopes

Certain types of medical equipment are more difficult to effectively clean than others. For example, endoscopes can be particularly challenging. They are used to diagnose and to treat medical conditions of the gastrointestinal tract, lungs, and other sites. The incidence of infections related to endoscope use is low,[1] but these devices have been linked to many health care–associated outbreaks.[1]

As with any medical device, it is important to follow the manufacturer's cleaning instructions, to train HCWs carefully about cleaning methods, and to test their competency before they perform the cleaning and disinfection. One competency review form is shown in Figure 6-3.

Detailed instructions are available on how to effectively clean endoscopes. Manufacturer guidelines and package directions for use of equipment and disinfecting or sterilizing agents should be followed at all times. The following are some helpful tips for manual processing:

- Meticulously clean the endoscope external and internal surfaces with an enzymatic detergent immediately after use.
- Test the endoscopes for leaks.
- Disconnect and immerse all endoscopic components and immerse in the enzymatic cleaner. Steam sterilize heat-stable parts.
- Flush and brush all accessible channels to remove organic materials.
- Brush all channels until no debris appears on the brush. Use disposable brushes for cleaning or make sure that brushes receive high-level disinfection or sterilization.
- Disinfect the endoscope in a high-level disinfectant or chemical sterilant, making certain the agent reaches all surfaces, channels, and crevices. Use approved chemical agents for high-level disinfection, including glutaraldehydes, orthophthaladelhydes, hydrogen peroxide, or hydrogen peroxide and peracetic acid.
- Rinse the endoscope with sterile water, filtered water, or tap water.
- Dry the insertion tube and channels with alcohol and forced air.
- Store the endoscopes in a vertical position so they dry effectively and in a manner to prevent contamination.

Reference

1. US Centers for Disease Control and Prevention. Guideline for Disinfection and Sterilization in Healthcare Facilities, 2008. Rutala WA, Weber DJ, Healthcare Infection Control Practices Advisory Committee, 2008. Accessed 17 Sep 2011. http://www.cdc.gov/hicpac/pdf/guidelines/Disinfection_Nov_2008.pdf.

In 1968 E. H. Spaulding devised a classification system for determining the appropriate cleaning strategy for equipment.[72] Organizations might want to use this system to determine the category and method for decontamination of equipment. Spaulding classified items for patient care into three categories: critical, semicritical, and noncritical. These terms refer to the intended use of the device and not the potential degree of contamination. For example, the noncritical category does not imply that items cannot carry contaminants but that their degree of causing harm to HCWs and patients is not critical. Examples of each category include the following:

- Critical—Items in this category need to be sterilized. They include devices that enter or come into contact with sterile tissues, such as instruments entering a surgical incision, cardiac and vascular catheters, implants, and needles placed into the vascular system.
- Semicritical—Items in this category generally require a high level of disinfection. These include items that come into contact with nonintact skin or mucous membranes, such as respiratory-therapy equipment, vaginal probes, anesthesia equipment, and flexible endoscopes.
- Noncritical—Items in this category require basic cleaning and low-level decontamination. Items that touch only intact skin would fall into this category because the skin acts as an effective barrier to most microorganisms. Such items can include crutches, bed boards, blood-pressure cuffs, bedpans and urinals, and a variety of other medical accessories as well as nonmedical accessories, such as recreational equipment.

When designing policies and procedures for equipment cleaning, organizations must make sure that such policies and procedures apply to all equipment within the organization, including equipment not owned by the organization, such as demonstration, substitute, loaner, or rental units. Because such equipment moves from person to person or organization to organization and is exposed to an unknown variety of potentially infectious agents, safe practices must include appropriate cleaning of equipment before it enters and exits the organization or is used on another patient.

Organizations can help remind HCWs which equipment should be cleaned, by what methods, and how frequently with noticeable, easy-to-read labels. Checklists can be used to help ensure that HCWs follow all the procedures necessary to effectively clean or disinfect the equipment. Logbooks that record the performance of decontamination procedures should be available and regularly monitored to document that proper cleaning procedures are being performed. *See* Sidebar 6-1 for more information about processing endoscopes.

University of North Carolina Health Care System
Endoscope Reprocessing Competency

I have read the University of North Carolina Hospitals Endoscope Infection Control Policy and the Safety Policy on Glutaraldehyde Control before presenting for competency review.

COMPETENCY CRITERIA:

Circle appropriate

outcome measure: **Competencies**

			Competencies
Met	Not Met	N.A.	Verbalizes knowledge of cleaning and disinfecting solutions used, labeling, length of effective use life and soak times.
Met	Not Met	N.A.	Documents concentration of glutaraldehyde appropriately (e.g., if used daily, test daily).
Met	Not Met	N.A.	Wears personal protective equipment, including gown, gloves, eyewear.
Met	Not Met	N.A.	Demonstrates initial gross decontamination of exterior of scope and accessories. Wipes exterior of scope with clean cloth soaked in detergent or enzymatic cleaner.
Met	Not Met	N.A.	Correctly tests scopes for leaks – "leak testing"
Met	Not Met	N.A.	Uses suction to fill channels with detergent or enzymatic cleaner.
Met	Not Met	N.A.	Demonstrates the process of manual washing and brushing of all channels, ports, and valves with appropriately prepared detergent or enzymatic cleaner.
Met	Not Met	N.A.	Brushes lip of biopsy port.
Met	Not Met	N.A.	Rinses exterior of scope, uses suction to rinse interior until fluid is clear, ends by suctioning air to clear fluid from scope.
Met	Not Met	N.A.	Fills interior channels with glutaraldehyde and immerses completely to prevent air bubbles. Utilizes 20-minute immersion time.
Met	Not Met	N.A.	Demonstrates the proper use of the automatic processor. Verbalizes knowledge of test cycles before and after use. Uses biological and chemical indicators.
Met	Not Met	N.A.	Avoids contaminating clean and/or disinfected items with dirty gloves. Washes hands after removing dirty gloves. Dons clean gloves prior to removing scope/accessories from glutaraldehyde.
Met	Not Met	N.A.	Rinses scope with sterile water, filtered water, or tap water. Uses "clean" suction.
Met	Not Met	N.A.	Uses forced air to dry the scope followed by alcohol to assist in drying, then purges scope with forced air.
Met	Not Met	N.A.	Demonstrates proper cleaning, high-level disinfection, rinsing, and drying of all accessories.
Met	Not Met	N.A.	Demonstrates proper cleaning and sterilization of biopsy forceps and other cutting instruments that enter sterile body sites.
Met	Not Met	N.A.	Labels or packages disinfected scopes/accessories to indicate disinfection has been done.
Met	Not Met	N.A.	Is able to state conditions indicating a scope has not been disinfected (e.g., if not labeled or packaged, scope is considered contaminated and requires high-level disinfection prior to use).
Met	Not Met	N.A.	Properly stores scope/accessories in a clean location.
Met	Not Met	N.A.	Empties and disinfects water bottles.
Met	Not Met	N.A.	Disinfects brushes.
Met	Not Met	N.A.	Empties and cleans pans.
Met	Not Met	N.A.	Removes personal protective equipment and discards appropriately.
Met	Not Met	N.A.	Washes hands before leaving reprocessing room.

I certify that this individual has met all competencies for reprocessing endoscopes.

Signature:_____   Date:_____

Print Name:_____   Title:_____

Figure 6-3. Endoscope Reprocessing Competency

Source: North Carolina Statewide Program for Infection Control and Epidemiology (SPICE) and William A. Rutala, PhD, MPH, CIC. Available online at http://www.unc.edu/depts/spice/dis/Endoscope.html. Used with permission.

Sterilization. Sterilization is used to meet Spaulding's criteria to render critical items free from organisms. Steam sterilization is highly reliable and is considered the first choice when a device is heat-tolerant. The steam conveys heat efficiently, but it is essential that the process reach all surfaces that must be sterile. Steam sterilizers are available using gravity displacement and prevacuum methods[73] Autoclaving for immediate use (flash sterilizing) should be used only when absolutely necessary, such as when an instrument is inadvertently contaminated during surgery and no replacement is available.[73] Immediate-use sterilization refers to short-duration high-temperature autoclaving without wrapping the device. When sterilized, the device must be transported to the operating table in a manner that maintains sterility.[73] Other methods of sterilization are described in Table 6-1.

A wide variety of chemical agents is useful for either disinfection or sterilization, including peracetic acid/hydrogen peroxide, glutaraldehyde, hydrogen peroxide, ortho-phthalaldehyde, and peracetic acid. All have advantages and disadvantages, as listed in Table 6-2, adapted from the US CDC *Guideline for Disinfection and Sterilization in Healthcare Facilities, 2008.*[70] The manufacturer's recommendations should be carefully followed, and the appropriate agent should be selected for the device to be processed.

Reuse of single-use devices. The reuse of single-use devices (SUDs) presents an infection and safety risk to patients. SUDs are constructed to be used one time, and repeated uses may result in breakage or changes in material from reprocessing or may involve complex cleaning and disinfection or sterilization that, if performed inadequately, may pose an infection risk. Countries that cannot afford disposable devices, are unable to obtain an adequate continual supply, or do not fully appreciate the risks may routinely or sporadically reuse SUDs. JCI has integrated several requirements into its standards to guide organizations in decision making and the process of using SUDs when necessary. *See* Chapter 3 and 4, as well as Appendix 1, for more information. Of great concern as related to resuse of SUDs are unsafe injection practices involving the reuse of syringes and needles. Box 6-1 describes some of these challenges and prevention strategies.

Laundry. Large amounts of linen are generated during the care of patients. This linen can be heavily contaminated with organisms ranging from those that are nonpathogenic to highly resistant MDROs. Thus, linen must be handled properly to minimize the dispersion of microorganisms and to protect the environment and HCWs from contact with the organisms. All organizations should have clear processes for the routine handling of soiled or contaminated linen. *Soiled linen* has been used or worn and is dirty or stained by perspiration, body oils, or other substances. *Contaminated linen* has been soiled by blood or has been in contact with potentially infectious materials.[74] Studies have demonstrated that linens can serve as vehicles for the transmission of organisms,[75,76] emphasizing the need for a safe and effective laundry process. Most organizations carefully separate dirty from clean linen. Linen generated during care should be contained (for example, placed in bags) at the point of use in a leak-resistant container. Any sorting of linen should be done with minimal agitation away from the patient care setting, preferably in a negative-pressure area and by HCWs wearing personal protective equipment (PPE). Laundry containers should be marked or color-coded for recognition.

To remove pathogens from soiled laundry, such as bedsheets and gowns, US CDC Environmental Guidelines recommend that laundering be performed for a minimum of 25 minutes in water with a temperature of at least 71°C (160°F) or with chlorine bleach.[77] Chemicals used in the laundry should be selected for the water temperature and the proper use concentration. After laundering, the linen should be packaged and stored or transported to prevent contamination. Clean laundry can be used for routine care and sterile linen for surgical procedures when required. Laundry from isolation rooms should be carefully collected by HCWs, preferably using a folding or rolling process, and placed in a single fluid-resistant container. Double bagging is not necessary unless the primary bag or container leaks.

Laundry workers who handle soiled or contaminated linen should be trained in the laundering process and should wear PPE. Food, drink, and smoking should not be permitted in the workplace. Clean linen should be stored at least six inches off the floor to avoid contamination by floor mopping or dirt on the floor. Even when linens are enclosed in plastic wrap, splash and splatter from mopping and other cleaning activities can contaminate the exterior surface and may pose an infection risk.[74,77]

The patient care environment. The environment can be a significant reservoir of microorganisms and has been implicated in transmission of HAIs.[78] Microbes are efficient in surviving and proliferating in moist and dry environments, and although it is relatively easy to culture and to identify them in the environment, the evidence linking them to HAIs, with few exceptions, is limited.[79] That being said, the prudent course is to maintain a clean and sanitary setting for patient care.

Air and water have been a concern as a means of transmitting infection. Only a few pathogens have been convincingly demonstrated to be transmitted by the airborne route, including varicella-zoster virus, influenza, measles,

Table 6-1. Summary of Advantages and Disadvantages of Commonly Used Sterilization Technologies

Sterilization Method	Advantages	Disadvantages
Steam	• Nontoxic to patient, HCWs, environment • Cycle easy to control and to monitor • Rapidly microbicidal • Least affected by organic/inorganic soils among sterilization processes listed • Rapid cycle time • Penetrates medical packing, device lumens	• Deleterious for heat-sensitive instruments • Microsurgical instruments damaged by repeated exposure • May leave instruments wet, causing them to rust • Potential for burns
Hydrogen peroxide gas plasma	• Safe for the environment • Leaves no toxic residuals • Cycle time is 28–75 minutes (varies with model type), and no aeration is necessary • Used for heat- and moisture-sensitive items because process temperature is < 50°C • Simple to operate, to install (208 V outlet), and to monitor • Compatible with most medical devices • Only requires electrical outlet	• Cellulose (paper), linens, and liquids cannot be processed • Sterilization chamber size from 1.8 to 9.4 ft.^{3} total volume (varies with model type) • Some endoscopes or medical devices with long or narrow lumens cannot be processed at this time in the United States (see manufacturer's recommendations for internal diameter and length restrictions) • Requires synthetic packaging (polypropylene wraps, polyolefin pouches) and special container tray • Hydrogen peroxide may be toxic at levels greater than 1 ppm TWA
100% ethylene oxide (ETO)	• Penetrates packaging materials, device lumens • Single-dose cartridge and negative-pressure chamber minimizes the potential for gas leak and ETO exposure • Simple to operate and to monitor • Compatible with most medical materials	• Requires aeration time to remove ETO residue • Sterilization chamber size from 4.0 to 7.9 ft.^{3} total volume (varies with model type) • ETO is toxic, carcinogenic, and flammable • ETO emission regulated by US states, but catalytic cell removes 99.9% of ETO and converts it to CO_2 and H_2O • ETO cartridges should be stored in flammable-liquid storage cabinet • Lengthy cycle/aeration time
ETO mixtures 8.6% ETO/91.4% HCFC 10% ETO/90% HCFC 8.5% ETO/91.5% CO_2	• Penetrates medical packaging and many plastics • Compatible with most medical materials • Cycle easy to control and to monitor	• Some US states (for example, CA, NY, MI) require ETO emission reduction of 90–99.9% • CFC (inert gas that eliminates explosion hazard) banned in 1995 • Potential hazards to HCWs and patients • Lengthy cycle/aeration time • ETO is toxic, carcinogenic, and flammable
Peracetic acid	• Rapid cycle time (30–45 minutes) • Low temperature (50–55°C liquid immersion sterilization • Environmentally friendly by-products • Sterilant flows through endoscope, which facilitates salt, protein, and microbe removal	• Point-of-use system, no sterile storage • Biological indicator may not be suitable for routine monitoring • Used for immersible instruments only • Some material incompatibility (for example, aluminum anodized coating becomes dull) • One scope or a small number of instruments processed in a cycle • Potential for serious eye and skin damage (concentrated solution) with contact

CFC = chlorofluorocarbon, HCFC = hydrochlorofluorocarbon.

Source: US Centers for Disease Control and Prevention. Guideline for Disinfection and Sterilization in Healthcare Facilities, 2008. Rutala WA, Weber DJ, Healthcare Infection Control Practices Advisory Committee, 2008. Accessed 17 Sep 2011. http://www.cdc.gov/hicpac/pdf/guidelines/Disinfection_Nov_2008.pdf.

Table 6-2. Summary of Advantages and Disadvantages of Chemical Agents Used as Chemical Sterilants* or as High-Level Disinfectants

Sterilization Method	Advantages	Disadvantages
Peracetic acid/ hydrogen peroxide	• No activation required • Odor or irritation not significant	• Materials compatibility concerns (lead, brass, copper, zinc) both cosmetic and functional • Limited clinical experience • Potential for eye and skin damage
Glutaraldehyde	• Numerous use studies published • Relatively inexpensive • Excellent materials compatibility	• Respiratory irritation from glutaraldehyde vapor • Pungent and irritating odor • Relatively slow mycobactericidal activity • Coagulates blood and fixes tissue to surfaces • Allergic contact dermatitis • Glutaraldehyde-vapor monitoring recommended
Hydrogen peroxide	• No activation required • May enhance removal of organic matter and organisms • No disposal issues • No odor or irritation issues • Does not coagulate blood or fix tissues to surfaces • Inactivates *Cryptosporidium* • Use studies published	• Material compatibility concerns (brass, zinc, copper, and nickel/silver plating) both cosmetic and functional • Serious eye damage with contact
Ortho-phthalaldehyde	• Fast-acting high-level disinfectant • No activation required • Odor not significant • Excellent materials compatibility claimed • Does not coagulate blood or fix tissues to surfaces claimed	• Stains skin, mucous membranes, clothing, and environmental surfaces • Repeated exposure may result in hypersensitivity in some patients with bladder cancer • More expensive than glutaraldehyde • Eye irritation with contact • Slow sporicidal activity
Peracetic acid	• Rapid sterilization cycle time (30–45 minutes) • Low-temperature (50–55°C) liquid-immersion sterilization • Environmentally friendly by-products (acetic acid, O_2, H_2O) • Fully automated • Single-use system eliminates need for concentration testing • Standardized cycle • May enhance removal of organic material and endotoxin • No adverse health effects to operators under normal operating conditions • Compatible with many materials and instruments • Does not coagulate blood or fix tissues to surfaces • Sterilant flows through scope, facilitating salt, protein, and microbe removal • Rapidly sporicidal • Provides procedure standardization (constant dilution, perfusion of channel, temperatures, exposure)	• Potential material incompatibility (for example, aluminum anodized coating becomes dull) • Used for immersible instruments only • Biological indicator may not be suitable for routine monitoring • One scope or a small number of instruments can be processed in a cycle • More expensive (endoscope repairs, operating costs, purchase costs) than high-level disinfection • Serious eye and skin damage (concentrated solution) with contact • Point-of-use system, no sterile storage

* All products are effective in presence of organic soil, are relatively easy to use, and have a broad spectrum of antimicrobial activity (bacteria, fungi, viruses, bacterial spores, and mycobacteria). The above characteristics are documented in the literature; contact the manufacturer of the instrument and sterilant for additional information. All products listed above are US Food and Drug Administration (FDA)–cleared as chemical sterilants except OPA, which is an FDA–cleared high-level disinfectant.

Source: US Centers for Disease Control and Prevention. Guideline for Disinfection and Sterilization in Healthcare Facilities, 2008. Rutala WA, Weber DJ, Healthcare Infection Control Practices Advisory Committee, 2008. Accessed 17 Sep 2011. http://www.cdc.gov/hicpac/pdf/guidelines/Disinfection_Nov_2008.pdf.

Box 6-1. Unsafe Injection Practices

Unsafe injection practices exist throughout the world and expose patients to unnecessary morbidity and mortality. Many outbreaks, infection clusters, or sporadic infections may not be recognized because of time delays from exposure to clinical manifestations and because many patients who develop hepatitis B (HBV) or hepatitis C (HCV) from unsafe injections may have only mild symptoms that do not raise suspicion or link to the injection.

One study in Africa examining immunization practices found that 15%–60% of clinics reported the reuse of needles and syringes without sterilization, leading to many abscesses at the injection site.[1] A study from rural China found that up to 55% of HCWs reported reusing needles and syringes during vaccinations. This practice resulted in 135 to more than 3,000 children per 100,000 population acquiring HBV.[2] Countries with more available resources may also engage in unsafe injection practices. In the United States, the US CDC identified 51 outbreaks of HBV and HCV infection that occurred in a variety of health care settings from July 1998 to June 2009. In this report, more than 75,000 patients were notified of a potential exposure, more than 600 patients were infected with HBV or HBC, and some died.[3]

In 2000 WHO established the Safe Injection Global Network (SIGN), an initiative that works with local communities to help them establish safe injection practices. This initiative has helped prevent millions of injection-related infections each year in the developing world.[4]

Infection practitioners should be vigilant about the reuse of needles and syringes in all care settings. The following selected principles may be helpful in guiding efforts to reduce or to eliminate unsafe injection practices[5]:

- Keep syringes and needles sterile and in their packaging until use and store them to prevent contamination.
- Ensure that each patient has a sterile syringe; do not use the same syringe on more than one patient, even if the needle is changed, and do not use the same syringe for injecting more than one patient, regardless of whether the plunger is pulled back before the injection. Different syringes should be used for drawing blood or infusing medications. Do not share syringes among patients.
- Ensure that sterile needles and syringes are used for all injections, regardless of whether the route is intravenous, intramuscular, or intradermal. Use a sterile needle for each patient, and use a needle only once for one process.
- Prepare the syringe with medication immediately before administration. Do not access a vial of medication with a used needle or syringe.
- Never prepare injectable medications in a contaminated workspace; use a clean, dry area with no dirty supplies, and do not prepare injectable medications in patient care areas where they might contact blood or body fluids.
- Do not store or save syringes that have been removed from their packaging for later use, and do not hold syringes in pockets of clothing.

More extensive guidance is found in the additional resources listed below.

Organizations may face challenges in implementing safe injection practices. It is important to identify barriers and to address them. A template is available to help organizations use such methods as direct observation, HCW interviews, questionnaires, and practice simulations to identify barriers.[6] WHO has developed a tool for organizations to assess their current statuses on safe injection practices.[7]

Additional Resources

Ambulatory Surgery Center Quality Collaboration

Safe Injection Practices Toolkit

http://www.ascquality.org/SafeInjectionPracticesToolkit.cfm

US Centers for Disease Control and Prevention

2007 Guideline for Isolation Precautions: Preventing Transmission of Infectious Agents in Healthcare Settings

http://www.cdc.gov/hicpac/pdf/isolation/isolation2007.pdf

The One & Only Campaign

http://www.cdc.gov/injectionsafety/1anOnly.html

World Health Organization

WHO Best Practices for Injections and Related Procedures Toolkit

http://whqlibdoc.who.int/publications/2010/9789241599252_eng.pdf

References

1. Dicko M, et al. Safety of immunization injections in Africa: Not simply a problem of logistics. *Bull World Health Organ*. 2000;78(2):163–169.
2. Murakami H, et al. Risk of transmission of hepatitis B virus through childhood immunization in northwestern China. *Soc Sci Med*. 2003 Nov;57(10):1821–1832.
3. Society for Healthcare Epidemiology of America. A Review of Hepatitis B and C Virus Infection Outbreaks in Healthcare Settings 2008–2009; Opening Our Eyes to Viral Hepatitis as a Healthcare-Associated Infection. Thompson ND, et al. Paper presented at Fifth Decennial International Conference on Healthcare-Associated Infections, Atlanta. 18–22 Mar 2010. Accessed 6 Oct 2011. http://shea.confex.com/shea/2010/webprogram/Paper1744.html.
4. World Health Organization. SIGN 2010: Annual Meeting of the Safe Injection Global Network, 9–11 Nov 2010, Dubai, United Arab Emirates. Accessed 5 Oct 2011. http://www.who.int/injection_safety/toolbox/sign2010_meeting.pdf.
5. Pennsylvania Patient Safety Authority. Prevent the occurrence of bloodborne disease transmission associated with unsafe injection practices. *Pennsylvania Patient Safety Advisory*. 2011 Jun;8(2):70–76.
6. Gurses AP, et al. A practical tool to identify and eliminate barriers to compliance with evidence-based guidelines. *Jt Comm J Qual Patient Saf*. 2009 Oct;35(10):526–532.
7. World Health Organization. A Guide for Supervising Injections. 12 Feb 2004. Accessed 5 Oct 2011. http://www.who.int/occupational_health/activities/3injsuper.pdf.

and *Mycobaterium tuberculosis*. *Staphylococcus aureus* and *Streptococcus pyogenes* have been linked to airborne spread in the operating theatre from dispersers and in newborn nurseries. There is also evidence that *Aspergilllus* spores and other fungal organisms are occasionally spread through the air.[79] Even with limited spread of organisms by air, infection-prevention programs should review and ensure that their facilities have the proper airflow throughout, including in special areas where either positive or negative pressure is required, such as the operating theatre, isolation rooms, laboratories, and other critical settings.

Water is used in diagnostic and therapeutic situations in hospitals, including dialysis, hydrotherapy pools and tubs, and eyewash stations. Patients in dialysis units, burn units, and other areas are susceptible to infections from contaminated water. *Legionella* has been transmitted from contaminated water sources, such as air-cooling towers and hot-water systems,[80,81] and extensive guidance has been published to help organizations ensure that water sources are not contaminated as well as methods to address contamination when it is identified, including the superheating of water, ultraviolet exposure, hyperchlorination, and ozonization[71,79,82] Other potential environmental reservoirs include carpets in patient care areas, air-fluidized beds, soaps, flowers, animals, and linens.[79]

Organizations should address how specific areas of the facility will be cleaned and disinfected. Cooling towers, air-ventilation systems, drains, ice machines, carpeting and flooring, elevator shafts, and garbage disposal areas can all support growth of microorganisms (for example, *Legionella* and *Aspergillus*[78,83,84]) that may serve as potential reservoirs for organisms. Policies and procedures should address these areas.

Waste Management

All health care organizations generate considerable waste from patient care and support services.[85] Each organization should have a solid waste disposal system that is managed by the housekeeping or environmental services. The process for waste management should account for biohazardous, nonbiohazardous, chemical, and other wastes. Policies should be written. Examples of contaminated waste from the health care setting include microbiological specimens; anatomical materials; blood and body fluids from routine patient care activities; contaminated dressings, surgical drapes, and sponges; sharps, including needles, scalpel blades, and phlebotomy equipment; isolation waste from persons with highly infectious diseases, such as viral hemorrhagic fevers; and other infectious materials. Various countries may define biohazardous wastes differently. One assessment of medical waste from Iran estimated that each occupied bed generated 6.67 kg of waste per day, of which 73% was considered infectious and 27% noninfectious.[86] In another study from Greece, of the total medical waste generated from selected hospitals, the infectious hospital wastes varied from 0.26 to 0.89 kg/bed/day.[87]

Box 6-2 summarizes the definition of biohazardous wastes from the US Occupational Safety and Health Administration.

HCWs who manage hazardous waste are at some risk for exposure to blood and bodily fluids, sharps injuries, and other events. Thus, the waste must be handled and disposed of properly to protect the HCWs who are containing, transporting, or disposing of the waste. The organization's process for waste management should begin at the point of generation and end with final disposal, whether in the hospital or externally by a contracted agent. The most common methods to safely dispose of waste that may be considered infectious or hazardous are to incinerate it, to sterilize it, or to bury it in a protected landfill.

HCWs who manage the waste should be trained and provided with PPE, such as gowns or aprons, gloves (sturdy), and (as needed) masks and eyewear. Training on the different types of waste and the appropriate management and disposal methods is critical.[88] Education on the handling of sharps is particularly important because of the potential for the transmission of infectious agents. HCWs involved in the disposal of sharps should also receive the appropriate vaccines and immunizations (for example, the hepatitis B vaccine). Specific methods are used for different types of waste management and disposal. Systems should be in place for HCWs to report adverse events related to waste management and methods for follow-up care.[89–91] Steps for managing health care waste safely are listed in Sidebar 6-2.

WHO promotes eight steps to manage the waste stream in health care from the point of generation "cradle" to final disposal "grave."[92] Additional guidance for organizations can be found in JCI's hospital Assessment of Patients (AOP) standards, particularly AOP.5.1, Measurable Element 3; and AOP.6.2, Measurable Element 4, which refer to the need to have written policies and procedures about "handling and disposal of infectious and hazardous materials." For more information on JCI standards, *see* Chapter 3 and Appendix 1.

Construction and Renovation

Nearly all health care organizations undertake renovation or construction at some time as buildings age and deteriorate or as new facilities are needed. Because of potential infection risks to patients, the infection-prevention team is critical to the renovation and construction process. The dust and debris generated during construction can contain microorganisms, such as *Aspergillus spp* and other fungi; ventilation systems may cease to function properly, causing decreased airflow and poor filtration; and storage areas for patient supplies and equipment and critical-support service areas and patient rooms may become contaminated. The most serious concern is the severe illness and death that can occur from *Aspergillus* in immunocompromised patients during construction.[93,94]

To ensure that care delivery processes can be carried out in a safe environment that supports best practices during construction, infection practitioners must be fully engaged in the decision processes for the construction or renovation project.[95]

The IPC team has a broad array of roles in planning, reviewing, overseeing, and completing construction,[96] including the following:

- Communicating with all parties about the essential procedures for IPC during construction
- Ensuring the necessary infection control education for internal and external contractors
- Performing or assisting with the infection control risk assessment (ICRA; see below)
- Supporting requirements for safe care of the patient populations served (for example, isolation rooms, hand-hygiene equipment, air and water quality, patient and supply flow, separation of clean and dirty laundry, appropriate design and space to prevent cross-transmission during the construction project)
- Determining environmental-monitoring needs
- Clarifying accountabilities for ensuring that infection-prevention expectations are carried out during the construction process

During the design phase, the IPC team should discuss with architects and the project team how they will build into

---

Sidebar 6-2. Steps for Safe Management of Health Care Waste

- Assess waste production in the health care setting to determine how much is generated, what type, how often, and in what areas.
- Determine categories of waste, such as general, hazardous (infectious), and highly hazardous.
- Evaluate treatment and disposal options in the local region—availability, effectiveness, risk to HCWs and environment, cost.
- Select optimal disposal option(s) for the health care setting.
- Assign responsibilities within the health care establishment, train HCWs, write policies and procedures, and provide PPE.
- Determine internal processes for waste handling by the type of waste category, segregation and containment at the point of care, identification (labeling), transportation and storage, collection frequency, and other activities as appropriate.
- Determine processes for waste handling if transporting to an external waste management site, such as a community incinerator.
- Monitor the process to ensure compliance.

---

the construction such items as the appropriate types and number of sinks and hand-washing stations, disposal of general and infectious wastes, types of surfaces used on surfaces and floors to eliminate infection reservoirs, materials for ceilings, and other items.[96] Discussion should also include the necessity of adequate soiled and clean utility rooms; methods for processing, storing, and transporting patient care supplies; and the flow of equipment, people, and supplies.

Before the project begins, an infection control risk assessment (ICRA) should be performed. An ICRA is a documented process that coordinates and weighs information about the type and extent of the construction and the potential for infectious agents to affect patients, and it combines this knowledge to allow the organization to anticipate the potential impact of the project on the risk of infection and safety of patients. The ICRA is used throughout all phases of the project, from planning and design to completion. Completing the ICRA can be a joint project between the construction manager, the safety manager, and the IPC team. The first step in any ICRA is indicated in Figure 6-4; all steps of the ICRA can be found online at http://www.premierinc.com /quality-safety/tools-services/safety/topics/construction/icra.jsp.

During the construction or renovation process, the IPC team and others are responsible for ensuring that barriers are in place, that construction workers are following procedures, that

Step 1: Using the following table, identify the type of construction-project activity.

TYPE A	**Inspection and Noninvasive Activities** Includes, but is not limited to: • Removal of ceiling tiles for visual inspection only (for example, limited to one tile per 50 square feet) • Painting (but not sanding) • Wall covering, electrical trim work, minor plumbing, and activities that do not generate dust or require cutting of walls or access to ceilings other than for visual inspection
TYPE B	**Small-scale, short-duration activities that create minimal dust** Includes, but is not limited to: • Installing telephone and computer cabling • Accessing chase spaces • Cutting walls or ceiling where dust migration can be controlled
TYPE C	**Work that generates a moderate to high level of dust or requires demolition or removal of any fixed building components or assemblies** Includes, but is not limited to: • Sanding of walls for painting or wall covering • Removal of floor coverings, ceiling tiles, and casework • New wall construction • Minor ductwork or electrical work above ceilings • Major cabling activities • Any activity that cannot be completed within a single work shift
TYPE D	**Major demolition and construction projects** Includes, but is not limited to: • Activities that require consecutive work shifts • Heavy demolition or removal of a complete cabling system • New construction

Step 2: Using the following table, identify the patient risk groups that will be affected. If more than one risk group will be affected, select the higher-risk group.

Low Risk	Medium Risk	High Risk	Highest Risk
• Office areas	• Cardiology • Echocardiography • Endoscopy • Nuclear Medicine • Physical Therapy • Radiology/MRI • Respiratory Therapy	• CCU • Emergency Room • Labor & Delivery • Laboratories (specimen) • Medical Units • Newborn Nursery • Outpatient Surgery • Pediatrics • Pharmacy • Postanesthesia Care Unit • Surgical Units	• Any area caring for immunocompromised patients • Burn Unit • Cardiac Cath Lab • Central Sterile Supply • Intensive Care Units • Negative-pressure isolation rooms • Oncology • Operating rooms, including C-section rooms

Figure 6-4. Infection Control Risk-Assessment Steps for Construction and Renovation

Source: Contributors to this matrix include V. Kennedy, B. Barnard, C. Fine, A. Streifel, and J. Bartley. Forms reviewed, revised, and copyright permission provided courtesy of Judene Bartley (Jbartley@ameritech.net). Last update 2009.

Step 3: Using the grid below, match the construction type to the patient risk group.

Construction Project Type

Patient Risk Group	TYPE A	TYPE B	TYPE C	TYPE D
LOW-Risk Group	I	II	II	III/IV
MEDIUM-Risk Group	I	II	III	IV
HIGH-Risk Group	I	II	III/IV	IV
HIGHEST-Risk Group	II	III/IV	III/IV	IV

Infection Control Committee approval will be required when the construction activity and risk level indicate that Class III or Class IV (shaded gray) control procedures are necessary.

See the Description of Required Infection Control Precautions by Class in Table 1, below.

Table 1. Description of Required Infection Control Precautions by Class

	During Construction Project	Upon Completion of Project
CLASS I	1. Execute work by methods to minimize raising dust from construction operations. 2. Immediately replace a ceiling tile displaced for visual inspection.	1. Clean work area upon completion of task.
CLASS II	1. Provide active means to prevent airborne dust from dispersing into atmosphere. 2. Water mist work surfaces to control dust while cutting. 3. Seal unused doors with duct tape. 4. Block off and seal air vents. 5. Place dust mat at entrance and exit of work area. 6. Remove or isolate HVAC system in area where work is being performed.	1. Wipe work surfaces with cleaner/disinfectant. 2. Contain construction waste before transport in tightly covered containers. 3. Wet mop or wet mop and vacuum with HEPA-filtered vacuum before leaving work area. 4. Upon completion, restore HVAC system where work was performed.
CLASS III	1. Remove or isolate HVAC system in area where work is being done to prevent contamination of duct system. 2. Complete all critical barriers (for example, sheetrock, plywood, plastic) to seal area from nonwork area or implement control-cube method (cart with plastic covering and sealed connection to work site with HEPA vacuum for vacuuming prior to exit) before construction begins. 3. Maintain negative air pressure within work site utilizing HEPA-equipped air-filtration units. 4. Contain construction waste before transport in tightly covered containers. 5. Cover transport receptacles or carts. Tape covering unless solid lid.	1. Do not remove barriers from work area until completed project is inspected by the owner's Safety Department and Infection Prevention & Control Department and thoroughly cleaned by the owner's Environmental Services Department. 2. Remove barrier materials carefully to minimize spreading of dirt and debris associated with construction. 3. Vacuum work area with HEPA-filtered vacuums. 4. Wet mop area with cleaner/disinfectant. 5. Upon completion, restore HVAC system where work was performed.
CLASS IV	1. Isolate HVAC system in area where work is being done to prevent contamination of duct system. 2. Complete all critical barriers (for example, sheetrock, plywood, plastic) to seal area from nonwork area or implement control-cube method (cart with plastic covering and sealed connection to work site with HEPA vacuum for vacuuming prior to exit) before construction begins. 3. Maintain negative air pressure within work site utilizing HEPA-equipped air-filtration units. 4. Seal holes, pipes, conduits, and punctures. 5. Construct anteroom and require all personnel to pass through this room so they can be vacuumed using a HEPA vacuum cleaner before leaving work site or they can wear cloth or paper coveralls that are removed each time they leave work site. 6. All personnel entering work site are required to wear shoe covers. Shoe covers must be changed each time the worker exits the work area.	1. Do not remove barriers from work area until completed project is inspected by the owner's Safety Department and Infection Prevention & Control Department and thoroughly cleaned by the owner's Environmental Services Department. 2. Remove barrier material carefully to minimize spreading of dirt and debris associated with construction. 3. Contain construction waste before transport in tightly covered containers. 4. Cover transport receptacles or carts. Tape covering unless solid lid. 5. Vacuum work area with HEPA-filtered vacuums. 6. Wet mop area with cleaner/disinfectant. 7. Upon completion, restore HVAC system where work was performed.

Figure 6-4. Infection Control Risk-Assessment Steps for Construction and Renovation *(Continued)*

Step 4. Identify the areas surrounding the project area, assessing potential impact.

Unit Below	Unit Above	Lateral	Lateral	Behind	Front
Risk Group	Risk Group	Risk Group	Risk Group	Risk Group	Risk Group

Step 5. Identify specific site of activity (for example, patient rooms, medication room, among others).

_____

Step 6. Identify issues related to ventilation, plumbing, and electrical in terms of the occurrence of probable outages.

_____

Step 7. Identify containment measures, using prior assessment. What types of barriers are needed (for example, solid wall barriers)? Will HEPA filtration be required?

_____

(Note: Renovation/construction area shall be isolated from the occupied areas during construction and shall be negative with respect to surrounding areas.)

Step 8. Consider potential risk of water damage. Is there a risk due to compromising structural integrity (for example, wall, ceiling, roof)?

Step 9. Work hours: Can or will the work be done during non-patient-care hours?

Step 10. Do plans allow for adequate number of isolation/negative-airflow rooms?

Step 11. Do the plans allow for the required number and type of hand-washing sinks?

Step 12. Do the IPC staff agree with the minimum number of sinks for this project? (Verify against FGI Design and Construction Guidelines or other local guidelines for types and area.)

Step 13. Do the IPC staff agree with the plans relative to clean and soiled utility rooms?

Step 14. Plan to discuss the following containment issues with the project team (for example, traffic flow, housekeeping, debris removal [how and when]).

_____

_____

_____

Figure 6-4. Infection Control Risk-Assessment Steps for Construction and Renovation *(Continued)*

Appendix: Identify and communicate the responsibility for project monitoring that includes infection prevention and control concerns and risks. The ICRA may be modified throughout the project. Revisions must be communicated to the Project Manager.

Infection Control Construction Permit

			Permit No:		
Location of Construction:			Project Start Date:		
Project Coordinator:			Estimated Duration:		
Contractor Performing Work			Permit Expiration Date:		
Supervisor:			Telephone:		

YES	NO	CONSTRUCTION ACTIVITY	YES	NO	INFECTION CONTROL RISK GROUP
		TYPE A: Inspection, noninvasive activity			GROUP 1: Low Risk
		TYPE B: Small-scale, short-duration, moderate to high levels			GROUP 2: Medium Risk
		TYPE C: Activity generates moderate to high levels of dust, requires more than one work shift for completion			GROUP 3: Medium/High Risk
		TYPE D: Major duration and construction activities Requiring consecutive work shifts			GROUP 4: Highest Risk

CLASS I	1. Execute work by methods to minimize raising dust from construction operations. 2. Immediately replace any ceiling tile displaced for visual inspection.	3. Minor Demolition for Remodeling
CLASS II	1. Provides active means to prevent air-borne dust from dispersing into atmosphere 2. Water mist work surfaces to control dust while cutting. 3. Seal unused doors with duct tape. 4. Block off and seal air vents. 5. Wipe surfaces with cleaner/disinfectant.	6. Contain construction waste before transport in tightly covered containers. 7. Wet mop or wet mop and vacuum with HEPA-filtered vacuum before leaving work area. 8. Place dust mat at entrance and exit of work area. 9. Isolate HVAC system in areas where work is being performed; restore when work is completed.
CLASS III **Date** **Initial**	1. Obtain infection control permit before construction begins. 2. Isolate HVAC system in area where work is being done to prevent contamination of the duct system. 3. Complete all critical barriers or implement control-cube method before construction begins. 4. Maintain negative air pressure within work site utilizing HEPA-equipped air-filtration units. 5. Do not remove barriers from work area until complete project is checked by Infection Prevention & Control and thoroughly cleaned by Environmental Services.	6. Vacuum work area with HEPA-filtered vacuums. 7. Wet mop with cleaner/disinfectant 8. Remove barrier materials carefully to minimize spreading of dirt and debris associated with construction. 9. Contain construction waste before transport in tightly covered containers. 10. Cover transport receptacles or carts. Tape covers. 11. Upon completion, restore HVAC system where work was performed.
CLASS IV **Date** **Initial**	1. Obtain infection-control permit before construction begins. 2. Isolate HVAC system in area where work is being done to prevent contamination of duct system. 3. Complete all critical barriers or implement control-cube method before construction begins. 4. Maintain negative air pressure within work site utilizing HEPA-equipped air-filtration units. 5. Seal holes, pipes, conduits, and punctures appropriately. 6. Construct anteroom and require all personnel to pass through this room so they can be vacuumed using a HEPA vacuum cleaner before leaving work site or they can wear cloth or paper coveralls that are removed each time they leave the work site. 7. All personnel entering work site are required to wear shoe covers.	8. Do not remove barriers from work area until completed project is checked by Infection Prevention & Control and thoroughly cleaned by Environmental. Services. 9. Vacuum work area with HEPA-filtered vacuums. 10. Wet mop with disinfectant. 11. Remove barrier materials carefully to minimize spreading of dirt and debris associated with construction. 12. Contain construction waste before transport in tightly covered containers. 13. Cover transport receptacles or carts. Tape covers. 14. Upon completion, restore HVAC system where work was performed.

Additional Requirements:

	_____Exceptions/Additions to this permit Date
Date Initials	Initials are noted by attached memoranda
Permit Request By:	Permit Authorized By:
Date:	Date:

Figure 6-4. Infection Control Risk-Assessment Steps for Construction and Renovation (Continued)

patients or services at risk are relocated or protected, that airflow at the construction site directs air away from patients, that dirt and debris are managed and disposed of appropriately, that traffic is restricted as needed, and that construction is stopped if infection control guidelines are not in place.[96] As the construction is nearing completion, the IPC professionals should be part of the team that approves or commissions the new area or facility before it is occupied. At this time, items on the final checklist include assessing appropriate airflow to general and special areas, ensuring that the filters and water system are working, and verifying that all expected equipment is in place.

Additional guidance for the role of the IPC team in construction and renovation and best-practice guidelines can be found in the following resources:

- Bartley JM, Olmsted RN, editors: *Construction & Renovation*, 3rd ed.: *Toolkit for Professionals in Infection Prevention and Control*. 3rd ed. Washington DC: Association for Professionals in Infection Control and Epidemiology, Inc., 2007.
- Sehulster L, Chinn RY, Healthcare Infection Control Practices Advisory Committee. Guidelines for environmental infection control in health-care facilities. Recommendations of CDC and the Healthcare Infection Control Practices Advisory Committee (HICPAC). *MMWR Recomm Rep*. 2003 Jun 6;52(RR-10):1–42.
- Facility Guidelines Institute. *Guidelines for Design and Construction of Health Care Facilities*, 2010 ed. Accessed 1 Oct 2011. http://www.fgiguidelines.org.

Food Handling

In hospitals, long term care organizations, and other health care organizations, food and its proper handling can present a significant IPC challenge, particularly in tropical climates. When developing policies regarding food services, organizations should examine their local, regional, and national regulations and create policies that maintain the quality of food from the kitchen to the patient[97] and address the following:

- Proper food storage, including location, temperature, and expiration
- Proper labeling of food and nonfood items
- Procurement of food from sources that process food under regulated quality and sanitation controls
- Storage of nourishments/food items that are accessible and available for patient and family use, including food brought from home
- Methods to prevent contamination while making, storing, and dispensing food and ice
- The use of separate or nonabsorbent and sanitized cutting boards for meat, poultry, fish, raw fruits and vegetables, and cooked foods

- Cleaning of work surfaces after each use
- Control of lighting, ventilation, and humidity to prevent moisture, condensation, and mold growth
- Appropriate employee health requirements, including the following:
  - Routine physical examinations
  - Prohibition of food preparation by any employee with an open, infected wound
  - Specific hand-washing techniques
  - Hairnets or caps and clean, washable garments
  - Absence of food, drink, or smoking in food-preparation areas
  - Methods for dishwashing and cleaning utensils
  - Appropriate discarding of plastic utensils and other disposables
  - Control of traffic in food-service areas
  - Garbage holding, transfer, and disposal

In some health care settings, families bring and prepare food for the patients. In these situations, the hospital or clinic should develop processes and guidelines that will keep the food and patients safe, including refrigerating, discarding leftover foods, washing cooking utensils, and other measures.

The IPC team should be cognizant of clusters of diarrheal illnesses in HCWs or patients that may indicate foodborne outbreaks in the health care setting. Guidelines are available for basic food safety and for the management of these outbreaks.[98]

One organization's experience with a food-borne *Salmonella* outbreak is detailed in Case Study 6-6.

CASE STUDY 6-6

Investigation of Salmonella *Group D Food-Borne Outbreak in Staff and Patients* (Qatar)

Mamoun Elsheikh, MD; J. A. Al–Ajmi, MD; Badriya Al Ali, PhD; Fatma Saleh Zayed Al Habshi RN, IP; M. Alishaq, PhD; E. Al Maslamani, MD; Joji C. Abraham RN, IP; Bency Lukose RN, IP; Bonnie George RN, IP; Josephine C. Okoli RN, IP; Ma. Leni Basco Garcia RN, IP; Rida Alkhdour RN, IP; Ancy George RN, IP; Ahmad Al Zubi RN, IP; Hosniyah Khalil RN, IP; Joane Nader RN, IP; Sanjay Doiphode, MD; Anand Deshmukh, MD; Jamal Mohd Saleh; Bakhita Rashid; William. J Pim; Joegi C. Rabos

Introduction

The Infection Prevention and Control Program (IPC section) of Hamad Medical Corporation (HMC) in Doha, Qatar, received informal reports of several staff who had eaten dinner on 6 December 2010 during an event catered by the hospital cafeteria. The HCWs had experienced gastrointestinal illness within 72 hours of finishing their meals. Following the development of a case definition, a retrospective case-control investigation was conducted among HCWs and patients who were served food from the hospital cafeteria by the catering department. A peer-matched control group that did not eat from the same source was selected. Clinical data were collected using a standardized questionnaire. Stool samples, food, and relevant environmental samples were microbiologically investigated for the presence of enteropathogens. Infection control practices within the catering department were reviewed, and relevant gaps were addressed. Objectives of the outbreak investigation were

- to investigate and to control the food-borne outbreak;
- to define the source and the mechanism of transmission; and
- to prevent future similar episodes by enhancing the implementation of effective infection control practices.

Figure 1. Food Poisoning Questionnaire

Methods

Case Definition

Any staff member or patient who consumed any kind of food served by HMC's catering department during the period 4 December 2010–21 December 2010 and developed clinical signs and symptoms of gastroenteritis, such as abdominal pain, nausea, vomiting, fever, or diarrhea, was defined as suspected case. A probable case included any clinically compatible case (that is, epidemiologically linked to a suspected case).

A control case was any HMC staff or patient who consumed the food from HMC's catering department during the same period and did not develop signs and symptoms of gastroenteritis during the same period.

Steps Followed

Investigation of the outbreak was performed by the following HMC departments:
- IPC Program
- Microbiology
- Risk Management
- Catering

An outbreak investigation team was formed and met on a daily basis. Quality Management, Microbiology, and Catering staff also met ad hoc to review and to evaluate the situation.

Action Plan

1. Exposed participants—those who consumed food served by HMC's catering department during the period 4 December–21 December 2010 and met the above-mentioned case definition—were asked to complete an e-mail-based questionnaire (see Figure 1, above).
2. Infection control practitioners reviewed patients' records, particularly those who met the case definition, their peer controls, and the results of the stool investigation.
3. A total of 130 HCWs from catering services—preparers, servers, food handlers, catering aides from housekeeping, and others—were microbiologically screened for the presence of enteropathogens.
4. Random raw-food samples were collected and sent to the food lab for relevant investigations. Additional swabs from the butchery section, such as cutting boards, cutting surface, meat grinder, freezers, preparation surfaces in dietetics, and blender, were also relevantly screened in the same lab.

Confidentiality of the data was strictly enforced. Staff and patients who were found to be infected or colonized were appropriately treated free of charge. Infected staff did not face any charges or accrue financial losses.

Results

The questionnaire was e-mailed to all 74 event participants; 40 participants responded, for a response rate of 54%. Seventeen HCWs developed gastroenteritis. Stool cultures were available for 11 HCWs. Seven cultures were positive for *Salmonella* group D. Stool cultures of 7 patients who met the case definition were also found to be positive for *Salmonella* group D. Screening of 130 staff from the catering department revealed that 6 were found to be positive for *Salmonella* group D, and 2 of them returned from vacation and resumed their duties prior to their clinical clearance as per the infection control policy.

A total of 20 stool samples was taken as controls. (Controls are those who consumed food from the hospital cafeteria but did not develop signs or symptoms of gastroenteritis.) None was found to be positive for *Salmonella*. Screening of different food samples, the kitchen's surfaces, and controls were all found to be negative for *Salmonella* and other enteropathogens.

DNA fingerprinting (PFGE) of the all *Salmonella* group D isolates revealed that all were genetically indistinguishable and belong to the *Salmonella* serotype Enteritidis.

Staff infected with *Salmonella* were immediately taken off duty and sent to the staff clinic for further investigation and treatment. All catering staff who were involved in the preparation and distribution of food (full diet and therapeutic diet) were screened for *Salmonella* group D and other enteric pathogens, and six were found to be positive. Regular environmental rounds were conducted in catering and the dietetics department to observe adherence to infection control practices.

The Infection Control Catering policy was amended as follows:

- Food handlers (including contract workers) should be screened for stool pathogens upon pre-employment, every six months thereafter, and upon return from leave and as needed (for example, having visited endemic areas).
- The Infection Control Department should be notified immediately if any catering staff develop potential symptoms or signs of gastroenteritis.
- Stool cultures should be included in the licensing screening program of food handlers.
- Reinforce infection-prevention practices, particularly hand hygiene and use of PPE.
- Train the supervisors to monitor staff-hygiene compliance, particularly during evening and night shifts.
- After returning from vacation, staff will not be assigned to catering to work until they are medically cleared, which includes screening for gastrointestinal pathogens according to Infection Control Department catering policy.
- Develop a checklist for monitoring the staff practice.
- Appoint dedicated or fixed housekeeping staff for the catering department.

Lessons Learned

This outbreak clearly demonstrates the great potential for food handlers working in health care settings and infected or colonized with *Salmonella* to be a source of infection transmission to patients and HCWs. Therefore, strict adherence to hand hygiene and standard precautions are recommended. Regular clinical clearance should include stool cultures of food handlers, especially those returning from vacations in endemic areas and those who develop symptoms of gastrointestinal disease. Educating HCWs on the proper hygienic practices is crucial to prevent such outbreaks in the future.

Preparing for Infection Prevention and Control Emergencies in the Health Care Setting

Similar to other disasters, an IPC emergency is usually unexpected and unpredictable and has the potential of overwhelming an organization's care capabilities over a significant period of time. JCI standards require that all types of organizations have emergency management plans that mitigate, prepare for, respond to, and recover from emergencies.

Preparation for emergencies is an essential part of any IPC program. Emergencies have implications for disease transmission from infectious pathogens; disruptions in the environment, such as from floods and earthquakes; and loss of basic services, such as water and electricity for refrigeration. An organization should prepare for potential emergencies that could increase the risk of infections, beginning with an analysis of the current state of preparedness.[99,100] JCI standards require that HCWs are trained and knowledgeable about their roles in the organization's plans for fire safety, security, hazardous materials, and emergencies. One method of preparation is to "practice" possible scenarios that might affect the organization and to develop a plan to deal with them. Facility staff, including infection practitioners, should be represented at emergency-management meetings that involve the hospital and the community.

Although basic strategies will be useful in any emergency, those related to infection risks have some specific requirements. To effectively prepare for an IPC emergency, organizations must answer many questions, including the following:

- What level of risk exists?

- How will the organization determine that an infection emergency is occurring? Who will initiate the emergency-management plan?

- Are IPC professionals, emergency departments, and others monitoring the usual and unexpected infections or infection syndromes and staying informed about emerging reports from public health departments and WHO or the US CDC?

- What will the chain of command be during an emergency? How will the organization communicate effectively? How will the IPC team be notified?

- What response options are available? For example, will the organization shut down, limit services, restrict access, or transfer patients off site? Or will the organization act as the primary emergency facility for the community? How will special services manage patients during an emergency?

- If the facility remains open, how will it manage the flow of people in and out of the building?

- If the organization must care for an unexpectedly large number of patients, how will these additional persons be accommodated—in other words, what is the organization's surge capacity?

- How will the organization deal with infected patients? If isolation is warranted, how will that be accomplished? How will the organization address the safety of isolated patients? Does the organization have adequate numbers of rooms for airborne infections or the capability to house these patients in a safe environment? If appropriate, how will the organization address a mass decontamination?

- In what situations will barrier precautions be necessary? How will HCWs be trained on the appropriate use of those precautions? Will training incorporate clinical and nonclinical HCWs?

- Should quarantine or evacuation be necessary, how will it be implemented? Where will patients go? What support systems will be in place for HCWs? How will they be protected from acquiring or transmitting disease?

- What occupational health considerations will be necessary for HCWs during an emergency?

- What community resources are available? Who should be contacted and how? Who from the organization has this responsibility?

- How will the IPC emergency plan be integrated with the community? What community resources can work together?

- How will the plan be tested? JCI requires periodic testing of an organization's emergency-management plan. It is important to test the IPC component of the plan to make sure that all issues are being addressed appropriately.

What is the role for the IPC practitioner in preparing for infectious-disease emergencies? Rebmann suggests nine areas to consider[101,102]:

1. Knowledge of disasters and emergency management
2. How to assess readiness and emergency-management plans
3. Planning for infection-prevention coverage
4. Participation in disaster response and recovery
5. Health care policy development
6. Surveillance
7. Patient management
8. Physical plant issues
9. The practitioner's role as an educator

Isolating Patients During an Emergency

When an organization makes the decision to isolate a patient, it might involve placing the patient in a private room, a segregated area, or a separate building; requiring visitors and HCWs to wear PPE, such as gowns, gloves, and masks; and restricting the movement of the patient outside the room or restricting visitors. In the emergency-management plan, organizations should identify how they will isolate large numbers of patients and make sure those patients receive prompt, safe, and documented care. The organization should keep meticulous records to keep track of patient's and HCWs' responses to isolation.[103]

Organizations should have systems in place to determine how such supplies as linens, eating utensils, and clothing are provided and managed for isolated patients and should have emergency supplies of these items in stores or have plans to obtain them before there is an influx of ill patients. It is important to examine current inventories of supplies, bedding, food, and water for a disaster, an epidemic of an infectious nature, or a biological attack to determine what needs to be added for care.

Mass Decontamination

In the event of an IPC emergency, health care organizations might be required to remove biological residue from first responders, victims, and families. This would involve isolating the contaminated persons; decontaminating or treating patients; protecting HCWs, other patients, visitors, and the facility itself; and effectively reestablishing normal service. In preparing for this type of emergency, organizations should identify where contaminated victims will be housed as well as how and where they will be decontaminated, regardless of the season. Organizations should also address how they will handle and store the contaminated materials.[104]

There are a few location options for decontaminating patients. Probably the most effective place is outside the main facility. By decontaminating patients in this area, organizations can protect HCWs, equipment, and other patients from being contaminated. If the weather is hot, tents or other temporary structures can be used to maintain privacy and to protect people from direct exposure to the elements. Decontamination showers can be set up, and individuals can be "cleaned" outside before being allowed into the facility. In this case, decontamination areas should be downwind of clean areas. When it is not possible to decontaminate patients, organizations should evaluate the layouts of their facilities to determine whether the air-handling systems can be isolated to prevent the spread of contaminants throughout the buildings and whether certain rooms, corridors, or entrances might be used to isolate or to quarantine HCWs and patients.[104]

Such equipment as fire-rated plastic sheeting, duct tape, and spring-loaded poles can be used to cordon off hallways or other areas and to separate contaminated areas from clean ones. In addition, large facilities might have decontamination rooms and showers that can be used to clean patients. Smaller organizations might determine that they are not appropriately equipped to handle emergencies involving large numbers of people and should work with the community to combine resources.

A decontamination area should be set up with a "dirty" side and a "clean" side. All contaminated personnel, equipment, and victims should stay on the dirty side until decontaminated. This side should consist of a triage station, treatment station, and decontamination area. The decontamination area should accommodate ambulatory and non-ambulatory patients. Patients should perform as much of the decontamination as possible to decrease cross-contamination.

Another consideration in the mass-decontamination process is the disposal of contaminated water. Runoff from showers must be controlled so the contaminant is not tracked into clean areas. A small tub attached to each decontamination shower area can serve as a temporary holding tank, and then contaminated water can be pumped out to a larger holding area for further testing and decontamination. If a disinfectant can neutralize a biological agent, then water runoff can be allowed to go down the drain.

In addition to decontaminating patients, organizations should have plans for decontaminating equipment. Some equipment is easy to clean and would not be too difficult to decontaminate. Others, such as permanent negative-air equipment, would present more challenges for decontamination.

Integrating with the Community

No matter what the size of an organization, it is important to create an emergency-management plan for IPC that is in harmony with the needs and resources of the community.[101,104] During an IPC emergency, organizations can and should work together to identify the problem, to isolate the issues, to treat the patients, and to return to normal operations. In creating an IPC emergency plan, organizations must meet with representatives from a variety of community agencies to make sure that any response plans capitalize on the unique strengths of the facilities and departments within the community and to outline the responsibilities of those organizations. For example, organizations should meet and coordinate response plans with the following groups:

- Other health care facilities in the area, such as acute care facilities, long term care facilities, ambulatory facilities, and behavioral health care centers
- Public service organizations, such as the police and fire services, the Red Cross, hazardous-materials enforcement organizations, and emergency-management agencies
- Local and regional public health departments or services
- Other organizations, such as schools (including colleges and universities), churches, and community centers
- Civil defense–coordinating centers
- Local and area industries and businesses
- Local and area government agencies involved with the following:
  - Housing
  - Utilities
  - Special-needs populations
  - Media
  - Civilian groups
  - Disaster-assistance nongovernmental organizations

In a communitywide effort, organizations can share resources. For example, organizations can share portable decontamination units or other buildings for child care, communications, holding areas, alternative care sites, and showers. In addition, organizations can assist each other so no organization is overwhelmed. For example, in a major catastrophe, Facility A could be designated as the hospital that will supply all emergency services; Facility B, which is smaller, will therefore not be overwhelmed. Facility A will transfer nonemergency patients to Facility B, send them to other local health care settings for care, or discharge them as appropriate.

When developing an integrated response plan, organizations should plan the responsibilities for each organization as well as the communication strategies between them. Following are some tips in creating such a plan:

- Include the IPC professional as an integral part of the planning from the beginning.
- Designate a representative from each organization and department to be a member of the overall emergency-coordinating body.
- Make sure that each organization maintains its own emergency response plan (for example, a health center may have a different plan from the acute care hospital).
- Identify to whom information about the emergency should be communicated, including public health organizations and a multiorganizational emergency-management team.
- Designate multiple means of communication in case standard methods are unavailable. For example, should phone or fax systems become disabled, organizations should have plans to use radio technology or wireless and Internet communication.
- Determine how temporary credentialing and privileging policies will be assigned so personnel can "float" between organizations if necessary.
- State to whom any volunteers are to report and outline a clear line of supervision.
- Identify ways of transporting patients to and from different facilities.

No one knows when, where, and whether a biological emergency will occur, but all organizations should take the time to effectively plan for one. Addressing issues of identification, isolation, and decontamination as well as identifying the resources within a community will help organizations preserve the safety of patients and the community as a whole.

Responding to Identified Risks and Performance Deficits: An Ongoing Process

One aspect of a successful IPC program is the ongoing identification of areas of risk and practices for improvement. During such IPC activities as surveillance, environmental rounds, and observations of care-delivery practices, IPC staff should pay close attention to positive and negative outcomes and examine the processes associated with high risks. Following are some questions organizations should ask to make sure that IPC policies and procedures are appropriate and that actual practices reflect best practices and requirements[105]:

- What systems/processes/policies currently put patients, HCWs, and others at risk for infections? Which systems have been effective in minimizing infections?
- Are the appropriate systems/processes/policies in place to help prevent infections?
- Have HCWs been oriented to policies and procedures, surveillance data, and reporting processes and procedures?

- Are HCWs following organizational IPC policies?
- Are there data to evaluate compliance with policies?
- Is information about infections reported internally (for performance improvement) and externally to public health or governmental agencies?

Based on the responses to these and other questions, organizations can evaluate system breakdowns or performance deficits and develop specific interventions to improve practices. This might involve creating a new program or education initiative, implementing a performance-improvement team, or updating, revising, and creating new policies as necessary. System issues can be addressed using performance-improvement tools and a team approach (*see* Chapter 5). For example, if surveillance identifies an increase in catheter-associated bloodstream infections (CABSIs) and additional, focused surveillance indicates that the appropriate sterile barriers are not being used during the insertion of central intravenous lines, or that the hub of the line is not being cleaned before entry, these observations may indicate the lack of a clear policy and procedure, lack of HCWs' knowledge or understanding of the policy, inadequate compliance with the stated requirements for the insertion of central lines, or lack of proper equipment for the procedure. Each of these factors should be considered when performance variation is identified and analyzed (*see* Sidebar 6-3).

In a continual process of improvement, and depending on the scope of the initiative, an organization might want to apply a quality-improvement methodology, such as Plan-Do-Study-Act (PDSA), Six Sigma, Robust Process Improvement™ (RPI), or failure mode and effects analysis (FMEA), to identify performance deficits and to guide the improvement process. PDSA is a four-step method for delineating quality issues, planning, implementing, testing, and integrating methods to improve the quality of processes. This method has been used to teach medical residents to sustain improvement through quality tools and can be applied to infection-prevention strategies.[106] PDSA might be used to improve care of a patient with an indwelling urinary catheter to reduce infections. Six Sigma is a data-driven improvement methodology that strives for near perfection by eliminating defects (driving toward six standard deviations between the mean and the nearest specification limit) in any process.[107] A Six Sigma approach could be helpful in working toward zero VAP infections in an ICU. FMEA is a systematic assessment that examines a process in detail before it is implemented. The evaluation includes the sequencing of events and actual and potential risks, failures, or points of vulnerability and the impact on clients (criticality). Areas for improvement are prioritized based on this

Sidebar 6-3. Analyzing Reasons for Performance Discrepancies

An important function of every IPC program is to understand the nature of performance discrepancies. When personnel do not follow approved practices, the result is a performance discrepancy that may increase infection risk. Such discrepancies need to be corrected or improved. The infection control committee or IPC professional may be responsible for recommending the corrective action. If the nature of the performance discrepancy is correctly identified and the system issues addressed, improvement is likely to follow.

Below are three common reasons for performance deficits:[1]

1. Lack of knowledge (personnel do not know how to perform the task correctly, or they do not understand the policy or process or why it is important)
2. Systems or system support, such as lack of equipment or barriers to using or not using the equipment (personnel know how to do the task, but the equipment does not support the task, is unavailable, or does not work), or other barriers in the system preventing the desired behavior
3. Lack of motivation or management reinforcement to perform the task correctly (personnel know how, and the equipment is appropriate, but they still do the task incorrectly)[1]

Developing skills to evaluate which of these reasons contribute to inadequate performance, along with looking at each as part of a system, will increase the likelihood that corrective action will be successful.[1] For example, flexible endoscopes are challenging to clean and to achieve high-level disinfection; the process is complex with many steps. The use of an improperly cleaned or disinfected endoscope can result in HAIs.[2,3] Providing instruction for personnel on how to do the job better will improve the situation only if the cleaning and disinfecting equipment is adequate, and personnel are given the time and support to perform the work correctly. If an automated endoscope washer fails to clean properly, an education program for HCWs will not improve the situation. Likewise, if personnel rush through the cleaning phase because there are too few endoscopes for the number of procedures, education and new cleaning brushes will not improve the situation. Therefore, careful analysis

and identification of the specific problem is critical before undertaking a solution.

Hand hygiene is another process with potential performance discrepancies. If HCWs know how to clean their hands and know when it is appropriate to do so, and if alcohol-based hand rub or soap and water and towels are available but personnel still do not wash their hands properly, they may not fully understand the importance of hand hygiene, they may lack incentive, or they may be "too busy" or perceive that they lack time.[4,5] There might also be an absence of insistence from the management that hand hygiene is expected for all employees. Lack of hand hygiene may go unnoticed, and compliance with the hand-hygiene policy may not be rewarded.

When a performance issue is identified and addressed, the organization should ensure that the desired performance is acknowledged and rewarded and that inadequate performance is corrected. Purposefully addressing performance issues using this simple framework with a focus on how the system supports or inhibits performance may help improve processes and outcomes and reduce infection risks for patients and HCWs.

References

1. Mager RF, Pipe P. *Analyzing Performance Problems*. Atlanta: Center for Effective Performance, 1997.
2. Wu H, Shen B. Health care-associated transmission of hepatitis B and C viruses in endoscopy units. *Clin Liver Dis*. 2010 Feb;14(1):61–68; viii.
3. Wendelboe AM, et al. Outbreak of cystoscopy related infections with *Pseudomonas aeruginosa*: New Mexico, 2007. *J Urol*. 2008 Aug;180(2):588–592; discussion 592.
4. Mathai AS, George SE, Abraham J. Efficacy of a multimodal intervention strategy in improving hand hygiene compliance in a tertiary level intensive care unit. *Indian J Crit Care Med*. 2011 Jan;15(1):6–15.
5. Hsu LY, et al. Hand hygiene and infection control survey pre- and peri-H1N1-2009 pandemic: Knowledge and perceptions of final year medical students in Singapore. *Singapore Med J*. 2011 Jul;52(7):486–490.

process. When implementing a new process for maintenance of central intravenous lines, FMEA may be helpful for advance planning.[108] RPI is a combination of methods and tools developed to improve the quality and safety of health care. The method was developed by the US-based Joint Commission Center for Transforming Healthcare The method uses Lean Methodology (an integrated system of principles, practices, tools, and techniques focusing on standardizing solutions to common organizational problems by reducing waste, increasing value, synchronizing work flow, and managing variability in production flow).[109] It also includes Six Sigma, the change-management process,

and other change-management methodologies and tools to move health care from its current state toward the same levels of high reliability found in the commercial-aviation and nuclear-energy industries.[110] RPI has been successfully employed to increase hand-hygiene compliance. For more details, *see* Chapter 3.

As with the development of the IPC program, specific interventions to improve patient care and to reduce infection risk should involve key players in the organization. It is helpful to have a multidisciplinary team to design, implement, and monitor specific interventions regarding IPC. For example, when creating an organizationwide MDRO prevention program, representatives from nursing, medical staff, pharmacy, microbiology, patient safety and quality, infection prevention, environmental services and administration can all provide valuable input and support for the design and implementation of the program.

As an initiative is being designed, HCWs should select metrics to be used to determine whether the initiative is meeting its objectives, the desired results are sustained, and new or revised IPC needs are identified. HCWs should regularly use these metrics to measure results during and after an initiative is implemented. An organization might want to use ongoing incidence data or a "point-prevalence" or "period-prevalence" study to periodically audit or monitor the success of a particular initiative. As described in Chapter 5, incidence data monitor new events during a given time period. For example, if the improvement objective is to increase the use of appropriate sterile barriers during insertion of central lines, incidence data would look at each new instance when these barriers were or were not used during the surveillance period. Although incidence or ongoing surveillance is a valuable way to evaluate effectiveness, it can be resource intensive. An alternative is to use the prevalence-survey method. Prevalence surveillance identifies *all* instances of inadequate barriers during a defined period of time (day, month). The findings from each measurement period are compared with the previous results. Consistent findings provide confidence that the situation is stable. If there are significant changes, further analyses are performed to understand why the rates have increased or decreased. Point- and period-prevalence surveillance is an efficient and cost-effective way to achieve ongoing performance monitoring.[111,112]

When a serious infection occurs that causes or contributes to permanent harm, unexpected serious illness, or unanticipated death, these infections and the events surrounding them should be considered sentinel events, and root cause analyses (RCAs) should be undertaken. For more information about deaths and injuries related to HAIs, please see the *Sentinel Event Alert* on this topic from the US-based Joint Commission at http://www.jointcommission.org/sentinel _event_alert_issue_28_infection_control_related_sentinel _events/. The RCA will help understand how the patient acquired an infection and why the patient died or had permanent disability. An RCA, sometimes called a sentinel event analysis, carefully analyzes the key or "root" factors that may have led to the outcome. Organizations accredited by JCI are required to perform RCAs and to report the results to JCI in some circumstances, including major permanent loss of function unrelated to the patient's natural illness course or underlying condition—information that clearly applies to an HAI.

For more information on JCI's sentinel event policy, consult a current JCI accreditation manual or contact JCI Accreditation at jciaccreditation@jcrinc.com.

See Box 6-3 for tips on conducting an RCA and a link to an online tool for conducting an RCA and action plan for IPC–related or other sentinel events. The Association for Professionals in Infection Control and Epidemiology (APIC) provides an excellent example of a sentinel event analysis method for infection issues at http://www.apic.org /AM/Template.cfm?Section=Search&section=Position _Statements1&template=/CM/ContentDisplay.cfm &ContentFileID=6148. For an example of how one organization used an RCA to reduce instances of MRSA bacteraemia, *see* Case Study 6-7.

CASE STUDY 6-7

Peripheral Line–Associated MRSA Bacteraemia (Malta)

Michael A. Borg, MD, MSc(Lond), DipHIC, FRCPath, PhD; Ermira Tartari, MSc

Introduction

Mater Dei Hospital in Msida, Malta, has had an active surveillance program for MRSA bacteraemia for many years. Although infection-prevention initiatives focusing on improved hand hygiene achieved a reduction in MRSA bacteraemia, incidence rates remained unacceptably high. As a result, RCA was started—every case was assessed by the IPC department, with the physicians and nurses involved, to identify possible contributory causes. Over the first 9 months of 2010, more than 30% of MRSA bacteraemia cases were linked to preceding inflammation at the peripheral venous catheter (PVC) insertion site or duration in excess of 72 hours.

Methods

A pilot project was launched in three medical wards, with the aim of introducing PVC standardized care. Personnel involved with the project included the IPC department, infection control committee members, hospital administrators, senior and junior physicians involved in cannulation, ward managers, and all nursing staff responsible for regular daily cannula assessment and documentation.

Baseline data on 132 peripheral catheters, in situ for more than 12 hours, were collected. Each catheter was assessed for documentation of insertion date, quality of dressing, number of days in situ, and evidence of inflammation. This was undertaken in the form of the standardized

Box 6-3. Conducting a Root Cause Analysis and Action Plan in Response to a Sentinel Event

This summary of tips will help in conducting a thorough and credible root cause analysis after a sentinel event occurs in an organization:

- Assign a team to assess the sentinel event. This team should include staff at all levels, including those closest to the issue(s) and those with decision-making authority.
- Communicate the team's progress and findings to senior leaders—keep them informed.
- Create a high-level work plan that includes target dates for accomplishing specific objectives and that thus provides a tool to guide and measure progress.
- Clearly define the issues surrounding the sentinel event and be sure that the team shares a common understanding of these issues.
- Brainstorm all possible or potential contributing factors. Focus on processes, not on people, until all possible questions and factors have been exhausted.
- Sort and analyze the list of contributing factors. Constructing a cause-and-effect diagram can be very helpful in this sorting process.
- Flowchart the processes involved to determine which process or system each factor is a part of.

- Search for common causes in support systems, which allow special causes in dependent processes to occur.
- Make intermediate changes as appropriate and necessary.
- Assess progress periodically.
- Be thorough. Do not end the analysis before identifying all the root causes and taking corrective actions.
- Redesign processes to reduce the likelihood of future sentinel events and to eliminate the root causes. This might involve changes in training, policies, procedures, forms, equipment, and so on.
- Focus improvement efforts on the larger systems to eliminate the common cause of the variation.
- Measure and assess to evaluate whether the redesign produced the expected results.

The US–based Joint Commission has a practical, comprehensive tool posted on its website at http://www.joint commission.org/Framework_for_Conducting_a_Root_Cause _Analysis_and_Action_Plan/ that helps organizations conduct a complete root cause analysis and construct an effective action plan for minimizing risk for or eliminating recurrences of the same or similar sentinel events. A brief sample of that form is below.

Level of Analysis		Questions	Findings	Root Cause?	Ask "Why?"	Take Action
What happened?	Sentinel Event	What are the details of the event? (Brief description)				
		When did the event occur? (Date, day of week, time)				
		What area/service was impacted?				

Visual Infusion Phlebitis (VIP) score as recommended by the Royal College of Nurses of the UK.[1] This method sets a standardized score for the various grades of inflammation at IV insertion sites ranging from 0 (perfectly healthy) to 5 (septic thrombophlebitis). A PVC insertion and maintenance form was designed that included an *aide-mémoire* checklist and documentation of bundle implementation. PVCs had to be changed (unless medically stated otherwise) in any of the following situations:

- PVC in site for more than 72 hours or intravenous treatment stopped
- Evidence of inflammation with VIP score > 1
- Deterioration or excessive dressing soiling

Physicians and nurses in the three wards were offered regular training on the new documentation requirements and postinsertion care of PVC lines. Other measures included daily assessment of PVC lines by the ward nurses.

The documentation was then assessed through weekly infection control audits and feedback constantly given to the wards involved. A total of 153 PVCs was then assessed in the postintervention phase.

Results

Phlebitis rates (VIP score > 1) fell from 22.7% in the preintervention to 6.5% in the postintervention phase (*see* Figure 1). There was also significant improvement in dressing quality and reduction of PVC duration days. The risk of developing phlebitis was 3.47 times higher in the preintervention phase than after intervention (95 confidence interval [CI]-1.77–6.84; p = 0.0001). After the intervention, several meetings were held with the medical and nursing staff in the pilot wards through which constructive feedback was received. This resulted in improvements and modifications to the original documentation for its subsequent adoption hospitalwide.

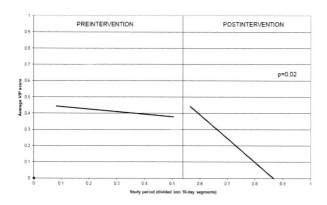

Figure 1. Time Series Graph Showing Average Documented VIP Score over the Duration of the Intervention (Grouped into 10-Day Intervals)

Results of the initiative were presented to the hospital's infection control committee as well as during hospital staff meetings, during which staff from the participating wards proved to be effective champions to convince their peers of the need to implement the initiative across the hospital and its feasibility, despite major challenges faced in bed occupancy and lack of nursing staff.

Lessons Learned

Surveillance of MRSA bacteraemia incidence and RCA were critical to identify incidence and to highlight potential causes. PVCs are a major factor contributing to MRSA bacteraemias occurring outside intensive care settings. A bundle of interventions that require PVCs to be removed after 72 hours unless medically contraindicated and immediately if no intravenous therapy is planned, to be covered by a sterile transparent dressing and to be monitored daily for inflammation using the VIP score method and removed if score exceeds 1, resulted in significant patient-safety improvement. Introduction of new initiatives must involve medical and nursing staff through educational sessions and group discussions to facilitate ownership and uptake.

Ward audits are vital to assess the impact of such measures. Most PVC–related complications, such as phlebitis, thrombosis, and bacteraemia, are preventable by simple and inexpensive interventions that can be undertaken in any setting, even in low-resource countries.

Case Study Reference

1. Royal College of Nursing. Standards for Infusion Therapy. Jan 2010. Accessed 5 Oct 2011. http://www.rcn.org.uk/__data/assets/pdf_file /0005/78593/002179.pdf.

Conclusion

This chapter has described some of the ongoing efforts to maintain and to continually improve care by reducing infection risk to patients and HCWs. It is incumbent on the IPC team to work with leaders and HCWs to look for new ways to reduce infections by staying current with best practices in the literature, assessing risks, developing evidence-based infection-prevention strategies, implementing them, and measuring accomplishments. Employing these methods will lead to improved patient safety and the quality of care.

References

1. US Centers for Disease Control and Prevention. Hand Hygiene Guidelines Fact Sheet. (Updated 25 Oct 2002.) Accessed 16 Sep 2011. http://www.cdc.gov/media/pressrel/fs021025.htm.
2. World Health Organization (WHO). *Who Guidelines on Hand Hygiene in Health Care*. Geneva: WHO, 2009.
3. Institute for Healthcare Improvement. What Zero Looks Like: Eliminating Hospital-Acquired Infections. Accessed 16 Sep 2011. http://www.ihi.org/knowledge/Pages/ImprovementStories/WhatZero LooksLikeEliminatingHospitalAcquiredInfections.aspx.
4. Cookson B, et al.: Comparison of national and subnational guidelines for hand hygiene. *J Hosp Infect.* 2009 Jul;72(3):202–210.
5. Pittet D. Improving adherence to hand hygiene practice: A multidisciplinary approach. *Emerg Infect Dis.* 2001 Mar–Apr;7(2):234–240.
6. Allegranzi B, et al. Successful implementation of the World Health Organization hand hygiene improvement strategy in a referral hospital in Mali, Africa. *Infect Control Hosp Epidemiol.* 2010 Feb;31(2): 133–141.
7. Allegranzi B., Pittet D.: Role of hand hygiene in healthcare-associated infection prevention. *J Hosp Infect.* 2009 Dec;73(4):305–315.
8. Allegranzi B, et al.: The First Global Patient Safety Challenge "Clean Care Is Safer Care": From launch to current progress and achievements. *J Hosp Infect.* 2007 Jun;65 Suppl 2:115–123.
9. Mathai E, et al.: Promoting hand hygiene in healthcare through national/ subnational campaigns. *J Hosp Infect.* 2011 Apr;77(4):294– 298.
10. World Health Organization. Clean Care Is Safer Care: Update no 32. 9 Jun 2011. Accessed 3 Oct 2011. http://www.who.int/gpsc/5may/news /no32/en.
11. Joint Commission Center for Transforming Healthcare. Hand Hygiene Project. Accessed 16 Sep 2011. http://www.centerfortransforming healthcare.org/projects/detail.aspx?Project=3.
12. Cummings KL, Anderson DJ, Kaye KS. Hand hygiene noncompliance and the cost of hospital-acquired methicillin-resistant *Staphylococcus aureus* infection. *Infect Control Hosp Epidemiol.* 2010 Apr;31(4):357– 364.
13. Stone PW, et al. Effect of guideline implementation on costs of hand hygiene. *Nurs Econ.* 2007 Sep–Oct;25(5):279–284.
14. Stiefel U, et al. Contamination of hands with methicillin-resistant Staphylococcus aureus after contact with environmental surfaces and after contact with the skin of colonized patients. *Infect Control Hosp Epidemiol.* 2011 Feb;32(2):185–187.
15. Perugini MR, et al. Impact of the reduction of environmental and equipment contamination on vancomycin-resistant *Enterococcus* rates. *Infection.* E pub 2011 Aug 17.
16. Otter JA, Yezli S, French GL. The role played by contaminated surfaces in the transmission of nosocomial pathogens. *Infect Control Hosp Epidemiol.* 2011 Jul;32(7):687-699.
17. Singh S, et al. Mobile phone hygiene: Potential risks posed by use in the clinics of an Indian dental school. *J Dent Educ.* 2010 Oct;74(10):1153– 1158.

18. Rutala B, et al. Bacterial contamination of keyboards: Efficacy and functional impact of disinfectants. *Infect Control Hosp Epidemiol.* 2006 Apr;27(4):372–377.

19. Lankford MG, et al. Assessment of materials commonly utilized in health care: Implications for bacterial survival and transmission. *Am J Infect Control.* 2006 Jun;34(5):258–263.

20. Brady RR, et al. Mobile phone technology and hospitalized patients: A cross-sectional surveillance study of bacterial colonization, and patient opinions and behaviours. *Clin Microbiol Infect.* 2011 Jun;17(6):830–835.

21. Patarakul K, et al. Cross-sectional survey of hand-hygiene compliance and attitudes of health care workers and visitors in the intensive care units at King Chulalongkorn Memorial Hospital. *J Med Assoc Thai.* 2005 Sep;88 Suppl 4:S287–293.

22. O'Boyle CA, Henly SJ, Larson E. Understanding adherence to hand hygiene recommendations: The theory of planned behavior. *Am J Infect Control.* 2011 Dec;29(6):352–360.

23. Marra AR, et al. Measuring rates of hand hygiene adherence in the intensive care setting: A comparative study of direct observation, product usage, and electronic counting devices. *Infect Control Hosp Epidemiol.* 2010 Aug;31(8):796–801.

24. Cheng VC, et al. Introduction of an electronic monitoring system for monitoring compliance with Moments 1 and 4 of the WHO "My 5 Moments for Hand Hygiene" methodology. *BMC Infect Dis.* 2011 May 26;11:151.

25. Saint S, et al. Improving healthcare worker hand hygiene adherence before patient contact: A before-and-after five-unit multimodal intervention in Tuscany. *Qual Saf Health Care.* 2009 Dec;18(6):429–433.

26. Doron SI, et al. A multifaceted approach to education, observation, and feedback in a successful hand hygiene campaign. *Jt Comm J Qual Patient Saf.* 2011 Jan;37(1):3–10.

27. Goldrick B, Gruendemann B, Larson E. Learning styles and teaching/learning strategy preferences: Implications for educating nurses in critical care, the operating room, and infection control. *Heart Lung.* 1993 Mar–Apr;22(2):176–182.

28. Gardner H. *Multiple Intelligences: The Theory in Practice.* New York: Basic Books, 1993.

29. Bagdasarian N, Malani PN. *Clostridium difficile* infection. In Lautenbach E, Woeltje KF, Malani PN, editors: *Practical Healthcare Epidemiology,* 3rd ed. Chicago: University of Chicago Press, 2010, 220–227.

30. Dubberke ER, et al.: Strategies to prevent *Clostridium difficile* infections in acute care hospitals. *Infect Control Hosp Epidemiol.* 2008 Oct;29 Suppl 1:S81–92.

31. Vernaz N, et al. Temporal effects of antibiotic use and hand rub consumption on the incidence of MRSA and Clostridium difficile. *J Antimicrob Chemother.* 2008; 62:601–607.

32. Sorra JS, Nieva VF. *Hospital Survey on Patient Safety Culture.* (Prepared by Westat, under Contract No. 290-96-0004.) AHRQ Publication No. 04-0041. Rockville, MD: Agency for Healthcare Research and Quality, Sep 2004.

33. Larson EL, et al. An organizational climate intervention associated with increased handwashing and decreased nosocomial infections. *Behav Med.* 2000 Spring;26(1):14–22.

34. Pittet D, et al. Hand hygiene among physicians: Performance, beliefs, and perceptions. *Ann Intern Med.* 2004 Jul 6;141(1):1–8.

35. Allegranzi B, et al. Religion and culture: Potential undercurrents influencing hand hygiene promotion in health care. *Am J Infect Control.* 2009 Feb;37(1):28–34.

36. Larson E. [Handwashing: It is essential even when gloves are used]. *Servir.* 1990 Nov–Dec;38(6):275–279.

37. Schneider J, et al. Hand hygiene adherence is influenced by the behavior of role models. *Pediatr Crit Care Med.* 2009 May;10(3):360–363.

38. Video gets patients more involved in hand hygiene. *Healthcare Benchmarks Qual Improv.* 2010 Mar;17(3):29–30.

39. Babík J, Bodnárová L, Sopko K. *Acinetobacter*—Serious danger for burn patients. *Acta Chir Plast.* 2008;50(1):27–32.

40. Matsumoto T, et al. [A case of hospital-acquired pneumonia caused by intermediately susceptible carbapenem *Acinetobacter baumannii*]. *Kansenshogaku Zasshi.* 2010 May;84(3):305–308.

41. Sarma JB, et al. Multidrug-resistant Enterobacteriaceae including metallo-β-lactamase producers are predominant pathogens of healthcare-associated infections in an Indian teaching hospital. *Indian J Med Microbiol.* 2011 Jan–Mar;29(1):22–27.

42. Croft CA, et al. Methicillin-resistant *Staphylococcus aureus* in a trauma population: Does colonization predict infection? *Am Surg.* 2009 Jun;75(6):458-61.

43. Huang SS, Platt R. Risk of methicillin-resistant *Staphylococcus aureus* infection after previous infection or colonization. *Clin Infect Dis.* 2003 Feb 1;36(3):281–285.

44. de Kraker ME, Davey PG, Grundmann H; on behalf of the BURDEN study group. Mortality and hospital stay associated with resistant *Staphylococcus aureus* and *Escherichia coli* bacteremia: Estimating the burden of antibiotic resistance in Europe. *PLoS Med.* 2011 Oct;8(10):e1001104.

45. Carmeli Y, et al. Health and economic outcomes of vancomycin-resistant enterococci. *Arch Intern Med.* 2002 Oct 28;162(19):2223–2228.

46. Cosgrove SE, et al. Comparison of mortality associated with methicillin-resistant and methicillin-susceptible *Staphylococcus aureus* bacteremia: A meta-analysis. *Clin Infect Dis.* 2003 Jan 1;36(1):53–59.

47. Huang SS, et al. Impact of routine intensive care unit surveillance cultures and resultant barrier precautions on hospital-wide methicillin-resistant *Staphylococcus aureus* bacteremia. *Clin Infect Dis.* 2006 Oct 15;43(8):971–978.

48. Robicsek A, et al. Universal surveillance for methicillin-resistant *Staphylococcus aureus* in 3 affiliated hospitals. *Ann Intern Med.* 2008 Mar 18;148(6):409–418.

49. Bode LG, et al. Sustained low prevalence of methicillin-resistant *Staphylococcus aureus* upon admission to hospital in The Netherlands. *J Hosp Infect.* 2011 Nov;79(3):198–201.

50. Wertheim HF, et al. Low prevalence of methicillin-resistant *Staphylococcus aureus* (MRSA) at hospital admission in the Netherlands: The value of search and destroy and restrictive antibiotic use. *J Hosp Infect.* 2004 Apr;56(4):321–325.

51. Harbarth S, et al. Universal screening for methicillin-resistant *Staphylococcus aureus* at hospital admission and nosocomial infection in surgical patients. *JAMA.* 2008 Mar 12;299(10):1149–1157.

52. Siegel JD, et al. 2007 Guideline for Isolation Precautions: Preventing Transmission of Infectious Agents in Health Care Settings. *Am J Infect Control.* 2007 Dec;35(10 Suppl 2):S65–164.

53. Agwu AL, et al. A World Wide Web-based antimicrobial stewardship program improves efficiency, communication, and user satisfaction and reduces cost in a tertiary care pediatric medical center. *Clin Infect Dis.* 2008 Sep 15;47(6):747-753.

54. Dellit TH, et al. Infectious Diseases Society of America and the Society for Healthcare Epidemiology of America guidelines for developing an institutional program to enhance antimicrobial stewardship. *Clin Infect Dis.* 2007 Jan 15;44(2):159–177.

55. Fishman N. Antimicrobial stewardship. *Am J Med.* 2006 Jun;119(6 Suppl 1):S53–61; discussion S62–70.

56. Agency for Healthcare Research and Quality. Glossary: Forcing Function. Accessed 17 Sep 2011. http://www.psnet.ahrq.gov/popup_glossary.aspx?name=forcingfunction.

57. Thursky K. Use of computerized decision support systems to improve antibiotic prescribing. *Expert Rev Anti Infect Ther.* 2006 Jun;4(3):491–507.

58. Maltezou HC, Tsakris A. Vaccination of health-care workers against influenza: Our obligation to protect patients. *Influenza Other Respi Viruses.* Epub 2011 Mar 21.

59. Johnson JG, Talbot TR. New approaches for influenza vaccination of healthcare workers. *Curr Opin Infect Dis.* 2011 Aug;24(4):363–369.

60. World Health Organization. Practical Guidelines for Infection Control in Health Care Facilities. 2004. Accessed 17 Sep 2011. http://www.wpro.who.int/nr/rdonlyres/006ef250-6b11-42b4-ba17-c98d413be8b8/0/practical_guidelines_infection_control.pdf.

61. US Centers for Disease Control and Prevention. Guidelines for Infection Control in Health Care Personnel. Bolyard EA, et al., Hospital Infection Control Practices Advisory Committee. Jun 1998. Accessed 17 Sep 2011. http://www.cdc.gov/hicpac/pdf/InfectControl98.pdf.

62. Sebazco S. Occupational health. In Carrico R, editor: *APIC Text of Infection Control and Epidemiology*, 3rd ed. Washington, DC: Association for Professionals in Infection Control and Epidemiology, 2009, 26-1–26-16.

63. National Center for Immunization and Respiratory Diseases. General recommendations on immunization: Recommendations of the Advisory Committee on Immunization Practices (ACIP). *MMWR Recomm Rep.* 2011 Jan 28;60(2):1-64.

64. Wu H, Shen B. Health care-associated transmission of hepatitis B and C viruses in endoscopy units. *Clin Liver Dis.* 2010 Feb;14(1):61–68; viii.

65. Seoane-Vazquez E, Rodriguez-Monguio R. Endoscopy-related infection: Relic of the past? *Curr Opin Infect Dis.* 2008 Aug;21(4):362–366.

66. Wendelboe AM, et al. Outbreak of cystoscopy related infections with *Pseudomonas aeruginosa*: New Mexico, 2007. *J Urol.* 2008 Aug;180(2):588–592; discussion 592.

67. Muscarella LF. The risk of disease transmission associated with inadequate disinfection of gastrointestinal endoscopes. *J Hosp Infect.* 2006 Jul;63(3):345–347.

68. Dohmae S, et al. *Bacillus cereus* nosocomial infection from reused towels in Japan. *J Hosp Infect.* 2008 Aug;69(4):361–367.

69. Fijan S, et al. Rotaviral RNA found on various surfaces in a hospital laundry. *J Virol Methods.* 2008 Mar;148(1–2):66–73.

70. US Centers for Disease Control and Prevention. Guideline for Disinfection and Sterilization in Healthcare Facilities, 2008. Rutala WA, Weber DJ, Hospital Infection Control Practices Advisory Committee. 2008. Accessed 17 Sep 2011. http://www.cdc.gov/hicpac/pdf/guidelines/Disinfection_Nov_2008.pdf.

71. Rutala WA, Weber DJ. How to assess risk of disease transmission to patients where there is a failure to follow recommended disinfection and sterilization guidelines. *Infect Control Hosp Epidemiol.* 2007 Feb;28(2):146–155.

72. Spaulding EH. Chemical disinfection of medical and surgical materials. In Lawrence CA, Block SS, editors: *Disinfection, Sterilization and Preservation.* Philadelphia: Lea and Febiger, 1968, 517–531.

73. Association for the Advancement of Medical Instrumentation (AAMI): *Comprehensive Guide to Steam Sterilization and Sterility Assurance in Health Care Facilities.* Arlington, VA: AAMI, 2010.

74. Belkin N. Laundry, patient linens, textiles, and uniforms. In Carrico R, editor: *APIC Text of Infection Control and Epidemiology*, 3rd ed. Washington, DC: Association for Professionals in Infection Control and Epidemiology, 2009, 101-1–101-7.

75. Neely AN, Maley MP. Survival of enterococci and staphylococci on hospital fabrics and plastic. *J Clin Microbiol.* 2000 Feb;38(2):724–726.

76. Muto CA, et al. SHEA guideline for preventing nosocomial transmission of multidrug-resistant strains of *Staphylococcus aureus* and *Enterococcus. Infect Control Host Epidemiol.* 2003 May;24(5):362–386.

77. Sehulster LM, et al. *Guidelines for Environmental Infection Control in Health-Care Facilities: Recommendations from the CDC and the Healthcare Infection Control Practices Advisory Committee (HICPAC).* Chicago: American Society for Healthcare Engineering/American Hospital Association, 2004.

78. Rutala WA, Weber DJ. The benefits of surface disinfection. *Am J Infect Control.* 2005 Sep;33(7):434–435.

79. Jarvis WR. The inanimate environment. In *Bennett and Brachman, Hospital Infections*, 5th ed. Philadelphia: Lippincott, 2007, 275–302.

80. Lin H, et al. *Legionella* pollution in cooling tower water of air-conditioning systems in Shanghai, China. *J Appl Microbiol.* 2009 Feb;106(2):606–612.

81. Anbumani S, Gururajkumar A, Chaudhury A. Isolation of *Legionella pneumophila* from clinical & environmental sources in a tertiary care hospital. *Indian J Med Res.* 2010 Jun;131:761–764.

82. Goetz AM, Yu V. *Legionella pneumophila.* In Carrico R, editor: *APIC Text of Infection Control and Epidemiology*, 3rd ed. Washington, DC: Association for Professionals in Infection Control and Epidemiology, 2009, 77-1–77-7.

83. Lass-Flörl C, et al. Epidemiology and outcome of infections due to *Aspergillus terreus*: 10-year single centre experience. *Br J Haematol.* 2005 Oct;131(2):201–207.

84. Warris A, Verweij PE. Clinical implications of environmental sources for *Aspergillus. Med Mycol.* 2005 May;43 Suppl 1:S59–65.

85. Prüss A, Giroult E, Rushbrook P, editors: *WHO Safe Management of Wastes from Healthcare Activities.* Geneva: World Health Organization, 1999.

86. Askarian M, Heidarpoor P, Assadian O. A total quality management approach to healthcare waste management in Namazi Hospital, Iran. *Waste Manag.* 2010 Nov;30(11):2321–2326.

87. Sanida G, et al. Assessing generated quantities of infectious medical wastes: A case study for a health region administration in Central Macedonia, Greece. *Waste Manag.* 2010 Mar;30(3):532–538.

88. Krisiunas E. Healthcare waste management. In: Friedman C, Newsom W, editors: *Infection Control: Basic Concepts and Practices*, 2nd ed. Portadown, UK: International Federation of Infection Control, 2011. 311–323.

89. Djeriri K, et al. [Occupational risk for blood exposure and staff behaviour: A cross-sectional study in 3 Moroccan healthcare centers]. *Med Mal Infect.* 2005 Jul–Aug;35(7–8):396–401.

90. Massrouje HT. Medical waste and health workers in Gaza governorates. *East Mediterr Health J.* 2001 Nov;7(6):1017–1024.

91. Akter N, et al. Hospital waste management and its probable health effect: A lesson learned from Bangladesh. *Indian J Environ Health.* 2002 Apr;44(2):124–137.

92. World Health Organization: The 8 Steps Along the Waste Stream. Accessed 17 Sep 2011 http://www.healthcarewaste.org/en/127_hcw_steps.html.

93. Garrett DO, Jochimsen E, Jarvis W. Invasive *Aspergillus spp* infections in rheumatology patients. *J Rheumatol.* 1999 Jan;26(1):146–149.

94. Chang CC, et al. Successful control of an outbreak of invasive aspergillosis in a regional haematology unit during hospital construction works. *J Hosp Infect.* 2008 May;69(1):33–38.

95. Bartley JM, Olmsted RN, editors: *Construction and Renovation: Toolkit for Professionals in Infection Prevention and Control*, 3rd ed. Washington DC: Association for Professionals in Infection Control and Epidemiology, 2007.

96. Bartley J, Olmsted R. Construction and renovation. In Carrico R, editor: *APIC Text of Infection Control and Epidemiology*, 3rd ed. Washington, DC: Association for Professionals in Infection Control and Epidemiology, Inc., 2009, 106-1–106-18.

97. Réglier-Poupet H, et al. Evaluation of the quality of hospital food from the kitchen to the patient. *J Hosp Infect.* 2005 Feb;59(2):131–137.

98. World Health Organization. Basic Food Safety for Health Workers. 1999. Accessed 17 Sep 2011. http://www.who.int/foodsafety/publications/capacity/healthworkers/en/.

99. Imai T, et al. Substantial differences in preparedness for emergency infection control measures among major hospitals in Japan: Lessons from SARS. *J Infect Chemother.* 2006 Jun;12(3):124–131.

100. Hui Z, et al. An analysis of the current status of hospital emergency preparedness for infectious disease outbreaks in Beijing, China. *Am J Infect Control.* 2007 Feb;35(1):62–67.

101. Rebmann T, 2008 APIC Emergency Preparedness Committee. APIC State-of-the-Art Report: The role of the infection preventionist in emergency management. *Am J Infect Control.* 2009 May;37(4):271–281.

102. Rebmann T. Assessing hospital emergency management plans: A guide for infection preventionists. *Am J Infect Control.* 2009 Nov;37(9):708–714.e4.

103. Hammond J. Mass casualty incidents: Planning implications for trauma care. *Scand J Surg.* 2005;94(4):267–271.

104. Braun BI, et al. Integrating hospitals into community emergency preparedness planning. *Ann Intern Med.* 2006, Jun 6;144(11):799–811.

105. The Joint Commission. *Meeting the Joint Commission's Infection Prevention and Control Requirements: A Priority Focus Area*, 2nd ed. Oak Brook, IL: Joint Commission Resources, 2009.

106. Oyler J, et al. Teaching internal medicine residents to sustain their improvement through the quality assessment and improvement curriculum. *J Gen Intern Med.* 2011 Feb;26(2):221–225.

107. Carboneau C, et al. A lean Six Sigma team increases hand hygiene compliance and reduces hospital-acquired MRSA infections by 51%. *J Healthc Qual.* 2010 Jul–Aug;32(4):61–70.

108. The Joint Commission. *Failure Mode and Effects Analysis in Health Care: Proactive Risk Reduction*, 3rd ed. Oak Brook, IL: Joint Commission Resources, 2010.

109. The Joint Commission. *Advanced Lean Thinking: Proven Methods to Reduce Waste and Improve Quality in Health Care.* Oak Brook, IL: Joint Commission Resources, 2009.

110. Joint Commission Center for Transforming Healthcare. Methodologies. Accessed 16 Sep 2011. http://www.centerfortransforming healthcare.org/about/methodologies.aspx.

111. Ustun C, et al. The accuracy and validity of a weekly point-prevalence survey for evaluating the trend of hospital-acquired infections in a university hospital in Turkey. *Int J Infect Dis.* Epub 2011 Jul 14.

112. Arias K. Surveillance. In Carrico R, editor: *APIC Text of Infection Control and Epidemiology*, 3rd ed. Washington, DC: Association for Professionals in Infection Control and Epidemiology, 2009, 3-1–3-17.

Future Issues in Infection Prevention and Control

By

Jaffar A. Al-Tawfiq, MD, DipHIC, FACP, FCCP
Prof. Ziad A. Memish, MD, FRCPC, FRCPE, FACP, FIDSA

Chapter Seven

Creating the Future of Infection Prevention and Control

The field of infection prevention and control (IPC) changes continually. New challenges alter priorities and often require intensified efforts to address new issues. Many IPC priorities discussed throughout the book continue to be critical for successful infection-prevention efforts. This chapter explores a few selected issues that will affect the future of the practice over the next years. Health care epidemiologists, IPC professionals, governments and other leaders, policy makers, and members of the public who are committed to infection prevention should consider these issues as they contemplate and plan for the future.

Setting the Target for Zero Infections

Since the initial publication of *To Err Is Human* by the Institute of Medicine in the United States in 1999, the patient-safety movement has taken a large leap. That publication estimated that between 44,000 and 98,000 Americans died each year from medical errors, including health care–associated infections (HAIs).[1] Today, the US Centers for Disease Control and Prevention (US CDC) estimates that in the United States, nearly 2 million persons develop HAIs each year, and approximately 99,000 die (equating to one death every six minutes).[2,3] Thus, it became clear that additional measures were needed to further reduce HAIs. In response, many organizations have adopted a "zero-tolerance" approach to patient safety in general and to infections in particular.[4,5]

HAIs exert significant impact on the life of patients, on their families, and on the health care services delivery system. Although prevention of HAIs is complex and challenging, it is the duty of each health care facility and its leaders to set a strategic organizational goal to eliminate HAIs. Efforts to minimize or to eliminate infections can be best achieved when implemented in a culture of patient safety through quality and performance-improvement methods. Using evidence to determine the potential impact of infections on the populations served by the organization and setting priorities that will ultimately lead to the greatest reduction in infections also means basing decisions on evidence from science and best practices, and carefully collected and analyzed surveillance data. Comparing data to other trusted resources through benchmarking can be helpful, but to achieve zero targets, organizations should not be satisfied with reaching "benchmarks" and remaining there. The ideal state is to continually improve and to strive for a zero-infection rate. This is a culture, a goal, an attitude, and a commitment that is endorsed by many authoritative groups and societies, such as Joint Commission International (JCI), the Society for Healthcare Epidemiology of America (SHEA), the World Health Organization (WHO), the US CDC, and the Association for Professionals in Infection Control and Epidemiology (APIC).[3,6,7]

Thus, in the future, each health care process and system should be designed to prevent and eliminate the occurrence of HAIs. As Donald Berwick, past CEO of the Institute for Healthcare Improvement, has said, "Every system is perfectly designed to achieve the results that it yields."[8(p.619)] Health care systems should be high-reliability organizations—that is, they should have exceptionally consistent systems in place that accomplish their goals of providing safe patient care as well as avoiding potentially catastrophic errors.[9] Yet, many health care systems are not reliable or dependable enough to provide safe care all the time. IPC professionals and other leaders should not tolerate practices that place patients and health care workers (HCWs) at risk for HAIs. The goal should always be to identify and to eliminate the risk for HAIs, whether from environmental hygiene, system design, HCW–related activities, or patient-related issues.

So, what does it mean to target zero infections? Although it may not be possible to eliminate every infection, IPC professionals and health care epidemiologists, with support from leadership, should establish the environment for this target by treating every infection as possibly preventable. When an infection occurs, the organization must investigate and analyze the reasons for the factors that led to it.

One strategy to move toward zero infections is to consider infection prevention a "system" that involves the coordination and integration of people and infrastructure designed to prevent infections. Some refer to the complex adaptive system (CAS) model as a preferred strategy.[10] A CAS model includes just a few simple rules for infection prevention, but they apply to all staff and are not negotiable (for example, the rule to always use sterile technique when appropriate). In a CAS, practice changes and improvements occur as closely as possible to the bedside by the staff who care for the patients. The staff share their learning and are allowed creativity to design better methods for infection prevention. Lastly, a CAS uses a "good-enough" design for infection-prevention practices to focus on the right amount of activity for such activities as surveillance balanced by leading or participating in interventions to reduce infections identified in the data.

For an effective strategy to work toward zero infections, it is important to involve a multidisciplinary, hospitalwide, or systemwide team committed to ensuring "zero tolerance for hospital-acquired infections." To be effective, this team must have the support of the leaders and engage them and all appropriate stakeholders in the change processes. The inter-professional (multidisciplinary) team might include a senior executive, the chief of nursing, a senior medical physician, the head of patient safety and quality, and leaders from specific clinical and support services, as well as staff nurses and support personnel. An important leadership role in helping to work toward zero infections is to ensure a safe environment for HCWs to report lapses in best practices and to communicate their ideas about how to improve care. Leaders should also support staff by empowering them to hold each other accountable for adherence to best practices. Thus, in a future state, the patient is at the center of all decisions and prevention activities, leaders and staff insist on safe practices that are embedded into practice and behaviors, and adherence to best practices is not negotiable.

The future road leading to "zero target for HAIs" could be achieved through the following steps:

1. Obtain leadership commitment to working toward zero infections.
2. Adapt "zero target" as a strategic plan in the organization.
3. Set an inspirational goal and gradually raise the bar. In this activity, the initial goal is set so the team can achieve the goals, and the bar is gradually raised and moved toward the target to ultimately achieve zero infections.
4. Incorporate the "zero" strategy into the organization's culture.
5. Set priorities based on surveillance data and best practices from the literature.
6. Create a safe environment for HCWs to speak up about adverse processes or outcomes.
7. Treat every infection as possibly preventable.
8. Investigate the reasons behind failure to prevent any infection.
9. Use an interprofessional team to investigate and to analyze infection cases.
10. Require that every HCW be accountable for the prevention of HAIs.
11. Educate HCWs through unit-specific or area-specific education.
12. Consider infection prevention as a system and consider all parts when designing care.

Reducing Blood and Body-Fluid Exposures

Worldwide, it is estimated that about three million HCWs are exposed to blood and body fluid (secondary to needlestick or sharps injuries each year).[11] In the United States, blood and body-fluid exposures resulted in 57 documented cases of HIV seroconversion through 2001.[12] In addition, it is estimated

that 80% of needlestick injuries are preventable.[13] Thus, for the future, it is imperative that each health care facility increase its efforts to design a program to prevent the occurrence of such accidents.

The development of such a program requires multiple approaches, including safer medical devices, improved techniques for safer handling of sharps, and the use of personal protective equipment. One of the most effective strategies is preexposure vaccination against hepatitis B virus (HBV) and postexposure prophylaxis for human immunodeficiency virus (HIV) and HBV. It is well known that the HBV vaccine is highly effective in the protection against HBV infection. The primary vaccine series produces a protective antibody level in > 95% of young adults and about 90% protection in adults after age 40. However, efficacy of HBV vaccine decreases in older adults.[14] The current literature shows that in certain countries, the compliance rate with the recommendation for HCWs to receive HBV vaccination is only about 50%.[15] Thus, as organizations plan for the future, it is important to have all HCWs receive the primary vaccination series for HBV as early as possible to maximize the benefit of such a vaccination program.

What can employers or the infection control committees do to improve low rates of vaccination compliance in the future? The use of a declaration form signed by any HCW who declines vaccination and including a statement that a worker declining HBV vaccination remains at risk of acquiring HBV infection is merely a release of liability rather than a true means of improving vaccination acceptance. What is needed to foster high compliance rates is a multifaceted program.[16] Surveillance data may lead to identification of the HCW groups at highest risk of exposure to blood and body fluid and what percentage accepted the vaccine. This information could be converted to an active action by designing targeted, specific interventions for high-risk groups that had declined vaccination. Because each health care setting is unique, local data are important for effective prevention planning. In addition to data collection and analysis, the selection of safer devices and training of HCWs play important roles in the prevention of sharps injuries.[17] A hands-on demonstration is very important, particularly when a new device is introduced into the health care facility. It is a trend now to use needleless devices to reduce percutaneous exposure to blood and body fluid. In a survey of 135 hospitals, half these hospitals used needleless intravenous systems.[18] The use of safety-engineered devices (SEDs), designed to limit blood contact or to shield the needle after use, was associated with a 75% reduction in percutaneous exposures.[19] The cost of the use of SEDs should be kept in mind when adopting this strategy. A study evaluating the use of SEDs showed a 49% reduction in hollow-bore needlestick injuries and a 57% reduction in high-risk injuries by retractable-syringe use. This reduction in injuries was associated with an overall budgetary increase of US$90,000 annually and was thought to be minimal in light of potential costs from needlestick injuries and follow-up care.[20] So in summary, future programs designed to reduce blood and body fluid exposure to near zero require the following steps for the success of this initiative:

1. Begin with surveillance data to perform a risk assessment
2. Identify high-risk behaviors and groups
3. Design an educational program for most frequently involved HCWs
4. Provide hands-on training for new injections, needles, and sharps-disposal practice
5. Use SEDs whenever possible
6. Promote single-use devices, disposing of sharps in puncture-proof containers, and disposing of rather than reusing containers when they are full to the approved level
7. Promote single-use vials rather than multidose vials

Implementing and Sustaining Evidence-Based Practices

Many guidelines of evidence-based practices to prevent HAIs have been introduced into clinical practice.[21] Some of these practices include the prevention of device-associated health care–associated infection, such as central line–associated bloodstream infections, ventilator-associated pneumonia, catheter-associated urinary tract infections, and surgical site infections (SSIs). However, practice in many health care facilities does not reflect adherence to these guidelines. In spite of education and organizational policy, compliance with certain procedures is less than optimal.[22] It is important for each facility to understand the obstacles and all potential causes of infection within its patient care processes and for IPC professionals to develop enhanced skills and use of performance-improvement tools to systematically assess the reasons for the failures. Figure 7-1 provides an example of a cause-and-effect diagram that surgical-services personnel can use to clearly define the potential causative variables for SSIs, look at less-than-optimal care system

and provide a high-level view of what potential improvement projects might promote evidence-based care that can lead to improved quality and decreased risk.

Infection prevention as a strategic priority for the organization will not be possible without a systematic methodology for addressing system breakdowns, sometimes called errors. It is primarily broken systems that unintentionally lead human beings to deliver less-than-optimal care. Performance-improvement initiatives are intended to eliminate errors by focusing on root causes of suboptimal care, one project at a time. Future problem analysis should incorporate these methods and tools.

The cause-and-effect diagram in Figure 7-1 can serve as a foundation for surgical-infection prevention teams to identify care breakdowns and highlight evidence-based projects such as correct IV–line placement, improved hand hygiene, preoperative patient-education redesign, and perioperative/postoperative glucose management as performance-improvement strategies.

Designing and embedding evidence-based guidelines into work flow requires the involvement of multifunctional and interprofessional teams, including frontline nurses, physicians, technicians, quality improvement, patient safety, infection control, and information technology (IT) staff. The team can use systematic methods to create change, such as Plan-Do-Study-Act, Six Sigma, Lean, and other performance-improvement methods and also can employ general "change-management" concepts to facilitate such changes. Senior leaders are critical to these efforts; without their engagement and support, these teams may not have the right resources (staff and time) to be able to effectively eliminate errors in the given processes.

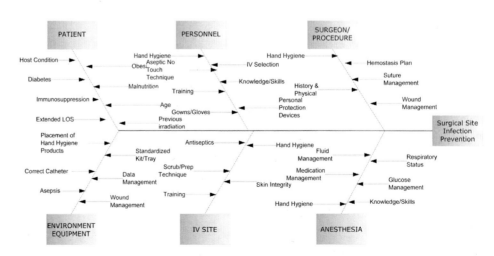

Figure 7-1. General Cause-and-Effect Diagram for Surgical Site Infection Prevention During Postoperative Care

Source: Joint Commission Resources.

When planning improvement strategies to implement and embed evidence-based practice it is important to ensure the following:

- Generated solutions are targeting the root cause.
- Actual interventions are being supported by senior leaders.
- All disciplines are engaged in solution generation.
- Solutions have eliminated error in the work flow processes.
- Solutions are implemented as a work flow redesign instead of added work, such as monitoring of a new policy and/or checklist.

Future efforts to ensure that evidence-based preventive measures are embedded into work flow processes require several approaches, including the following:[23]

1. Understand the culture of the organization and leaders with respect to change
2. Define barriers and challenges in the care system
3. Form an interprofessional team to get input from appropriate staff
4. Describe the current state of the event and the desired or future state using techniques such as high-level maps, identifying risk points, and then drawing the desired or ideal state. For one such map, *see* Figure 7-2. These steps will help identify gaps and errors in the process generate root causes.
5. Use change-management and performance-improvement methods for the process
6. Empower frontline staff to speak up
7. Institute pilot tests before fully deploying a large change process
8. Develop support and collaboration across clinical and support units within a service
9. Provide data feedback to HCWs
10. Utilize a variety of solution types to monitor and to sustain new processes

Reducing Multidrug-Resistant Organisms and Antimicrobial Resistance

As organizations prepare for the future, one of the most critical efforts of any successful IPC program is the reduction of multidrug-resistant organisms (MDROs). Monitoring and controlling these epidemiologically significant organisms helps staff continually assess the endemic level, work toward reducing the incidence, and quickly identify any cluster or outbreak to initiate early intervention and prevent their spread. Three important future areas for reducing MDROs and antimicrobial resistance are discussed below.

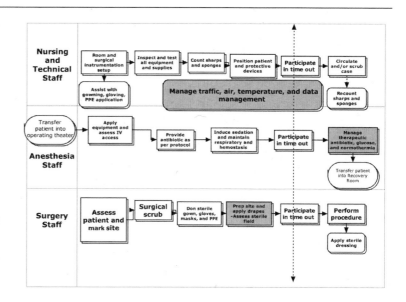

Figure 7-2. High-Level Process Map

This figure shows a high-level process map of responsibilities for nursing, technical, anesthesia, and surgical staff to prevent surgical site infections.

Antimicrobial Resistance: Metrics for Monitoring MDROs

Different health care organizations use different metrics for such monitoring, which limits the usefulness of these monitoring activities in comparing rates among different health care settings. To standardize MDRO metrics, SHEA/HICPAC developed guidelines and recommendations for metrics for MDROs in health care settings.[24] Because these guidelines are not risk adjusted, the guidelines should not be used for interhospital comparison.[24] In addition, labeling patients as life-long carriers of particular MDROs would significantly increase the cumulative prevalence of these organisms in any given health care setting. It has also been noted that the application of SHEA/HICPAC guidelines requires significant support from IT and the use of electronic records. In addition, these metrics are challenging to construct and require a considerable amount of time.[25] Another difficulty is the potential inclusion of data from active surveillance cultures in the calculation of the metrics. This type of data would significantly increase the calculated metrics if active surveillance cultures are practiced widely in any setting. The question of whether any metric could be utilized in the IPC activities depends on the ability of that specific metric to address the need of the organization. Detailed examination of the clinical and economic impact of MDROs on the institution (risk assessment) is an essential first step. The optimal MDRO–control program will also include a clear statement of goals and deliverables and a plan to communicate new initiatives up and down the organizational hierarchy.[26] Joint Commission Resources has published a toolkit for leaders that addresses the clinical and economic consequences of antibiotic resistance and MDROs (*see* Chapter 6, page 99).[26]

To achieve the goal of preventing and controlling MDROs, the following steps are recommended:

1. Use validated metrics for evaluating use of antimicrobial agents.
2. Identify process and outcome measures to be able to track processes such as those inherent in the implementation of bundle procedures and the actual outcome measure, such as the rate of a specific infection under question.
3. Participate in data validation to ensure that the data are accurate and usable.
4. Use information technology for alerts regarding isolation of patients with organisms of epidemiologically significant importance, such as vancomycin-resistant *Enterrococcus* (VRE) and methicillin-resistant *Staphylococcus aureus* (MRSA).
5. Wisely use active surveillance data (*see* Chapter 6 for more information) collected through screening procedures to determine colonization with an MDRO.
6. Gather data from all available resources.
7. Assign qualified personnel to calculate and to analyze data.
8. Develop an effective method for dissemination of information to appropriate staff.

Antimicrobial Resistance: Proactive Measures to Reduce Rates

One of the ominous signs in health care is the progressive increase in the rate of antimicrobial resistance with diminished production and discovery of new antimicrobial agents. In fact, it is estimated that about 70% of HAIs are due to a resistant bacteria for at least one commonly used drug.[27] In 2004 the Infectious Disease Society of America (IDSA) drew attention to six emerging bacteria responsible for two thirds of all HAIs with the acronym "ESKAPE"[28]: *Enterococcus faecium*, *Staphylococcus aureus*, *Klebsiella species*, *Acinetobacter baumannii*, *Pseudomonas aeruginosa*, and *Enterobacter* species. However, recognizing the importance of *Clostridium difficile* as one of the problematic pathogens, IDSA changed "ESKAPE" to "ESCAPE" to include this organism.[28] As a result of this increasing antimicrobial resistance, it is important for health care facilities to develop and to implement proactive programs to combat the development of resistance. Although this practivity may seem to be simple to adapt in the health care setting, it is very complicated, as the prevalence of MDROs from the community may be significant. A collabo-

rative approach among health care sectors in the community is important to facilitate such an activity, and each organization must choose the strategies that fit its culture and will lead to early and sustained success.

Influencing antimicrobial resistance and trends should be proactive and incorporate some of the measures through the following activities:

- Use passive and active surveillance.
- Maximize isolation precautions and incorporate these activities into a daily routine.
- Implement antimicrobial prescribing audits and feedback to clinicians.
- Use formulary restriction and preauthorization.
- Standardize medication order sets and clinical pathways (to foster evidence-based prescribing).
- Use antimicrobial order forms.
- Implement de-escalation of therapy (review culture and susceptibility pattern with on-going review of therapy).
- Optimize dose (right dose for site of infection; renal dose adjustment).
- Convert from IV to oral dose as appropriate.
- Provide real-time feedback to improve antimicrobial use;
- Form an interprofessional team for monitoring and improving antimicrobial prescribing practices.
- Develop and tailor guidelines for treating infections based on local sensitivity patterns.

Antimicrobial Resistance: New Technology for Detecting Multidrug-Resistant Pathogens

With the increasing pressure of multidrug resistance as well as the need for rapid and accurate detection of antibiotic-resistant organisms to determine proper placement and isolation of patients, there is an increased need for new methodologies for the identification of these organisms. Recently, rapid molecular detection methods for selective organism have been developed. These tests include the detection of MRSA and multidrug-resistant tuberculosis (MDR-TB). It is well known that several molecular typing systems are used for determining microbial clonality and to assess the presence of an outbreak.[29] In addition, these techniques are important tools in identifying the source (environmental or personnel) of an outbreak, distinguishing infectious from noninfectious strains, and distinguishing relapses from reinfections.[30]

However, it is increasingly important to have rapid diagnosis of the presence of multidrug resistance. Culture methods may result in a delay of 2 to 3 days before results are available and thus may delay the isolation process.[31] For the detection of MRSA, two polymerase chain reaction (PCR)–based assays are used to detect the mecA methicillin-resistance gene in *S. aureus* by targeting the junction of staphylococcal cassette chromosome mec (SCCmec).[32] The use of rapid molecular testing is thought to be cost effective.[33] However, the mecA gene could also be detected in coagulase-negative *Staphylococcus*. Thus, it is important to have other genes detected to differentiate these organisms from S. aureus.[34] In contrast, the presence of vanA and vanB is unique to enterococci, and thus rapid detection of these genes would signify VRE.[34] Some important issues should be kept in mind, including the high sensitivity of these assays as well as the possible presence of inhibitors in clinical samples that may give rise to false-negative results.

Immunizing Health Care Workers

Immunization of HCWs plays a major role in the reduction of HAIs, such as outbreaks of influenza and pertussis.[35] In addition, such immunization adds to the protection of the HCW from HBV or hepatitis C virus as potential infections secondary to blood or body-fluid exposure.. Thus, it is imperative that, for the future, all medical facilities formulate and implement comprehensive immunization policies for HCWs. Despite the well-known benefits of these vaccines, the immunization rates of HCWs for some vaccines fall short of adequate levels. For example, the average immunization rate for influenza is often low, at about 40%.[36] Moreover, low vaccination rates in health care settings that rely on voluntary vaccination programs continue, despite strong immunization recommendations made since 1984 by such authorities as the US CDC and the Advisory Committee on Immunization Practices. It is important to have at least 90% of HCWs immunized with influenza vaccine to have effective coverage to prevent HAIs.[37]

Should health care organizations depend on the incentive of HCWs to raise the compliance rates, or should they take more active roles? Historically, relying on HCW incentive has not yielded the required coverage, and thus it has been proposed by many health care institutions to mandate such vaccines.[38] The policy of mandated immunization requires HCWs who do not receive a vaccine to have unpaid leave during their influenza illness or to wear masks throughout their shifts and identifying marks on their badges. Such measures have been challenged by some HCW labor unions. Although these unions support voluntary vaccination and strongly encourage compliance with these recommendations, they support an individualized decision by each HCW regarding whether to receive a particular vaccination. It has also been argued that HCWs should accept the decision to receive vaccines, as it is embodied in the Hippocratic Oath that new physicians

take—first, do no harm—and that not receiving such vaccines poses significant risk and harm to the patients.[39]

In the future, how can health care organizations and IPC programs intensify efforts to improve immunization rates among HCWs? What are the needed strategies to increase vaccination rates and thus to reduce the burden of the disease and associated costs? Some health care organizations have "raised the bar" by achieving more than 95% compliance with influenza vaccination.[40] In the past, the main tools to achieve this goal were based on education of HCWs, access to available resources, and providing information on best practices, guidelines, and recommendations. Educational programs should be directed toward promoting immunization and removing misconceptions about vaccines that might interfere with the institution of effective HCW–immunization programs. Although these general tools have been successful in increasing the rate of influenza vaccines in certain health care settings, it is unlikely that these interventions would be enough to provide sustainable improvement. Thus, health care policy makers need to depend on other strategies for the promotion of staff immunization.

The US-based Joint Commission released a monograph to improve influenza vaccination, including evidence-based guidelines, published studies, legislative and regulatory efforts, accreditation considerations, and practical strategies and tools to improve influenza-vaccination rates among HCWs.[41] These strategies can be used to improve immunization rates for other recommended vaccines. JCI standards require organizations to periodically offer preventive immunizations, and SHEA and APIC have more specific recommendations. In its position paper, APIC recommends that influenza vaccine be required annually as part of a comprehensive strategy to reduce HAIs for all HCWs with direct patient care.[42] Moreover, SHEA endorses a policy in which annual influenza vaccination is a condition of initial and continued HCW employment or professional privileges.[43] In a mandatory program of influenza vaccination for HCWs, influenza vaccination rates of > 98% were achieved and sustained over the subsequent four years.[33] Mandating employees who have patient contact to either be vaccinated annually against influenza or to sign a declination specifying the reason(s) for refusal and augmenting this policy with the requirement that those who fail to comply appear before the Medical Executive Committee resulted in an 88% rate of vaccination.[44] Some organizations had mandated influenza vaccination; employees who were neither vaccinated nor exempted were not scheduled for work, and if they were still not vaccinated or exempt, they were terminated. This strict policy resulted in an overall compliance rate of 98.4%.[45]

The issue of mandatory vaccination is a controversial strategy, and the issue of HCW autonomy against patient safety is a challenging balance to achieve.[46–50] However, the evidence for reduction in influenza infection when the vaccine is administered is strong. Thus, for the future, IPC programs should consider the following strategies to increase compliance with influenza immunizations:

1. Provide incentives for HCWs to participate in the immunization programs.
2. Mandate vaccination through a regional or local agency.
3. Prepare the organization and the recipients for the mandatory policy before implementation with education, benefits, rules, and consequences.
4. Use compliance data in the annual credentialing process as possible.
5. Utilize mobile clinics to bring the vaccine to HCWs, particularly during influenza-vaccine campaigns.
6. Provide vaccinations free of charge to the staff.
7. Adopt educational programs specifically targeting myths, misconceptions and benefits of vaccines.
8. Utilize available monographs and guidelines from local, regional, and international organizations.
9. Consider a policy mandating influenza vaccination with the appropriate local and national laws.
10. Monitor compliance with a mandated policy and provide feedback.

One organization's influenza-vaccination initiative is detailed in Case Study 7-1.

CASE STUDY 7-1

Improving Influenza Vaccination Among Health Care Workers (Saudi Arabia)

Hanan H. Balkhy, MD; Badria M. Alotaibi, MPH; Amnah Al Aawwam, BSN; Bassem Abukhzam, BSN

Introduction

Every winter, King Abdulaziz Medical City (KAMC), a tertiary care center in Riyadh, Saudi Arabia, is faced with major delays in admitting patients due to full occupancy of hospital beds. This is mainly due to the large number of patients presenting with influenza and other respiratory illnesses. The hospital has no way of diverting patients to other hospitals and is committed to serve the National Guard population. Hence, HCWs are faced with the risk of acquiring respiratory illnesses from caring for their patients. Many of the HCWs prefer to work while sick, enhancing the cycle of disease transmission between HCWs and patients, but many others take

off when ill, which negatively impacts the workforce. One of the solutions is to maintain a healthy workforce by providing the annual influenza vaccine to all HCWs and high-risk patients free of charge. When this vaccination was presented to the HCWs as a voluntary solution, no more than 29% complied. Further measures were needed to improve the influenza-vaccine acceptance among HCWs.

Methods

Since 2003 the IPC department has led an annual campaign that makes it a priority to immunize, free of charge, all HCWs and high-risk patients with the annual influenza vaccine. These campaigns were administered by the public health nurses in the IPC department. The campaigns were preceded by hospitalwide educational campaigns using the hospital's intranet as well as brochures, pamphlets, and posters. These materials provided information on influenza and its symptoms, preventive strategies, cough etiquette, vaccine importance, and ways to get free vaccination.

During the first four campaigns, special clinics were arranged for HCWs. Special visits were conducted to bring vaccinations to high-risk areas, such as the critical-care units, emergency room, hemodialysis unit, and organ-transplant units. HCWs from those areas who missed those visits, as well as HCWs from all other hospital departments, were able to receive their influenza vaccines at the employee health clinic. Despite using multiple overlapping announcements and extending the clinic hours for more than three weeks, vaccine coverage in the first four campaigns ranged between 21% and 29% (*see* Figure 1).

During the winter of 2007–2008, KAMC adapted a major methodological change by engaging the nursing department in its efforts to enhance the vaccine coverage. The nursing department, an umbrella of all nurses at all KAMC departments, administratively covers more than 40% of clinical HCWs at KAMC. Every year before starting the campaign, infection control staff, together with the nursing-department staff, nominate a champion nurse from each department to be responsible for immunizing all HCWs in his or her area under the supervision of infection control staffs. After engaging the nursing department, vaccine coverage more than doubled, as can be seen in Figure 1.

A second major methodological change was adopted in 2009 as an extra precautionary step to the H1N1 influenza pandemic. Precampaign advertisements and announcements stressed the mandatory rather than voluntary nature of the 2009–2010 seasonal influenza vaccination. However, HCWs' anxiety during the pandemic probably masked any benefit of this methodological change, and instead KAMC experienced

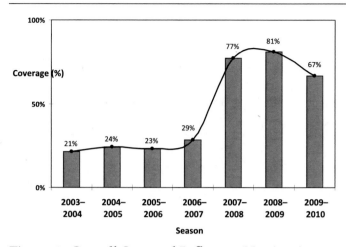

Figure 1. Overall Seasonal Influenza Vaccination Coverage Among Health Care Workers

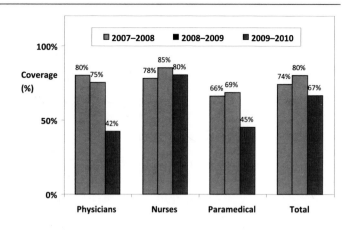

Figure 2. Seasonal Influenza Vaccination Coverage Among the Different Disciplines at King Abdualziz Medical City, Riyadh, Saudi Arabia

a 17% drop in coverage compared to the previous season. Interestingly the drop was observed only among physicians and paramedical personnel but not nurses. Analysis of the signed waiver for those who refused to receive their vaccines showed that the majority had had bad vaccine experiences, including previous reactions to influenza vaccine (55%) and allergy to eggs (13%). Moreover, 2% refused to receive the vaccine because they had PCR–proven H1N1 disease during the pandemic, which was an acceptable reason to decline vaccination.

Analysis of vaccine coverage by job category during the last three seasons (*see* Figure 2) showed that nurses had the highest coverage (80%, $p < 0.001$), followed by physicians (74%), and paramedical personnel (67%). This is in contrast with some reports that showed that physicians had the highest coverage. KAMC leaders believe that engaging nurses from all hospital departments may have contributed to this high influenza-vaccine coverage.

Results

The annual influenza campaign has been a major challenge every year. It seems that the fears and concerns about vaccine side effects remain a major hindrance to its acceptance by HCWs, specifically physicians. KAMC leadership believes that engaging the nurses will dramatically improve the uptake of the vaccine, but not to the highest level possible. Making the vaccine mandatory rather than voluntary improved vaccination rates even further.

Lessons Learned

The biggest lesson learned is that the engagement of other HCWs, specifically nurses, in the influenza campaign had a major positive impact on immunization rates. KAMC leaders

need to be creative when engaging physicians in future campaigns and identifying and engaging champions among the different disciplines for the coming years.

Using Social Marketing in Health Care Worker Behavior Change

The tradition of infection prevention and control dictates dissemination of information through multiple levels of staff and leaders to all HCWs. Effective communication will help to achieve desired behaviors and improvements in infection control activities, such as hand hygiene, isolation procedures, management of devices, and other practices. Often education is seen as the primary method of communication, but many studies show that simple education alone does not improve behavior.[51–54] Numerous approaches have been used to change HCW behavior. Pittet showed that improving compliance with hand hygiene required a multifactorial approach, including education, visual reminders, feedback, administrative rewards, and availability of alcohol-based hand rubs.[55] Many researchers have employed change-management or behavioral-change theory techniques to promote effective infection control behaviors.[56] According to the theory of planned behavior, the immediate cause of compliance with hand hygiene is *intention* to perform hand hygiene. This intention is anticipated by attitude, subjective norm (a person's perception of the social pressure), and the perception of the ease or difficulty in performing hand hygiene.[57] When, despite enormous effort, IPC hand-hygiene behaviors have not improved, some organizations have attempted to enforce policy compliance by denying merit increases, using discipline, or even terminating employees for policy violations. Others have implemented nonreimbursement or noncompensation for sick days. However, such disciplinary actions may interfere with the employee-employer cooperative relationship, decrease morale and trust, create anxiety, and interfere with an effective care team.[57]

Social marketing has been explored as a tool for creating change in staff behavior. In 2008 the American Marketing Association defined *marketing* as "the activity, set of institutions, and processes for creating, communicating, delivering, and exchanging offerings that have value for customers, clients, partners, and society at large."[58] Social marketing is concerned with a few concepts to drive change, including the following[59]:

- Voluntary behavioral change is a key component relying on change that is not correctional in nature.
- Behavior change is driven by the needs of HCWs and the benefits or disadvantages they perceive will be gained from such a change.
- Techniques such as segregation, custom-made techniques, and concentration on the welfare of the individual and the society and not of the organization are other important components of social marketing.

In infection prevention, the population of HCWs may be "segmented" into subgroups with unique perspectives on accepting influenza vaccine. For these subgroups, the social marketer may develop communication strategies that are custom designed for each particular group. In social marketing, the concept of marketing is used to establish an environment that will drive a change in behavior rather than to endorse or support a commercial product. In the social-marketing process, different concepts are taken together to promote an infection control behavior, specifically addressing the needs of HCWs and the stage of readiness for change and compliance.[60] In addition, social marketing considers how staff perceive benefits of compliance with a specific policy that could be related to personal gain, such as protecting self or family members from MDROs or influenza. In one study about influenza vaccination, 89% of those who received the vaccine stated that they did so to protect themselves.[36] Looking at compliance with infection control measures or recommendations shows that noncompliance is a competitive activity. Competition in social marketing means that HCWs may not comply with hand hygiene, because not washing hands is more convenient and faster.[57] Social marketing is a way of looking at IPC promotion through the eyes of the customers (HCWs) and planning for activities that promote compliance with infection control measures through the use of multiple techniques and tactics.

The role of social marketing has not been utilized well in the field of infection control. However, with the explosion of tools and technology is this area, it should be considered for future planning directed at behavior change. This technique can provide IPC professionals with methods to complement education and policies and to reduce barriers to change while offering opportunities for improvement, and it offers a multi-faceted approach to change that has proven to be effective.[58] Practical steps to using social marketing include

- employing change-management theory to drive a change in behavior;
- utilizing behavior-change theories to understand health care dynamics and to promote hand hygiene;
- developing interdisciplinary action plans to improve compliance with infection control;
- customizing infection-prevention activities to address individuals and institutional needs;
- relating improved compliance rates to personal gains; and
- looking at infection prevention and control activities through the eyes of HCWs.

Developing Future Infection Prevention and Control Staffing Resources

In the 1980s the US CDC performed the SENIC study, which proposed that staffing infection control programs with 1 infection control practitioner for every 250 occupied acute care beds was adequate based on the practice in many health care facilities in the United States at that time.[61] However, increasing demands on infection control, expansion of the role, and lack of adequate resources were cited as the most frequent reasons for the lack of optimal infection control performance.[62] Thus, a Delphi study was performed that showed that a ratio of 0.8–1.0 infection control practitioners for every 100 occupied acute care beds would be necessary to perform the essential functions of the role.[63] Many health care systems may find these staffing ratios a challenge in the face of increasing health care costs and the need to optimize manpower.

Many health care facilities in the international community have inadequately staffed infection-prevention programs. When increasing numbers of staff, the IPC team should review the several published studies[64–67] to identify formulas for staffing that have been tested. The team should also evaluate the infection control needs of the populations they serve in the organization to determine the level of required resources. With this information in hand, they can make the business case to the leaders to obtain staff based on enhancing patient safety and reducing infection risk to patients, eliminating harm to staff, or avoiding lost revenue. In addition to considering increased staff, senior management could establish a performance-improvement team to develop and implement strategies to reduce HAIs. Using a focused surveillance approach could also save money and resources. These surveillance activities should concentrate on high-volume, high-risk, or problem-prone infections. Of course, tracking MDROs is of great importance for any organization and could be done through the microbiology laboratory followed by clinical assessment done by the IPC staff. The infection control practitioner could use data on the number of prevented HAIs and the estimated costs avoided to build the case for more resources when appropriate.[68] Having a lower infection rate—or a no-infection "zero target"—should always be the organization's goal, and it is also important for health care leaders to be educated about these issues so they can make decisions about allocating the needed budget and resources.

Designing the Environment for Infection Prevention and Control

With the increasing popularity of patient- and family-centered care and the recognition that the design of the environment can influence infection risk, there is an increasing demand on changing the design of newly built or renovated acute care hospitals and other care settings. Recently, the concept of "evidence-based design" was introduced.[69] Single-occupancy rooms provide many benefits, including enhanced privacy, support for patient-centered care, fewer room-to-room transfers, flexibility with adaptable acuity, and spatial separation, to mitigate cross-transmission of pathogens. Studies have shown that single-room design was associated with a lower risk of acquiring epidemiologically significant organisms, such as MRSA, *Pseudomonas spp*, and *Candida spp*.[70,71] Although single-room design is associated with higher costs compared with multibed rooms, benefits for safety and comfort of the patients outweigh this increased cost.[70,71]

Thus, in the future, as new construction or renovation is being planned, IPC professionals and health care epidemiologists should be involved in facility design from a building's inception. They are critical to providing guidance to reduce the risk of infection,[72] particularly from aspergillosis.[73] They should lead or participate in a formal assessment of infection risk during construction, as described in Chapter 6.[73] As IPC professionals become more involved in healthy environments, they must become proficient in safe design features that can be incorporated into a building and also knowledgeable about how patients and supplies move through the environment. While there are many considerations, the three aspects that should be considered in all future safe environmental design are flow of supplies, patient flow, and ventilation.

Appropriate Flow of Supplies

Materials should flow from contaminated areas to clean areas with no back-and-forth activity; for example, in areas such as procedure areas (including wound-care management), surgical units where major and minor procedures are performed (including day surgery, excision clinics, preoperative and recovery rooms), and work areas where instruments are processed (central sterilization and disinfection units). The operating rooms should be walled and be in one area to minimize dust and to eliminate flies or rodents, particularly in resource-poor countries, and to have central air-conditioning. The operating rooms should be located away from areas of the hospital heavily traveled by staff, patients, and visitors. Areas for processing instruments should be designed to have at least three sections: decontamination, packaging, and sterilization and storage. Physical barriers should separate the decontamination area from the other sections to contain contamination on used items.[74] The challenge is containing contamination and reminding staff to move in one direction.

Patient Flow

The flow of patients with MDROs and other pathogens or infections may pose a risk for other patients if colonized or infected patients are not identified within the organization. Some hospitals rely on written lists to identify and to communicate to other staff which patients are placed in isolation. However, this process requires vigilance and manpower, and patients may be transferred with contaminated equipment or without notice. To overcome this difficulty in the future, it would be helpful to have a computerized flagging system rather than paper lists, particularly in this era of electronic medical records. This is of particular importance for patients with infectious tuberculosis (TB and other airborne infections).

Ventilation

It is important to note that rooms with variable ventilation (meaning they can be manually switched between positive and negative pressure) are not permitted in newly constructed facilities or in renovated areas of the facility.[72] The number of rooms required for airborne-infection isolation should be determined by a risk assessment of the health care facility.[35] Hospital management is challenged with the logistics of securing sufficient numbers of airborne-infection isolation rooms (AIIRs) or of providing designated areas for patient cohorts when the number of AIIRs is insufficient.[35]

Using Data Mining and Information Technology

Surveillance of HAIs relies heavily on the quality of surveillance data to assist IPC professionals to focus their activities on specific types of infections, epidemiologically important microorganisms, and wards and locations where HAIs are high. This important aspect of the infection control program has historically relied on manual collection, sorting, and analysis of data. With current and future advances in information technology, IPC professionals should expect to have technological systems that provide accurate and reliable data in a more timely manner and to use this capability to more rapidly identify potential endemic HAIs and outbreaks. Studies of data-mining systems have found that IPC programs that use automated-surveillance technology are more likely to implement evidence-based practices to control and to prevent HAIs,[75] that the use of an electronic surveillance system decreases the time spent conducting surveillance by up to 61%,[76] and that the use of an automated surveillance system may allow more time for data analysis and interventions to improve patient care.[77] However, despite these advantages, few hospitals currently have data-mining technology. In one survey, only 23% of 192 organizations had electronic surveillance systems.[75]

In the future, technology will be employed to provide a number of more refined opportunities for data analysis. For example, electronically linking bacteriology databases with hospital mortality records can be a simple and reproducible tool for identifying the number of deaths attributable to HAIs. One study of linking these two databases found that HAIs were the cause of 0.9% of all patients' mortalities and a contributory cause in another 8.0% of patients.[78] With the current state of technology, it is now possible to link data from the clinical-laboratory and hospital-information systems, thus creating association rules linking patients, sample types, locations, organisms, and antibiotic susceptibilities.[79] In the future, it is proposed that this technology will become more sophisticated and useful to IPC staff. Of importance, the estimated sensitivity of automated-surveillance systems ranges from 0.65 to 0.943, with a specificity ranging from 0.72 to 0.999.[80] As technology improves and the sensitivity of automated-surveillance system approaches 100%, this will be an important characteristic to save infection control practitioners' time.[81] Thus, better utilizing the infection control practitioners' time in the future will include doing the following:

1. Use automated-surveillance systems
2. Use IT systems for data mining to identify potential infections and outbreaks

3. Link multiple systems, such as microbiology, health information, and pharmacy data, to extract information related to antibiotic utilization and clusters of drug-resistant organisms

Planning for Emerging Diseases and Pathogens

The emergence of new infections and the reemergence of old diseases keep infectious diseases as a leading cause of morbidity and mortality throughout the world. Reemerging infectious diseases usually reappear after a significant reduction in the number of cases, such as Enterovirus, *Clostridium difficile*, and enterotoxigenic *Eschericia coli*. On the other hand, emerging diseases include outbreaks of previously unknown diseases, such as NDM (New Delhi metallo-beta-lactamase [NDM-1]), or an increased incidence in the past two decades of known diseases. It was noted in 2005 that there were about 1,400 recognized infectious pathogens, and 180 (12.9%) were emerging or reemerging.[82]

Recently, there was an emergence of NDM and *Escherichia coli* (EHEC) O104:H4. NDM-1 was first detected in 2008 in a Swedish patient of Indian origin with *Klebsiella pneumoniae* infection; the organism was subsequently reported in many patients from India, Pakistan, the United Kingdom, 13 European countries, and Canada.[83] This new strain poses several challenges: the need for vigilance, the ease of spreading a resistant strain throughout the globe, and the risk of plasmid-mediated transfer of this carbapenemase enzyme blaNDM-1 between different bacteria.[83]

Emerging and reemerging infections will occur in the future. As these occur, IPC programs will need to maintain effective surveillance systems within their own organizations, to link with global surveillance databases, and to design creative and unique methods to manage patients' infections with new diseases. It is also important to have early warning systems for the emergence of new infectious diseases. The collaboration between public health and infection control is very crucial. They should work together to develop surveillance systems for early recognition of diseases and effective responses to limit the spread of these diseases. In addition, better predictive capabilities are needed for the detection of emerging infectious diseases. We should not depend on crisis management but develop a strategic plan for these diseases. Having a regional, a local, and an international surveillance activity coupled with an accurate database for emerging and reemerging infectious diseases also would be very helpful. Sidebar 7-1 describes one country's efforts to coordinate infection prevention efforts at the national level through the Ministry of Health.

Sidebar 7-1. Developing a National Infection Prevention and Control Policy: The Ministry of Health, Kenya

Ndegwa Linus, MPHE, HCS, PhD (SHEA International Ambassador)

Gathari Ndirangu, MBChB, MMed

Rachel Kamau, BDS, NASCOP

Susan Otieno, MPHE

Introduction

Health care in Kenya includes public and private sectors. In 2008, the government's Ministry of Health (MOH) was split into two ministries—the Ministry of Medical Services and Ministry of Public Health and Sanitation. The private sector consists of private for-profit, faith-based, and nongovernmental organization facilities. Health services are provided through a network of more than 6,000 health facilities nationwide, with the public-sector system accounting for about 51% of these facilities.

The Kenyan government, through the MOH, recognized that HAIs were a problem within the health care system and had put in place various policies addressing aspects of IPC in the country. However, the country lacked a comprehensive IPC policy to guide HCWs on the issues of infection control practices.

The Process

In 1998 some MOH staff were sensitized on IPC concept through various workshops organized by WHO. These staff started the process of developing IPC policy but faced many challenges, including transfers, retirements, and the lack of a well-coordinated team to spearhead the process. This led to collapse of the process until 2004, when a US President's Emergency Plan for AIDS Relief (PEPFAR)–funded project (making medical injection safe, or MMIS) was implemented by an outside consultant. MMIS worked with the MOH to establish an injection-safety task force, which revived interest in the IPC with a bias on injection-safety practice in the country. The task force developed a policy and standard guidelines on injection safety.

In August 2009 the MOH began the process of developing the National IPC Policy and Guidelines for Health Care Services in Kenya. This process began with a situational analysis to determine IPC practices and to identify the gaps for such practices. The analysis was made through interviews and direct observation of practice with policy makers and health care workers in public, private, and faith-based health sectors across various regions of the country. The analysis identified a need for simple, user-friendly IPC policies and guidelines for all types of staff at all levels of the health care system. The situational analysis revealed that few facilities had active IPC committees, while others were inactive, having not met for more than six months prior to the situational analysis. The need to set up active IPC committees in all health care facilities was identified as critical to strengthen IPC. A subsequent stakeholder forum agreed on the need for a national policy on IPC as well as guidelines for all health care services in the country to help the facilities practice IPC uniformly.

Results

In September 2009 a national committee to spearhead development of the IPC Policy and Guidelines was formed, with members drawn from the national MOH office and health care providers from public, private, and faith-based health sectors, medical training institutions, and nongovernmental organizations. This committee conducted a technical appraisal of a draft of National IPC Policy and Guidelines that had been prepared by a consultant contracted to lead the process. The draft was later reviewed by national and international IPC experts during a regional IPC workshop in November 2009.

The committee met regularly to review the inputs from various experts. The National IPC Policy was also reviewed by the MOH departmental heads, who gave their input and took ownership of the policy and guidelines development. The National IPC Policy and Guidelines for Health Care Services in Kenya were subsequently edited and finalized. The final document was later printed, launched, and disseminated to HCWs in the country.

The National IPC Policy for Health Care Services in Kenya aims to promote high standards of IPC to reduce the risk of HAIs and to improve the safety of patients, clients, HCWs, and the general public in Kenya. It identifies the roles and responsibilities of the various players in promoting IPC practice, the legal and regulatory framework for best IPC practice, continuous quality improvement, promotion of HCW safety, and advocacy and resource mobilization for IPC. The National IPC Guidelines for Health Care Services in Kenya aim to standardize IPC practice in the country by using evidence-based best practices. The guidelines provide the procedures for carrying out standard and transmission-based precautions, including isolation, environmental management practices, traffic flow, instrument and equipment processing, laboratory safety and precautions, laundry and linen processing, HCW occupational safety, and prevention of HAIs.

These documents were developed through the collaborative efforts of the MOH, the US CDC, other implementing partners, and other key stakeholders demonstrating genuine public-private partnership in the improvement of health care in Kenya toward achievement of the United Nations' Millennium Development Goals (MDGs) and national health goals. Through these efforts, HCWs now have documents that allow them to practice IPC in a standard way; to define the procedures, roles, and responsibilities for IPC committees; and to provide a platform for continuous quality improvement.

Lessons Learned

Developing a national infection control policy requires MOH commitment, collaboration, and partnership with key stakeholders. Qualitative data from the situational analysis were used to inform the process of developing the documents.

Conclusion

This chapter describes some of the future issues and looming challenges that may alter priorities and require intensified efforts in practice during the next several years. Health care epidemiologists, infection control practitioners, governments and other leaders, policy makers, and members of the public who are committed to infection prevention should consider these issues as they contemplate and plan for the future. Employing effective solutions to future challenges will lead to improved patient safety and quality of care.

References

1. Kohn LT, Corrigan JM, Donaldson MS. *To Err Is Human: Building a Safer Health System.* Washington, DC: National Academy Press, 2000. Accessed 13 Oct 2011. http://books.nap.edu/books/0309068371/html/index.html

2. Klevens RM, et al. Estimating health care–associated infections and deaths in U.S. hospitals, 2002. *Public Health Rep.* 2007 Mar–Apr; 122:160–166.

3. Edwards JR, et al. National Healthcare Safety Network (NHSN) report: Data summary for 2006 through 2008, issued December 2009. *Am J Infect Control.* 2009 Dec;37(10):783–805.

4. Warye KL, Murphy DM. Targeting zero health care-associated infections. *Am J Infect Control.* 2008 Dec;36(10):683–684.

5. Raad II. Commentary: Zero tolerance for catheter-related bloodstream infections: The unnegotiable objective. *Infect Control Hosp Epidemiol.* 2008 Oct;29(10):951–953.

6. Jarvis WR. The Lowbury Lecture. The United States approach to strategies in the battle against healthcare-associated infections, 2006: Transitioning from benchmarking to zero tolerance and clinician accountability. *J Hosp Infect.* 2007 Jun;65 Suppl 2:3–9.

7. APIC Position Statement. Targeting Zero Healthcare Associated Infections. 18 Jul 2008. Accessed 13 Oct 2011. http://www.apic.org/AM/CM/ContentDisplay.cfm?ContentFileID=11707.

8. Berwick DM. A primer on leading the improvement of systems. *BMJ.* 1996 Mar 9;312(7031):619–622.

9. McKeon LM, Oswaks JD, Cunningham PD. Safeguarding patients: Complexity science, high reliability organizations, and implications for team training in healthcare. *Clin Nurse Spec.* 2006 Nov–Dec;20(6):298–304.

10. Murphy D, Carrico R, Warye K. Building the infection prevention system of tomorrow: Proceedings of the 2007 APIC Futures Summit. *Am J Infect Control.* 2008 May;36(4):232–240.

11. Prüss-Ustün A, Rapiti E, Hutin Y. Estimation of the global burden of disease attributable to contaminated sharps injuries among health-care workers. *Am J Ind Med.* 2005 Dec;48(6):482–490.

12. Do AN, et al. Occupationally acquired human immunodeficiency virus (HIV) infection: National case surveillance data during 20 years of the HIV epidemic in the United States. *Infect Control Hosp Epidemiol.* 2003 Feb;24(2):86–96.

13. US Centers for Disease Control and Prevention. Evaluation of safety devices for preventing percutaneous injuries among health-care workers during phlebotomy procedures—Minneapolis-St. Paul, New York City, and San Francisco, 1993–1995. *MMWR Morb Mortal Wkly Rep.* 1997 Jan 17;46(2):21–25.

14. Poland GA. Hepatitis B immunization in health care workers. Dealing with vaccine nonresponse. *Am J Prev Med.* 1998 Jul;15(1):73–77.

15. Rachiotis G, et al. Vaccination against hepatitis B virus in workers of a general hospital in Athens. *Med Lav.* 2005 Jan–Feb;96(1):80–86.

16. Hood J, Smith A. Developing a "best practice" influenza vaccination program for health care workers—An evidence-based, leadership-modeled program. *AAOHN J.* 2009 Aug;57(8):308–312.

17. Looijmans-van den Akker I, et al. Effects of a multi-faceted program to increase influenza vaccine uptake among health care workers in nursing homes: A cluster randomised controlled trial. *Vaccine.* 2010 Jul 12;28(31):5086–5092.

18. Beekmann SE, et al. Hospital bloodborne pathogens programs: Program characteristics and blood and body fluid exposure rates. *Infect Control Hosp Epidemiol.* 2001 Feb;22(2):73–82.

19. Lamontagne F, et al. Role of safety-engineered devices in preventing needlestick injuries in 32 French hospitals. *Infect Control Hosp Epidemiol.* 2007 Jan;28(1):18–23.

20. Whitby M, McLaws ML, Slater K. Needlestick injuries in a major teaching hospital: The worthwhile effect of hospital-wide replacement of conventional hollow-bore needles. *Am J Infect Control.* 2008 Apr;36(3):180–186.

21. Yokoe DS, et al. A compendium of strategies to prevent healthcare-associated infections in acute care hospitals. *Infect Control Hosp Epidemiol.* 2008 Oct;29 Suppl 1:S12–21.

22. Ranji SR, et al. *Closing the Quality Gap: A Critical Analysis of Quality Improvement Strategies.* Vol. 6: Prevention of Healthcare–Associated Infections. Technical Reviews, No. 9.6. Rockville, MD: US Agency for Healthcare Research and Quality, Jan 2007.

23. The Joint Commission. *Advanced Lean Thinking: Proven Methods to Reduce Waste and Improve Quality in Health Care.* Oak Brook, IL: Joint Commission Resources, 2009.

24. Cohen AL, et al. Recommendations for metrics for multidrug-resistant organisms in healthcare settings: SHEA/HICPAC position paper. *Infect Control Hosp Epidemiol.* 2008 Oct;29(10):901–913.

25. Furuya EY, et al. Challenges of applying the SHEA/HICPAC metrics for multidrug-resistant organisms to a real-world setting. *Infect Control Hosp Epidemiol.* 2011 Apr;32(4):323–332.

26. The Joint Commission: *What Every Health Care Executive Should Know: The Cost of Antibiotic Resistance.* Oak Brook, IL: Joint Commission Resources, 2009.

27. Collins AS. Preventing health care–associated infections. In Hughes RG, editor: *Patient Safety and Quality: An Evidence-Based Handbook for Nurses.* Rockville, MD: US Agency for Healthcare Research and Quality, 2008. Accessed 13 Oct 2011. http://www.ahrq.gov/qual/nurseshdbk/docs/CollinsA_PHCAI.pdf.

28. Peterson LR. Bad bugs, no drugs: No ESCAPE revisited. *Clin Infect Dis.* 2009 Sep 15;49(6):992–993.

29. Peterson LR, Noskin GA. New technology for detecting multidrug-resistant pathogens in the clinical microbiology laboratory. *Emerg Infect Dis.* 2001 Mar–Apr;7(2):306–311.

30. Singh A, et al. Application of molecular techniques to the study of hospital infection. *Clin Microbiol Rev.* 2006 Jul;19(3):512–530.

31. Siegel JD, et al. Management of multidrug-resistant organisms in health care settings, 2006. *Am J Infect Control.* 2007 Dec;35(10 Suppl 2):S165–193.

32. Malhotra-Kumar S, et al. Evaluation of molecular assays for rapid detection of methicillin-resistant *Staphylococcus aureus. J Clin Microbiol.* 2010 Dec;48(12):4598–4601.

33. Rakita RM, et al. Mandatory influenza vaccination of healthcare workers: A 5-year study. *Infect Control Hosp Epidemiol.* 2010 Sep;31(9):881–888.

34. Diekema DJ, et al. Rapid detection of antimicrobial-resistant organism carriage: An unmet clinical need. *J Clin Microbiol.* 2004 Jul;42(7):2879–2883.

35. US Centers for Disease Control and Prevention. 2007 Guideline for Isolation Precautions: Preventing Transmission of Infectious Agents in Health Care Settings. Siegel JD, et al., Healthcare Infection Control Practices Advisory Committee. 2007. Accessed 13 Oct 2011. http://www.cdc.gov/hicpac/pdf/isolation/isolation2007.pdf

36. Al-Tawfiq JA, Antony A, Abed MS. Attitudes towards influenza vaccination of multi-nationality health-care workers in Saudi Arabia. *Vaccine.* 2009 Sep 4;27(40):5538–5541.

37. Centers for Diseases Control and Prevention. 2010–11 Influenza Prevention & Control Recommendations: Additional Information About Vaccination of Specific Populations. 15 Aug 2010. Accessed 13 Oct 2011. http://www.cdc.gov/flu/professionals/acip/specificpopulations.htm.

38. Poland GA. Mandating influenza vaccination for health care workers: Putting patients and professional ethics over personal preference. *Vaccine*. 2010 Aug 16;28(36):5757–5759.

39. Field RI. Mandatory vaccination of health care workers: Whose rights should come first? *P T*. 2009 Nov;34(11):615–618.

40. Iowa Healthcare Collaborative: Immunizations. Accessed 13 Oct 2011. http://www.ihconline.org/aspx/general/page.aspx?pid=10

41. The Joint Commission. Providing a Safer Environment for Health Care Personnel and Patients Through Influenza Vaccination: Strategies from Research and Practice. 2009. Accessed 13 Oct 2011. http://www.jointcommission.org/assets/1/18/Flu_Monograph.pdf.

42. Association for Professionals in Infection Control and Epidemiology. APIC Position Paper: Influenza Immunization of Healthcare Personnel. 1 Oct 2008. Accessed 13 Oct 2011. http://www.apic.org/AM/Template.cfm?Section=Home1&TEMPLATE=/CM/ContentDisplay.cfm&CONTENTFILEID=11049

43. Talbot TR, et al. Revised SHEA position paper: Influenza vaccination of healthcare personnel. *Infect Control Hosp Epidemiol*. 2010 Oct;31(10):987–995.

44. Palmore TN, et al. A successful mandatory influenza vaccination campaign using an innovative electronic tracking system. *Infect Control Hosp Epidemiol*. 2009 Dec;30(12):1137–1142.

45. Babcock HM, et al. Mandatory influenza vaccination of health care workers: Translating policy to practice. *Clin Infect Dis*. 2010 Feb 15;50(4):459–464.

46. van Delden JJ, et al. The ethics of mandatory vaccination against influenza for health care workers. *Vaccine*. 2008 Oct 16;26(44):5562–5566.

47. Talbot TR. Improving rates of influenza vaccination among healthcare workers: Educate; motivate; mandate? *Infect Control Hosp Epidemiol*. 2008 Feb;29(2):107–110.

48. Tilburt JC, et al. Facing the challenges of influenza in healthcare settings: The ethical rationale for mandatory seasonal influenza vaccination and its implications for future pandemics. *Vaccine*. 2008 Sep 12;26 Suppl 4:D27–30.

49. Helms CM, Polgreen PM. Should influenza immunisation be mandatory for healthcare workers? Yes. *BMJ*. 2008 Oct 28;337:a2142.

50. Isaacs D, Leask J. Should influenza immunisation be mandatory for healthcare workers? No. *BMJ*. 2008 Oct 28;337:a2140.

51. World Health Organization. WHO Guidelines on Hand Hygiene in Health Care. 2009. Accessed 13 Oct 2011. http://whqlibdoc.who.int/publications/2009/9789241597906_eng.pdf.

52. Conly JM, et al. Handwashing practices in an intensive care unit: The effects of an educational program and its relationship to infection rates. *Am J Infect Control*. 1989 Dec;17(6):330–339.

53. Dubbert PM, et al. Increasing ICU staff handwashing: Effects of education and group feedback. *Infect Control Hosp Epidemiol*. 1990 Apr;11(4):191–193.

54. Mayer JA, et al. Increasing handwashing in an intensive care unit. *Infect Control*. 1986 May;7(5):259–262.

55. Pittet D. Improving adherence to hand hygiene practice: A multidisciplinary approach. *Emerg Infect Dis*. 2001 Mar–Apr;7(2):234–240.

56. O'Boyle CA, Henly SJ, Larson E. Understanding adherence to hand hygiene recommendations: The theory of planned behavior. *Am J Infect Control*. 2001 Dec;29(6):352–360.

57. Mah MW, Deshpande S, Rothschild ML. Social marketing: A behavior change technology for infection control. *Am J Infect Control*. 2006 Sep;34(7):452–457.

58. American Marketing Association. Definition of Marketing. Accessed 13 Oct 2011. http://www.marketingpower.com/AboutAMA/Pages/DefinitionofMarketing.aspx.

59. Stead M, Hastings G, McDermott L. The meaning, effectiveness and future of social marketing. *Obes Rev*. 2007 Mar;8 Suppl 1:189–193.

60. World Health Organization. Issues in Health Services Delivery. Discussion Paper 1, Strategies for Assisting Health Workers to Modify and Improve Skills: Developing Quality Health Care—A Process of Change. Woodward CA. 2000. Accessed 13 Oct 2011. http://www.who.int/hrh/documents/en/improve_skills.pdf.

61. Haley RW, Shachtman RH. The emergence of infection surveillance and control programs in US hospitals: An assessment, 1976. *Am J Epidemiol*. 1980 May;111(5):574–591.

62. Wright SB, et al. Expanding roles of healthcare epidemiology and infection control in spite of limited resources and compensation. *Infect Control Hosp Epidemiol*. 2010 Feb;31(2):127–132.

63. O'Boyle C, Jackson M, Henly SJ. Staffing requirements for infection control programs in US health care facilities: Delphi project. *Am J Infect Control*. 2002 Oct;30(6):321–333.

64. Morrison J, Health Canada, Nosocomial and Occupational Infections Section. Development of a resource model for infection prevention and control programs in acute, long term, and home care settings: Conference proceedings of the Infection Prevention and Control Alliance. *Am J Infect Control*. 2004 Feb;32(1):2–6.

65. van den Broek PJ, et al. How many infection control staff do we need in hospitals? *J Hosp Infect*. 2007 Feb;65(2):108–111.

66. Richards C, et al. Characteristics of hospitals and infection control professionals participating in the National Nosocomial Infections Surveillance System 1999. *Am J Infect Control*. 2001 Dec;29(6):400–403.

67. Stevenson KB, et al. Assessing the status of infection control programs in small rural hospitals in the western United States. *Am J Infect Control*. 2004 Aug;32(5):255–261.

68. Stone PW, et al. The economic impact of infection control: Making the business case for increased infection control resources. *Am J Infect Control*. 2005 Nov;33(9):542–547.

69. Ulrich RS, et al. A review of the research literature on evidence-based healthcare design. *HERD*. 2008 Spring;1(3):61–125.

70. Bartley JM, Olmsted RN, Haas J. Current views of health care design and construction: Practical implications for safer, cleaner environments. *Am J Infect Control*. 2010 Jun;38(5 Suppl 1):S1–12.

71. Bracco D, et al. Single rooms may help to prevent nosocomial bloodstream infection and cross-transmission of methicillin-resistant *Staphylococcus aureus* in intensive care units. *Intensive Care Med*. 2007 May;33(5):836–840.

72. Facility Guidelines Institute. *2010 Guidelines for Design and Construction of Health Care Facilities*. Washington, DC: American Institute of Architects/Facility Guidelines Institute, 2010.

73. Kyriakides GK, et al. Immunologic monitoring and aspergillosis in renal transplant patients. *Am J Surg*. 1976 Feb;131(2):246–252.

74. US Centers for Disease Control and Prevention. Guideline for Disinfection and Sterilization in Healthcare Facilities, 2008. Rutala WA, Weber DJ, Hospital Infection Control Practices Advisory Committee. 2008. Accessed 17 Sep 2011. http://www.cdc.gov/hicpac/pdf/guidelines/Disinfection_Nov_2008.pdf

75. Halpin H, et al. Hospital adoption of automated surveillance technology and the implementation of infection prevention and control programs. *Am J Infect Control*. 2011 May;39(4):270–276.

76. Leal J, Laupland KB. Validity of electronic surveillance systems: A systematic review. *J Hosp Infect*. 2008 Jul;69(3):220–229.

77. Burke JP. Surveillance, reporting, automation, and interventional epidemiology. *Infect Control Hosp Epidemiol*. 2003 Jan;24(1):10–12.

78. Hautemanière A, et al. Identifying possible deaths associated with nosocomial infection in a hospital by data mining. *Am J Infect Control*. 2011 Mar;39(2):118–122.

79. Brossette SE, Hymel PA Jr. Data mining and infection control. *Clin Lab Med*. 2008 Mar;28(1):119–126, vii.

80. Wright MO. Automated surveillance and infection control: Toward a better tomorrow. *Am J Infect Control*. 2008 Apr;36(3 Suppl):S1–6.

81. Chiou SF, Chuang JH. Only automated surveillance with 100% sensitivity can save ICPs' time. *Am J Infect Control*. 2011 May;39(4):346.

82. Greenfield RA, Bronze MS. Emerging pathogens and knowledge in infectious diseases. *Am J Med Sci*. 2010 Sep;340(3):177–180.

83. Moellering RC Jr. NDM-1—A cause for worldwide concern. *N Engl J Med*. 2010 Dec 16;363(25):2377–2379.

Appendix 1

JCI Infection Prevention and Control Requirements

The following is a list of all Joint Commission International (JCI) requirements specific to the area of infection prevention and control (IPC). Also indicated is whether JCI requires written documentation of compliance and whether that documentation should be provided in the English language. Please note that only standards pertaining to IPC are included. Although the complete text of all IPC–related standards is provided, only the IPC–related applicability text (in italics) is included—when the applicability is not stated directly in the standard text—due to space limitations. For a complete list of all current JCI standards, see JCI's accreditation and certification Web page at http://www.jointcommissioninternational.org/Accreditation-and-Certification-Process/.

Ambulatory Care

Standard *Including applicability to IPC, when necessary*	Type of Written Documentation Needed	Documentation in English Required
International Patient Safety Goals (IPSG)		
IPSG.5 The ambulatory care organization develops an approach to reduce the risk of health care–associated infections.	Policy and Procedure	Yes
Infection Control and Facility Safety (IFS)		
IFS.1 The organization designs and implements a comprehensive program to reduce the risks of organization-acquired infections in patients and staff.	Program	No
IFS.2 One or more individuals oversee all infection prevention and control activities. This individual(s) is qualified in infection control practices through education, training, experience, or certification.	None	No
IFS.3 There is a designated coordination mechanism for all infection prevention and control activities that involves clinical and managerial staff as appropriate to the size and complexity of the organization.	None	No
IFS.4 The infection prevention and control program is based on current scientific knowledge, accepted practice guidelines, and applicable law and regulation.	None	No
IFS.5 The ambulatory care organization identifies the procedures and processes associated with the risk of infection and implements strategies to reduce infection risk.	Process Policies	No

Standard *Including applicability to IPC, when necessary*	Type of Written Documentation Needed	Documentation in English Required
IFS.7 The ambulatory care organization's facility is designed to provide accessible, efficient, and safe clinical care in a secure and supportive environment. *Facilities that house ambulatory care organizations have a number of design features that make them accessible to all types of patients and facilitate care that is personal, safe, and secure. Such features include the following:...* *c) Adequate hand hygiene methods are located in or adjacent to the office/exam rooms.* *e) The premises, fittings, and furniture are kept clean and in good repair, meeting standards for lighting, heating, ventilation, and infection prevention and control.* *f) A special, separate waiting area with separate ventilation is available for patients who may have an infectious disease.* *g) Safe storage and disposal for clinical waste and potentially infectious waste that require special disposal, such as sharps/needles and other disposable equipment that may have come in contact with body fluids, is available.*	None	No
IFS.10 The ambulatory care organization has a plan for the inventory, handling, storage, and use of hazardous materials and the control and disposal of hazardous materials and waste. *The ambulatory care organization identifies and safely controls hazardous materials and waste according to a plan. ... The plan provides processes for* *a) handling, storage, and use of hazardous materials;* *b) the inventory of hazardous materials and waste;* *c) reporting and investigation of spills, exposures, and other incidents;* *d) proper disposal of hazardous waste;* *e) proper protective equipment and procedures during use, spill, or exposure;* *f) documentation, including any permits, licenses, or other regulatory requirements; and* *g) proper labeling of hazardous materials and waste.*	Plan	No
Patient Access and Assessment (PAA)		
PAA.1.1 Patient flow in the ambulatory care organization is designed to provide uniform access based on the needs of the patient. *Patients with or without an appointment, patients who are obviously ill and possibly infectious to other patients and staff, patients with emergency needs that require stabilization and transfer, and other types of patients all need to be managed efficiently.*	None	No
PAA.8 Pathology and clinical laboratory services and consultation are readily available to meet patient needs.	None	No
PAA.8.1 Laboratory services provided within the ambulatory care organization meet applicable local and national standards, laws, and regulations; are directed and staffed by qualified individuals; are organized with adequate supplies; and have a quality control program.	Policy and Procedure	No
PAA.8.2 Current written policies and procedures are readily available and address, at a minimum • specimen collection; • specimen preservation; • instrument calibration; • quality control and remedial action; • equipment performance evaluation; and • test performance. *Laboratory services provided within the ambulatory care organization meet the following requirements:* *• They participate in the organization's infection prevention and control program.*	Written Quality Control Program Program Document Policy and Procedure	No No No

Standard *Including applicability to IPC, when necessary*	Type of Written Documentation Needed	Documentation in English Required
PAA.3.1 The scope and content of initial assessments conducted by different clinical disciplines is defined in writing and is based on applicable laws and regulations. *Each ambulatory care organization identifies those patients who may require additional assessment and appropriately modifies the assessment process. For example, the assessment process may be modified for patients who have special needs, such as… patients with infectious or communicable diseases.*	Written Criteria	Yes
Patient Care and Continuity of Care (PCC)		
PCC.3.1 Policies and procedures guide the care of emergency patients.	Policy and Procedure	Yes
PCC.3.2 Policies and procedures guide the use of resuscitation services throughout the organization.	Policy and Procedure	Yes
PCC.3.3 Policies and procedures guide the handling, use, and administration of blood and blood products.	Policy and Procedure	Yes
PCC.3.4 Policies and procedures guide the use of restraint.	Policy and Procedure	Yes
PCC.3.5 Policies and procedures guide the care of those at-risk populations identified by the organization. *Ambulatory care organizations may treat a wide variety of at-risk patient populations. The organization identifies such at-risk populations they serve, including populations such as… patients with infectious or communicable diseases.*	Policy and Procedure	Yes
PCC.5 Medications available within the ambulatory care organization for dispensing to patients or for practitioner administration are organized efficiently and effectively, and use is guided by policies and procedures. *As applicable to the situation, the policies and procedures are developed by qualified and relevant practitioners and address… (d) the medication recall process, including patient notification and the inadvertent use of medications known to be expired.*	Policy and Procedure	No
Patient Rights and Responsibilities (PRR)		
PRR.2.2 Patients and, when appropriate, families are informed of their responsibilities in the care process. *The ambulatory care organization identifies those responsibilities for patients and, when appropriate, families in the care process. Each organization identifies those responsibilities through a collaborative process involving patients, health care practitioners, and other appropriate individuals.* *The responsibilities identified include at least… d) respecting the organization's policies and procedures related to smoking, infection prevention and control, and environmental care.*	None	No
Patient Record and Information Flow (PRI)		
PRI.9 The ambulatory care organization collects and analyzes aggregate data to support patient care, effective management, and the quality and patient safety program. *The ambulatory care organization collects and analyzes aggregate data to support patient care and ambulatory care organization management. … In particular, aggregate data from risk management, utility system management, infection prevention and control, and utilization review can help the ambulatory care organization understand its current performance and identify opportunities for improvement.*	None	No

Standard *Including applicability to IPC, when necessary*	Type of Written Documentation Needed	Documentation in English Required
Improvement in Quality and Patient Safety (IQS)		
IQS.3 Quality monitoring includes both clinical and managerial processes and outcomes as selected by the ambulatory care organization's leaders. *Clinical monitoring areas include [as applicable to the organization]... infection.*	Plan	No
Human Resource Management (HRM)		
HRM.2 New staff orientation provides initial job training and assessment of capability to perform job responsibilities. *The orientation includes, as appropriate, the reporting of medical errors, infection prevention and control practices, the organization's policies on medication orders, and so on. ... Any contract workers and volunteers are also oriented to the ambulatory care organization and their specific assignment or responsibilities, such as patient safety and infection prevention and control.*	None	No
HRM.2.1 Ongoing in-service or other education and training maintain and improve staff competence. *To maintain acceptable staff performance, teach new skills, and provide training on new equipment and procedures, the ambulatory care organization provides or arranges for facilities, educators, and time for ongoing in-service and other education. ... For example, medical staff members may receive education on infection prevention and control, advances in medical practice, or new technology.*	None	No
HRM.4 Health professional training and education, when provided within the ambulatory care organization, are guided by policies that ensure adequate supervision. *The ambulatory care organization provides the required level of supervision for each type and level of trainee or community worker. The trainees and community workers are integrated into the organization's orientation, quality, patient safety, and infection prevention and control programs.*	None	No

Clinical Care Program Certification

Standard *Including applicability to IPC, when necessary*	Type of Written Documentation Needed	Documentation in English Required
International Patient Safety Goals (IPSG)		
IPSG.5 The clinical care program develops an approach to reduce the risk of health care–associated infections.	Policy and Procedure	Yes
Delivering or Facilitating Clinical Care (DFC)		
DFC.2 All clinical and nonclinical staff are oriented to the program and to their specific job responsibilities. *The orientation includes, as appropriate, the reporting of medical errors; infection prevention and control practices; the program's policies, procedures, and guidelines; and any other necessary information and training.*	None	No

Clinical Laboratories

Standard *Including applicability to IPC, when necessary*	Type of Written Documentation Needed	Documentation in English Required
International Patient Safety Goals (IPSG)		
IPSG.5 The clinical laboratory develops an approach to reduce the risk of health care–associated infections.	Policy and Procedure	Yes
Resource Management and Laboratory Environment (RSM)		
RSM.4.4 The laboratory follows written guidelines for the periodic evaluation of all reagents, including water, to provide for accuracy and precision of results. *f) The laboratory does not use materials of substandard reactivity or outdated or deteriorated materials.*	Document	No
RSM.6 The laboratory has a plan for inventory, handling, storage, and use of hazardous materials and the control and disposal of hazardous waste.	Document	No
RSM.6.1 The laboratory uses a coordinated process to reduce the risks of infection as a result of exposure to biohazardous materials and waste.	Document	No
Management and Leadership (MGT)		
MGT.4.2.1 Quality measurement includes those aspects of the following that are selected by leaders: a) The laboratory's safety and infection control programs	None	No
MGT.4.6 Data are analyzed when undesirable trends and variation are evident from the data. *When the laboratory detects or suspects undesirable change from what is expected, it initiates intense analysis to determine where best to focus improvement. In particular, intense analysis is initiated when levels, patterns, or trends vary significantly and undesirably from* *• what was expected;* *• those of other laboratories; or* *• recognized standards.* *Analyses are conducted for* *• all confirmed transfusion reactions, if applicable to the laboratory; and* *• other events, such as infectious disease outbreaks.*	None	No
Quality Control Processes (QCP)		
QCP.11.1.1 A detailed history of a donor is performed prior to selection for blood donation. *The history performed is adequate to screen out unsuitable donors. It includes providing donors with educational materials explaining the risks of infectious disease, unusual antibodies, and, as feasible, drugs.* *The history of the donor includes the following:* *• drug use; history of infectious disease, such as malaria or hepatitis; positive blood test for HBsAg; or, during the preceding 12 months,* *• receipt of a transfusion of blood or blood components;* *• receipt of hepatitis immunoglobulin;* *• skin penetrations, such as tattoos or acupuncture; and/or* *• history of incarceration for at least 72 hours in a correctional institution.*	Document	No

Standard *Including applicability to IPC, when necessary*	Type of Written Documentation Needed	Documentation in English Required
QCP.11.1.2 An adequate physical examination is performed prior to approving the individual as a blood donor. *A proper physical examination is necessary to ensure the health of the donor and safety of the blood. The physical examination is performed by a qualified individual and documented. It should include the following, with defined criteria for acceptance of the donor:* *...d) Arm inspection to ensure the absence of skin punctures or scars indicating injection of narcotics, and no infectious skin diseases that would become a risk of contamination of the blood*	Document	No
QCP.11.10.3 The director has defined criteria for recognition of transfusion reactions, as well as steps to take when symptoms occur. *The following are defined and implemented:* *k) When faulty components have or might have caused a potential adverse reaction, there is a process for notifying the blood donor service that provided the component and for follow-up for transfusion-transmitted disease, including a procedure that describes how recipients who have been transfused with potentially infectious blood or components are to be notified and counseled.*	Document	No
QCP.14 The laboratory follows written policies and procedures for molecular testing.	Document	No
QCP.14.1 Validation studies include representatives from each specimen type expected to be tested in the assay and specimens representing the scope of reportable results.	Document	No
QCP.14.2 The laboratory establishes quality control limits, reference ranges, and reportable ranges.	Document	No
QCP.14.3 The laboratory verifies each test run of patient samples in molecular pathology, using quality controls.	Document	No
QCP.14.4 Molecular testing reports include specific testing information.	Document	No
QCP.14.5 The laboratory follows written policies and procedures for molecular genetic testing.	Document	No
QCP.14.6 Molecular genetic testing reports include specific testing information. *Molecular testing is the analysis or the detection of nucleic acids by hybridization, with or without amplification.* *Molecular testing has become an area of rapid growth and change in the laboratory. This is due to the tremendous potential that molecular testing has for improving the prediction, prevention, detection, and treatment of disease. It promises to be extremely useful in diagnosis, therapy, epidemiologic investigations, and infection control.* *While molecular testing shows great promise, like any other medical testing, it also has the potential to cause great harm if errors occur. Inaccurate results can lead to misdiagnosis or inappropriate treatment or counseling. Therefore, standards are used to sufficiently support the safeguards required for molecular testing.*	Document	No

Home Care*

Standard *Including applicability to IPC, when necessary*	Type of Written Documentation Needed	Documentation in English Required
International Patient Safety Goals (IPSG)		
IPSG.5 The home care organization develops an approach to reduce the risk of health care–associated infections.		
Infection Prevention and Control (IPC)		
IPC.1 One or more individuals, qualified in infection control practices through education, training, experience, or certification, oversee all infection prevention and control activities.		
IPC.2 The home care organization designs, implements, and designates a coordination mechanism for a comprehensive program to reduce the risks of organization-acquired infections in patients and staff.		
IPC.3 The infection prevention and control program is based on current scientific knowledge, accepted practice guidelines, and applicable law and regulation.		
IPC.4 The home care organization uses a risk-based approach in establishing the focus of the health care–associated infection prevention and reduction program.		
IPC.4.1 The home care organization implements and supports an evidence-based immunization program.		
IPC.5 The home care organization identifies the procedures and processes associated with the risk of infection and implements strategies to reduce infection risk.		
IPC.6 Gloves, masks, eye protection, other protective equipment, soap, and disinfectants are available and used correctly when required.		
IPC.7 The home care organization provides education on infection control practices to family, patients, and all care providers.		
Patient Access and Assessment (PAA)		
PAA.2.2 The home care organization conducts individualized initial assessments for special populations cared for by the organization. *In particular, if present in the patient population, the assessment process may be modified for high-risk patients, such as… infectious patients….*		
Patient Medication Management (PMM)		
PMM.2.3 The home care organization has a medication recall system. *There is a policy or procedure that addresses any use of or the destruction of medications known to be expired or outdated.*		
Improvement in Quality and Patient Safety (IQS)		
IQS.3 The organization's leaders identify key measures in the organization's structures, processes, and outcomes to be used in the organizationwide quality improvement and patient safety plan.		
IQS.3.1 The organization's leaders identify at least five (5) key measures for each of the organization's clinical structures, processes, and outcomes.		
IQS.3.2 The organization's leaders identify at least five (5) key measures for each of the organization's managerial structures, processes, and outcomes.		
IQS.3.3 The organization's leaders identify key measures for each of the International Patient Safety Goals that are applicable to the home care surveys provided. *The measures selected related to the important clinical areas include [when applicable to services provided]…antibiotic or other medication use; use of blood/blood products; infection prevention and control, surveillance, and reporting.*		

*JCI Home Care survey requirements were not finalized at the time of this publication; however, the standards language represented above is official as of 1 January 2011. Go to http://www.jointcommissioninternational.org/Accreditation-and-Certification-Process/ for updated information.

Standard *Including applicability to IPC, when necessary*	Type of Written Documentation Needed	Documentation in English Required
IQS.7 Data are analyzed when undesirable trends and variation are evident from the data. *An analysis is conducted for… other events, such as infectious disease outbreaks.*		
Management and Safety of the Environment (MSE)		
MSE.4 The home care organization has a plan for the identification of, handling, storage, and use of hazardous materials and the control and disposal of hazardous materials and waste. *The plan addresses the patient's environment and provides processes for* *• handling, storage, and use of hazardous materials;* *• the identification of hazardous materials and wastes stored in the home;* *• a process for managing spills, exposures, and other incidents;* *• proper disposal of hazardous wastes;* *• proper protective equipment and procedures during use, spill, or exposure; and* *• proper labeling of hazardous materials and wastes.*		

MSE.5.1 Equipment that is received and stored by the home care organization for use in the patient's home is stored appropriately.
The home care organization's receipt and storage of equipment includes
• clearly identifying and separating areas for
  – clean equipment and dirty equipment,
  – cleaning and disinfecting equipment,
  – equipment requiring maintenance or repair,
  – obsolete inventory, and
  – equipment ready for use;
• maintaining the cleanliness of equipment ready for use;
• maintaining warehouse and storage areas cleanliness; and
• other considerations, such as temperature requirements, expiration dates, and maintaining battery charge requirements (per the manufacturer's guidelines).		

Staff Qualifications and Education (SQE)		
SQE.7 Upon appointment to the staff, all clinical and nonclinical staff members are oriented to the home care organization and the services to which they are assigned and to their specific job responsibilities. *The orientation includes the reporting of errors, patient safety, infection prevention and control practices, the home care organization's policies on telephone medication orders, and so on. Contract workers, volunteers, and students/trainees are also oriented to the home care organization and their specific assignments or responsibilities, such as patient safety and infection prevention and control. The orientation also includes the organization's mission, values, and code of conduct.* *Contract workers, volunteers, and students/trainees are also oriented to the home care organization and their specific assignments or responsibilities, such as patient safety and infection prevention and control.*		
SQE.8 Each staff member receives ongoing in-service and other education and training to maintain or to advance his or her skills and knowledge. *This education is relevant to each staff member as well as to the continuing advancement of the home care organization in meeting patient needs. For example, clinical staff may receive education on infection prevention and control, advances in practice, or new technology. Each staff member's educational achievements are documented in his or her personnel record.* **SQE.8.4** The home care organization provides a staff health and safety program. *Whatever the staffing and structure of the program, staff understand how to report, to be treated for, and to receive counseling and follow-up for such injuries as needlesticks, exposure to infectious diseases, the identification of risks and hazardous conditions in the environment, and other health and safety matters.*		

Standard *Including applicability to IPC, when necessary*	Type of Written Documentation Needed	Documentation in English Required
Governance and Leadership (GAL)		
GAL.5.4 The home care organization's leaders provide orientation and training for all staff of the duties and responsibilities for the service to which they are assigned. *The orientation includes the home care organization's mission, the service's mission, the scope of services provided, and the policies and procedures related to providing services. For example, all staff understand the infection prevention and control procedures within the home care organization and within the service provided. When new or revised policies or procedures are implemented, staff are trained.*		
Communication and Information Management (CIM)		
CIM.19 Aggregate data and information support patient care, organization management, and the quality management program. **CIM.19.1** The home care organization has a process to aggregate data and has determined which data and information are to be regularly aggregated to meet the needs of clinical and managerial staff in the home care organization and agencies outside the organization. **CIM.19.2** The home care organization has a process for using or participating in external databases. *In particular, aggregate data from risk management, infection prevention and control, and utilization review can help the home care organization understand its current performance and identify opportunities for improvement.*		

Hospitals

Standard *Including applicability to IPC, when necessary*	Type of Written Documentation Needed	Documentation in English Required
International Patient Safety Goals (IPSG)		
IPSG.5 The hospital develops an approach to reduce the risk of health care–associated infections.	Policy and Procedure	Yes
Prevention and Control of Infections (PCI)		
PCI.1 One or more individuals oversee all infection prevention and control activities. This individual(s) is qualified in infection prevention and control practices through education, training, experience, or certification.	None	No
PCI.2 There is a designated coordination mechanism for all infection prevention and control activities that involves physicians, nurses, and others as based on the size and complexity of the organization.	None	No
PCI.3 The infection prevention and control program is based on current scientific knowledge, accepted practice guidelines, applicable laws and regulations, and standards for sanitation and cleanliness.	None	No
PCI.4 The organization's leaders provide adequate resources to support the infection prevention and control program.	None	No
PCI.5 The organization designs and implements a comprehensive program to reduce the risks of health care–associated infections in patients and health care workers.	Policy and Procedure	Yes
PCI.5.1 All patient, staff, and visitor areas of the organization are included in the infection prevention and control program.	None	No

Standard *Including applicability to IPC, when necessary*	Type of Written Documentation Needed	Documentation in English Required
PCI.6 The organization uses a risk-based approach in establishing the focus of the health care–associated infection prevention and reduction program.	Risk Assessment	No
PCI.7 The organization identifies the procedures and processes associated with the risk of infection and implements strategies to reduce infection risk.	Processes Policy and Procedure	No No
PCI.7.1 The organization reduces the risk of infections by ensuring adequate equipment cleaning and sterilization and the proper management of laundry and linen.	None	No
PCI.7.1.1 There is a policy and procedure in place that identifies the process for managing expired supplies and defines the conditions for reuse of single-use devices when laws and regulations permit.	Policy and Procedure	Yes
PCI.7.2 The organization reduces the risk of infections through proper disposal of waste.	None	No
PCI.7.3 The organization has a policy and procedure on the disposal of sharps and needles.	Policy	No
PCI.7.4 The organization reduces the risk of infections in the facility associated with operations of the food service and of mechanical and engineering controls.	None	No
PCI.7.5 The organization reduces the risk of infection in the facility during demolition, construction, and renovation.	None	No
PCI.8 The organization provides barrier precautions and isolation procedures that protect patients, visitors, and staff from communicable diseases and protect immunosuppressed patients from acquiring infections to which they are uniquely prone.	Policy and Procedure	No
PCI.9 Gloves, masks, eye protection, other protective equipment, soap, and disinfectants are available and used correctly when required.	Guideline	No
PCI.10 The infection prevention and control process is integrated with the organization's overall program for quality improvement and patient safety.	None	No
PCI.10.1 The organization tracks infection risks, infection rates, and trends in health care–associated infections.	None	No
PCI.10.2 Quality improvement includes using measures related to infection issues that are epidemiologically important to the organization.	None	No
PCI.10.3 The organization uses risk, rate, and trend information to design or to modify processes to reduce the risk of health care–associated infections to the lowest possible levels.	None	No
PCI.10.4 The organization compares its health care–associated infection rates with other organizations through comparative databases.	None	No
PCI.10.5 The results of infection prevention and control measurement in the organization are regularly communicated to leaders and staff.	None	No
PCI.10.6 The organization reports information on infections to appropriate external public health agencies.	None	No
PCI.11 The organization provides education on infection prevention and control practices to staff, physicians, patients, families, and other caregivers when indicated by their involvement in care.	Program	Yes
Assessment of Patients (AOP)		
AOP.1.8 The organization conducts individualized initial assessments for special populations cared for by the organization. *In particular, when the organization serves one or more of the special-needs patients or populations listed below, the organization conducts individualized assessments of the following:* *…• Patients with infectious or communicable diseases* *…• Patients whose immune systems are compromised.*	Criteria	No

Standard *Including applicability to IPC, when necessary*	Type of Written Documentation Needed	Documentation in English Required
AOP.5.1 A laboratory safety program is in place, followed, and documented. *The laboratory safety management program includes… written policies and procedures for the handling and disposal of infectious and hazardous materials.*	Policy and Procedure	Yes
AOP.6.2 A radiation safety program is in place, followed, and documented. *The radiation safety program reflects the risks and hazards encountered. The program addresses safety practices and prevention measures for radiology and diagnostic imaging staff, other staff, and patients. The program is coordinated with the organization's safety management program. The radiation safety management program includes …• written policies and procedures for handling and disposal of infectious and hazardous materials; and • availability of safety protective devices appropriate to the practices and hazards encountered.*	Program Policy and Procedure	Yes No
Medication Management and Use (MMU)		
MMU.3.3 The organization has a medication recall system. *There is a policy or procedure that addresses any use of or the destruction of medications known to be expired or outdated.*	Policy and Procedure	No
MMU.5 Medications are prepared and dispensed in a safe and clean environment. *The pharmacy or pharmaceutical service prepares and dispenses medications in a clean and safe environment that complies with law, regulation, and professional practice standards. The organization identifies the standards of practice for a safe and clean preparation and dispensing environment. Medications stored and dispensed from areas outside the pharmacy (for example, patient care units) comply with the same safety and cleanliness measures). Staff preparing compounded sterile products (such as IVs and epidurals) are trained in the principles of aseptic technique. Similarly, hooded vents are available and used when indicated by professional practices (for example, cytotoxic medications).*	None	No
Quality Improvement and Patient Safety (QPS)		
QPS.1.1 The organization's leaders collaborate to carry out the quality improvement and patient safety program. *Leaders ensure the program addresses coordination among the multiple organizational units concerned with quality and safety, such as the infection prevention and control program….*	None	No
QPS.3 The organization's leaders identify key measures in the organization's structures, processes, and outcomes to be used in the organizationwide quality improvement and patient safety plan. **QPS.3.1** The organization's leaders identify key measures for each of the organization's clinical structures, processes, and outcomes. **QPS.3.2** The organization's leaders identify key measures for each of the organization's managerial structures, processes, and outcomes. **QPS.3.3** The organization's leaders identify key measures for each of the International Patient Safety Goals. *The measures selected related to the important clinical areas include, among others, infection prevention and control, surveillance, and reporting.*	None None None None	No No No No
QPS.7 Data are analyzed when undesirable trends and variation are evident from the data. *An analysis is conducted for several types of occurrences, including infectious disease outbreaks.*	None	No

Standard *Including applicability to IPC, when necessary*	Type of Written Documentation Needed	Documentation in English Required
Governance, Leadership, and Direction (GLD)		
GLD.5.4 Directors provide orientation and training for all staff of the duties and responsibilities for the department or service to which they are assigned. *For example, all staff understand the infection prevention and control procedures within the organization and within the department or service.*	Program	No
Management of Communication and Information (MCI)		
MCI.20.2 The organization has a process for using or participating in external databases. *In particular, aggregate data from risk management, utility system management, infection prevention and control, and utilization review can help the organization understand its current performance and identify opportunities for improvement.*	None	No
Staff Qualifications and Education (SQE)		
SQE.7 All clinical and nonclinical staff members are oriented to the organization, the department, or unit to which they are assigned and to their specific job responsibilities at appointment to the staff. *The orientation includes the reporting of medical errors, infection prevention and control practices, the organization's policies on telephone medication orders, and so on.*	None	No
SQE.8.4 The organization provides a staff health and safety program. *How an organization orients and trains staff, provides a safe workplace, maintains biomedical and other equipment, prevents or controls health care–associated infections, and many other factors determine the health and well-being of staff.*	None	No
Facility Management and Safety (FMS)		
FMS.2 The organization develops and maintains a written plan(s) describing the processes to manage risks to patients, families, visitors, and staff. *Processes include managing the infection prevention and control risks of the buildings, grounds, and equipment; hazardous materials; medical equipment; and utility systems.*	Plans	Yes
FMS.3 One or more qualified individuals oversee the planning and implementation of the program to manage the risks in the care environment.	None	No
FMS.3.1 A monitoring program provides data on incidents, injuries, and other events that support planning and further risk reduction. *The risk management program, including infection prevention and control, is managed by a qualified person(s) and monitored through data collection and analysis.*	None	No
FMS.8 The organization plans and implements a program for inspecting, testing, and maintaining medical equipment and documenting the results.	None	No
FMS.8.1 The organization collects monitoring data for the medical equipment management program. These data are used to plan the organization's long-term needs for upgrading or replacing equipment.	None	No
FMS.8.2 The organization has a product/equipment recall system. *Medical equipment is inventoried, inspected, tested, maintained, and monitored for optimal performance, including preventing infections.*	Policy	No

Standard *Including applicability to IPC, when necessary*	Type of Written Documentation Needed	Documentation in English Required
FMS.9 Potable water and electrical power are available 24 hours a day, 7 days a week, through regular or alternate sources, to meet essential patient care needs.	None	No
FMS.9.1 The organization has emergency processes to protect facility occupants in the event of water or electrical system disruption, contamination, or failure.	None	No
FMS.9.2 The organization tests its emergency water and electrical systems on a regular basis appropriate to the system and documents the results.	None	No
Water and electric power, key factors in maintaining infection prevention and control, are available at all times.		
FMS.10 Electrical, water, waste, ventilation, medical gas, and other key systems are regularly inspected, maintained, and, when appropriate, improved.	None	No
FMS.10.1 Designated individuals or authorities monitor water quality regularly.	None	No
FMS.10.2 The organization collects monitoring data for the utility system management program. These data are used to plan the organization's long-term needs for upgrading or replacing the utility system.	None	No
All utilities are maintained, monitored, and, if necessary, improved to avoid or mitigate infection.		
FMS.11 The organization educates and trains all staff members about their roles in providing a safe and effective patient care facility.	None	No
FMS.11.1 Staff members are trained and knowledgeable about their roles in the organization's plans for fire safety, security, hazardous materials, and emergencies.	None	No
FMS.11.2 Staff are trained to operate and to maintain medical equipment and utility systems.	None	No
FMS.11.3 The organization periodically tests staff knowledge through demonstrations, mock events, and other suitable methods. This testing is then documented.	None	No
Staff are trained, and that training is maintained and documented to keep patients, staff, and others safe from infection and other adverse outcomes.		

Long Term Care*

Standard *Including applicability to IPC, when necessary*	Type of Written Documentation Needed	Documentation in English Required
International Patient Safety Goals (IPSG)		
IPSG.5 The long term care organization develops an approach to reduce the risk of health care–associated infections.		
Infection Prevention and Control (IPC)		
IPC.1 One or more individuals, qualified in infection control practices through education, training, experience, or certification, oversee all infection prevention and control activities.		
IPC.2 The long term care organization designs, implements, and designates a coordination mechanism for a comprehensive program to reduce the risks of organization-acquired infections in residents and staff.		
IPC.3 The infection prevention and control program is based on current scientific knowledge, accepted practice guidelines, and applicable law and regulation.		

* JCI Long Term Care survey requirements were not finalized at the time of this publication; however, the standards language represented above is official as of 1 January 2011. Go to http://www.jointcommissioninternational.org/Accreditation-and-Certification-Process/ for updated information.

Standard *Including applicability to IPC, when necessary*	Type of Written Documentation Needed	Documentation in English Required
IPC.4 The long term care organization uses a risk-based approach in establishing the focus of the health care–associated infection prevention and reduction program. **IPC.4.1** The home care organization implements and supports an evidence-based immunization program.		
IPC.5 The long term care organization identifies the procedures and processes associated with the risk of infection and implements strategies to reduce infection risk. **IPC.5.1** The organization reduces the risk of infections by ensuring adequate equipment cleaning and sterilization and the proper management of laundry and linen. **IPC.5.1.1** There is a policy and procedure in place that identifies the process for managing expired supplies and defines the conditions for reuse of single-use devices when laws and regulations permit. **IPC.5.2** Food preparation, handling, storage, and distribution are safe and comply with laws, regulations, and current acceptable practice. **IPC.5.3** The organization reduces the risk of infections through proper disposal of waste and the disposal of sharps and needles. **IPC.5.4** The organization reduces the risk of infection in the facility during demolition, construction, and renovation.		
IPC.6 The organization provides barrier precautions and isolation procedures that protect residents, visitors, and staff from communicable diseases and protects immunosuppressed residents from acquiring infections to which they are uniquely prone.		
IPC.7 Gloves, masks, eye protection, other protective equipment, soap, and disinfectants are available and used correctly when required.		
IPC.8 The long term care organization provides education on infection control practices to family, residents, and all care providers.		
Resident Access and Assessment (RAA)		
RAA.2.2 The long term care organization conducts individualized initial assessments for special populations cared for by the organization. *In particular, if present in the resident population, the assessment process may be modified for high-risk residents, such as… infectious residents; and… residents whose immune systems are compromised.*		
Resident Medication Management (RMM)		
RMM.2.3 The long term care organization has a medication recall system. *There is a policy or procedure that addresses any use of or the destruction of medications known to be expired or outdated.*		
Improvement in Quality and Resident Safety (IQS)		
IQS.3 The organization's leaders identify key measures in the organization's structures, processes, and outcomes to be used in the organizationwide quality improvement and resident safety plan. **IQS.3.1** The organization's leaders identify at least five (5) key measures for each of the organization's clinical structures, processes, and outcomes. **IQS.3.2** The organization's leaders identify key measures for each of the organization's managerial structures, processes, and outcomes. **IQS.3.3** The organization's leaders identify key measures for each of the International Patient Safety Goals that are applicable to the long term care surveys provided. *The measures selected related to the important clinical areas include [when applicable to services provided]… antibiotic or other medication use;… use of blood/blood products;… [and] infection prevention and control, surveillance, and reporting.*		

Standard *Including applicability to IPC, when necessary*	Type of Written Documentation Needed	Documentation in English Required
IQS.7 Data are analyzed when undesirable trends and variation are evident from the data. *An analysis is conducted for the following:… Other events, such as infectious disease outbreaks.*		
Management and Safety of the Environment (MSE)		
MSE.7 The long term care organization has a plan for the inventory, handling, storage, and use of hazardous materials and the control and disposal of hazardous materials and waste. *Hazardous materials and waste need to be managed in the long term care environment. Hazardous materials and waste are identified by the long term care organization and safely controlled according to a plan. Such materials and waste include chemicals, chemotherapeutic agents, hazardous gases and vapors, and other regulated medical and infectious waste.*		
Staff Qualifications and Education (SQE)		
SQE.7 Upon appointment to the staff, all clinical and nonclinical staff members are oriented to the long term care organization and the service to which they are assigned and to their specific job responsibilities. *The orientation includes the reporting of errors, resident safety, infection prevention and control practices, the long term care organization's policies on telephone medication orders, and so on. The orientation also includes the organization's mission, values, and code of conduct.* *Contract workers, volunteers, and students/trainees are also oriented to the long term care organization and their specific assignments or responsibilities, such as resident safety and infection prevention and control.*		
SQE.8 Each staff member receives ongoing in-service and other education and training to maintain or to advance his or her skills and knowledge. *For example, clinical staff may receive education on infection prevention and control, advances in practice, or new technology. Each staff member's educational achievements are documented in his or her personnel record.* **SQE.8.4** The long term care organization provides a staff health and safety program. *How an organization orients and trains staff, provides a safe workplace, maintains biomedical and other equipment, prevents or controls health care–associated infections, and many other factors determine the health and well-being of staff.*		
Governance and Leadership (GAL)		
GAL.5.4 The long term care organization's leaders provide orientation and training for all staff of the duties and responsibilities for the services to which they are assigned. *For example, all staff understand the infection prevention and control procedures within the long term care organization and within the services provided.*		
Communication and Information Management (CIM)		
CIM.19 Aggregate data and information support resident care, organization management, and the quality management program. **CIM.19.1** The long term care organization has a process to aggregate data and has determined which data and information are to be regularly aggregated to meet the needs of clinical and managerial staff in the long term care organization and agencies outside the organization. **CIM.19.2** The long term care organization has a process for using or participating in external databases. *In particular, aggregate data from risk management, infection prevention and control, and utilization review can help the long term care organization understand its current performance and identify opportunities for improvement.*		

Medical Transport

Standard *Including applicability to IPC, when necessary*	Type of Written Documentation Needed	Documentation in English Required
Biologic and Chemical Agents (BCA)		
BCA.1 The organization designs and implements a coordinated program to reduce the risks of infections.	Plan	Yes
BCA.1.1 All patient, staff, vehicles, and other areas of the organization are included in the infection control program.	Plan	Yes
BCA.2 The organization establishes the focus of the infection prevention and reduction program.	Plan	Yes
BCA.3 The medical transport organization identifies the policies and processes associated with the risk of infection and implements strategies to reduce infection risk.	Policy and Procedure Plan	Yes Yes
BCA.4 Gloves, masks, protective clothing, soap, and disinfectants are available and used correctly when required.	Plan	Yes
BCA.5 The organization has a plan for the inventory, handling, storage, and use of stocked hazardous materials and the control and disposal of self-generated hazardous materials and waste.	Plan	Yes
BCA.6 The organization develops and implements a plan for response and mitigation of hazardous materials incidents.	Plan	Yes
BCA.6.1 The organization develops and implements a plan that protects rescue staff and minimizes their exposure to hazardous materials.	Plan	Yes
BCA.6.2 Rescue personnel are monitored during a hazardous materials incident.	Plan	Yes
BCA.7 One or more individuals oversee all infection, biologic, and chemical agent control activities. This individual(s) is qualified in BCA control practices through education, training, experience, or certification.	Plan	Yes
BCA.8 The BCA control program is based on current scientific knowledge, accepted practice guidelines, and applicable law and regulation.	Plan	Yes
BCA.9 The organization's information management systems support the BCA control program.	Plan	Yes
BCA.10 The organization provides education on BCA control practices to staff, patients, and, as appropriate, family and other caregivers.	Plan	Yes
BCA.10.1 All staff receive an orientation to the organization's BCA control procedures and practices.	Plan	Yes
BCA.10.2 All staff are educated in BCA control when new procedures are implemented and when significant trends are noted in surveillance data.	Plan	Yes
Quality Management and Improvement (QMI)		
QMI.3.7 Monitoring includes infection, biologic, hazardous materials control, surveillance, and reporting.	None	No

Standard *Including applicability to IPC, when necessary*	Type of Written Documentation Needed	Documentation in English Required
Governance, Leadership, and Direction (GLD)		
GLD.5.1 Organization leaders plan with community leaders and the leaders of other organizations to meet the community's emergency and medical transport system needs.	None	No
GLD.5.1.1 Organization leaders develop a plan to respond to likely community emergencies, epidemics, and natural or other disasters. *Sudden changes, such as natural disasters and outbreaks of infectious diseases, will precipitate rapid change. An organization needs to plan to respond quickly and effectively to an emergency, disaster, or epidemic in the community (for example, floods, earthquakes, worker injuries from a factory explosion, flu outbreaks).*	Plan	Yes
Staff Qualifications and Education (SQE)		
SQE.5 All staff members are oriented to the organization and to their specific job responsibilities upon appointment to the staff. *The orientation includes, as appropriate, safety, infection control, documentation requirements, error reporting, medical and administrative protocols, disaster response, and so forth.*	None	No
SQE.6 Each staff member receives ongoing in-service and other education and training to maintain or advance his or her skills and knowledge. *This education is relevant to each staff member as well as to the continuing advancement of the organization in meeting patient needs. For example, staff may receive education on safety, infection control, advances in medical practice, or new technology.*	None	No
Management of Information (MOI)		
MOI.4 Aggregate data and information support patient care, organization management, and the quality management program. **MOI.4.1** The organization has a process to aggregate data and has determined what data and information are to be regularly aggregated to meet the needs of medical direction and managerial staff in the organization and agencies outside the organization. **MOI.4.2** The organization contributes to external databases in accordance with law or regulation. **MOI.4.3** The organization uses external reference databases for comparative purposes. **MOI.4.3.1** The security and confidentiality of patient-specific data and information are maintained when contributing to or using external databases. *In particular, aggregate data from risk management, utility system management, infection control, and utilization review can help the organization understand its current performance and identify opportunities for improvement.*	None None None None None	No No No No No
Care of Patients (COP)		
COP.9.4.1 The organization has a medication recall system. *There is a policy or procedure that addresses any use of or the destruction of any known expired or outdated medications.*	Policy and Procedure	No

Primary Care

Standard *Including applicability to IPC, when necessary*	Type of Written Documentation Needed	Documentation in English Required
International Patient Safety Goals (IPSG)		
IPSG.5 The primary care center develops an approach to reduce the risk of health care–associated infections.	None	No
Patient-Centered Services (PCS)		
PCS.1 Basic and essential services, as needed by the primary care center's population, are provided. *The center determines which basic and essential services it will provide, including… management of chronic infections/diseases using protocols and collaborative management and consultation, as indicated by the patient's condition.*	None	No
PCS.2 Additional primary care services and procedures are provided by the primary care center or through agreements with outside organizations and agencies. *The center provides these additional primary care services and procedures or arranges the services with outside sources, including… screening and management of sexually transmitted diseases and related infectious diseases… [and] vaccinations and immunizations.*	None	No
PCS.14.1 Medications available within the primary care center for dispensing to patients or for practitioner administration are organized efficiently and effectively, and their use is guided by policies and procedures. *As applicable to the center's situation, the policies and procedures are developed by qualified and relevant practitioners and address the following:* *d) the medication recall process, including patient notification and the inadvertent use of medications known to be expired.*	None	No
Organization and Delivery of Services (ODS)		
ODS.14 The primary care center collects and analyzes aggregate data to support patient care, primary care center management, and the quality management and patient safety program. *Such databases may include those for infectious diseases, cancer, or research.*	None	No
ODS.16 The primary care center facility is designed to provide accessible, efficient, and safe clinical care in a secure and supportive environment. *Facilities that house primary care centers have a number of design features that make them accessible to all types of patients and facilitate care that is personal, safe, and secure. Such features include the following:* *• Adequate hand hygiene facilities are located in or adjacent to the office/exam room.* *• The premises, fittings, and furniture are kept clean and in good repair, meeting standards for lighting, heating, ventilation, and infection control.* *• A special, separate waiting area with separate ventilation is available for patients who may have an infectious disease.* *• The center provides for safe storage and disposal of clinical waste and potentially infectious waste that require special disposal, such as sharps/needles and other disposable equipment that may have come in contact with body fluids.*	None	No

Standard *Including applicability to IPC, when necessary*	Type of Written Documentation Needed	Documentation in English Required
ODS.19 The primary care center has a plan for the inventory, handling, storage, and use of hazardous materials and the control and disposal of hazardous materials and waste. *The center identifies and safely controls hazardous materials and waste according to a plan. Such materials and waste include chemicals, medications supplies and reagents, radioactive materials and waste, hazardous gases and vapors, and other regulated medical and infectious waste. The plan provides processes for* *a. handling, storage, and use of hazardous materials;* *b. the inventory of hazardous materials and waste;* *c. reporting and investigation of spills, exposures, and other incidents;* *d. proper disposal of hazardous waste;* *e. proper protective equipment and procedures during use, spill, or exposure;* *f. documentation, including any permits, licenses, or other regulatory requirements; and* *g. proper labeling of hazardous materials and waste.*	Plan	Yes
ODS.24.1 New staff orientation provides initial job training and assessment of capability to perform job responsibilities. *The orientation includes, as appropriate, the reporting of medical errors, infection control practices, the center's policies on medication orders, and so on. The orientation period also allows the evaluation of the new staff member's capability to perform his or her job responsibilities. Any contract workers and volunteers are also oriented to the center and their specific assignment or responsibilities, such as patient safety and infection control.*	None	No
ODS.24.2 Ongoing in-service or other education and training maintain and improve staff competence. *For example, medical staff members may receive education on infection control, advances in medical practice, or new technology.*	None	No
ODS.24.3 All staff/practitioners/students/volunteers/contract workers understand and can demonstrate their role relative to safety. *The education can include hand hygiene practices, common medication administration errors, clear communication of critical information among caregivers, and how to involve the patient in the safety program.*	None	No
ODS.24.5 Health professional training and education, when provided within the primary care center, are guided by policies that ensure adequate supervision. *The trainees and community workers are integrated into the primary care center's orientation, quality, patient safety, and infection control programs.*	None	No
ODS.27 The primary care center uses a coordinated process to reduce the risks of endemic and epidemic infections in patients and health care workers.	None	No
ODS.27.1 Case findings and identification of demographically important infections provide surveillance data and data for reporting, when appropriate, within the primary care center and to public health agencies.	None	No
ODS.28 The primary care center identifies the procedures and processes associated with the risk of infection and implements strategies to reduce infection risks.	None	No
ODS.29 Management systems support the infection control process to ensure adequate data analysis, interpretation, and presentation.	None	No

Standard *Including applicability to IPC, when necessary*	Type of Written Documentation Needed	Documentation in English Required
Improvement in Quality and Safety (IQS)		
IQS.1 Those responsible for governing and leading the primary care center plan and oversee a quality improvement and patient safety program and set measurement priorities and priorities for improvement. *As most primary care centers are complex operations, with many structures (for example, committees, teams), processes (for example, patient registration, blood drawing, initial exams, referrals), and outcomes (for example, children are immunized, patients are educated regarding medications, infections are resolved), a center has more opportunities to monitor than it has time and resources.*	Plan	No
IQS.3 Quality monitoring includes both clinical and managerial processes and outcomes, as selected by the primary care center's leaders. *Clinical monitoring areas include… use of science-based tests and treatments (for example, ACE inhibitors, BP control, A1C hemoglobin for diabetes, vaccination rates);… use of antibiotics;… [and] infection control, surveillance, and reporting….* *Managerial monitoring areas include… surveillance, control, and prevention of events that jeopardize the safety of patients, families, and staff.*	None	No
IQS.7 Data are analyzed when undesirable trends and variation are evident from the data. *An analysis is considered for the following:… other events, such as infectious disease outbreaks.*	None	No

Appendix 2

Infection Prevention and Control Web Resources

Compiled and edited by:
Nizam Damani
MBBS, MSc, MRCPI, FRCPath, CIC, DipHIC
Clinical Director, Infection Prevention and Control,
Craigavon Area Hospital, Portadown, UK

Evidence-Based Practice

Cochrane Collaboration (UK)	http://www.cochrane.org/
Joanna Briggs Institute (Australia)	http://www.joannabriggs.edu.au/
National Guideline Clearinghouse (US)	http://www.ngc.gov
National Institute for Health and Clinical Excellence (NICE; UK)	http://www.nice.org.uk
National Resource for Infection Control (NIRC; UK)	http://www.nric.org.uk/
Scottish Intercollegiate Guidelines Network (SIGN; UK)	http://www.sign.ac.uk/

Journals and Newsletters

American Journal of Infection Control	http://www.ajicjournal.org/
Australian Infection Control	http://www.aica.org.au/
Canadian Journal of Infection Control	http://www.chica.org/inside_cjic_journal.html
Communicable Disease and Public Health	www.hpa.org.uk/cdph/
Communicable Disease Newsletter (WHO)	http://www.searo.who.int/en/Section10_12935.htm
Communicable Disease Report Weekly	www.hpa.org.uk/cdr/
Emerging Infectious Diseases	http://www.cdc.gov/ncidod/EID/
Eurosurveillance	http://www.eurosurveillance.org/
Infection Control and Hospital Epidemiology	http://www.journals.uchicago.edu/ICHE/home.html
Infection Control Resource	http://www.infectioncontrolresource.org/
International Journal of Infection Control	http://www.ijic.info/
Joint Commission Journal on Quality and Patient Safety™	http://www.jointcommissioninternational.org/Periodicals /THE-JOINT-COMMISSION-JOURNAL-ON-QUALITY -AND-PATIENT-SAFETY/903/
Journal of Hospital Infection	http://www.journalofhospitalinfection.com/
Journal of Infection Prevention	http://bji.sagepub.com/
CDC *Morbidity & Mortality Weekly Report* (*MMWR*)	http://www.cdc.gov/mmwr/
WHO *Weekly Epidemiological Record*	http://www.who.int/wer/

Organizations and Regulatory Bodies

American College of Occupational and Environmental Medicine (US)	http://www.acoem.org/
American Society for Microbiology (US)	http://www.asm.org/
Asia Pacific Society of Infection Control (APSIC)	http://apsic.info/
Asociación Argentina de Enfermeros en Control de Infecciones (ADECI)	http://www.adeci.org.ar/
Association for Professionals in Infection Control and Epidemiology (APIC; US)	http://www.apic.org
Association of PeriOperative Registered Nurses (AORN; US)	http://www.aorn.org
Australian Infection Control Association	http://www.aica.org.au/
Baltic Network for Infection Control and Containment of Antibiotic Resistance (Estonia, Latvia, Lithuania, and northwest Russia)	http://www.balticcare.org/Links.htm
British Travel Health Association (UK)	http://www.btha.org
Centers for Disease Control and Prevention (CDC; US)	http://www.cdc.gov
Certification Board of Infection Control and Epidemiology, Inc. (US)	http://www.cbic.org/
Chilean Society of Infection Control and Hospital Epidemiology	http://www.sociedad-iih.cl/
Danish Society for Infection Control Nurses (DSICN)	http://www.hygiejnesygeplejerske.dk/
Dutch Working Party on Infection Prevention (WIP)	http://www.wip.nl/UK/
European Centre for Disease Prevention and Control (ECDC)	http://www.ecdc.europa.eu/
European Operating Room Nurses Association (EORNA)	http://www.eorna.eu
European Society of Clinical Microbiology and Infectious Diseases (ESCMID)	http://www.escmid.org
Finnish Society for Hospital Infection Control	http://www.sshy.fi/
German Society for Hospital Hygiene	http://www.dgkh.de/
Global Alert and Response (GAR; WHO)	http://www.who.int/csr/en/
Global Infectious Disease and Epidemiology Network (US)	http://www.gideononline.com/
Health and Safety Executive (UK)	http://www.hse.gov.uk
Health Protection Agency (HPA; UK)	http://www.hpa.org.uk/
Health Protection Scotland	http://www.hps.scot.nhs.uk/
Health Protection Surveillance Centre (HPSC; Republic of Ireland)	http://www.hpsc.ie/hpsc/
Healthcare Infection Society (UK)	http://www.his.org.uk
Hellenic Society for the Control of the Nosocomial Infections and Healthcare Quality Assurance	http://www.infection.gr/DesktopDefault.aspx
Hong Kong Infection Control Nurses' Association	http://www.hkicna.org/
Hospital in Europe Link for Infection Control Through Surveillance (HELICS)	http://helics.univ-lyon1.fr/helicshome.htm
Hospital Infection Society of India	http://hisindia.org/

Infection Control Africa Network (ICAN)	http://www.ipcan.co.za/
Infection Control Society Pakistan (ICSP)	http://infectioncontrolsociety.org
Infection Prevention Society (IPS; UK)	http://www.ips.uk.net
Infectious Disease Research Network (IDRN; UK)	http://www.idrn.org/
Infectious Diseases and Clinical Microbiology Specialty Society of Turkey	http://www.ekmud.org/tr/mainPage.asp
Infectious Diseases Society of America (US)	http://www.idsociety.org/
Infectious Diseases Society of Pakistan (IDSP)	http://www.idspak.org/
Institute for Healthcare Improvement (US)	http://www.ihi.org/
Institute of Decontamination Sciences (IDSc; UK)	http://www.idsc-uk.co.uk/
International Federation of Infection Control (IFIC; UK)	http://www.theific.org
International Nosocomial Infection Control Consortium (INICC; Argentina)	http://www.inicc.org/
International Scientific Forum on Home Hygiene (IFH; UK)	http://www.ifh-homehygiene.org/
International Sharps Injury Prevention Society (US)	http://www.isips.org/
International Society for Infectious Diseases (ISID; US)	http://www.isid.org
International Society of Travel Medicine (ISTM; US)	http://www.istm.org
The Joint Commission (US)	http://www.jointcommission.org/
Joint Commission International (US)	http://www.jointcommissioninternational.org/
L'Association des infirmières en prévention des infections (AIPI; Canada)	http://www.aipi.qc.ca/
Medicine and Healthcare Products Regulatory Agency (MHRA; UK)	http://www.mhra.gov.uk
National Division of Infection Control Nurses (NDICN; New Zealand)	http://www.infectioncontrol.co.nz/home/
National Electronic Library of Infection (NELI; UK)	http://www.neli.org.uk/
National Foundation for Infectious Diseases (US)	http://www.nfid.org/
Occupational Safety & Health Administration (OSHA; US)	http://www.osha.gov
Pan American Health Organization (US)	http://www.paho.org
Public Health Agency (PHA), Northern Ireland	http://www.publichealth.hscni.net/
Public Health Agency of Canada	http://www.phac-aspc.gc.ca/
Robert Koch Institute	http://www.rki.de/
Society for Healthcare Epidemiology of America (SHEA; US)	http://www.shea-online.org
Society of Professionals of Infection Control of Egypt (SPIC; Egypt)	http://www.spicegypt.org/joomla/
Swedish Association for Infection Control (SAIC)	http://www.sfvh.se/
UK Dept. of Health (reducing HCAI)	http://hcai.dh.gov.uk/
US Food and Drug Administration	http://www.fda.gov/
World Forum for Hospital Sterile Supply	http://www.wfhss.com
World Health Organization (WHO)	http://www.who.int/

Index